a LANGE medical book

Medical Epidemiology

Population Health and Effective Health Care

Fifth Edition

Edited by

Raymond S. Greenberg, MD, PhD
Executive Vice Chancellor for Health Affairs
The University of Texas System
Austin

WITH CO-AUTHORS

New York   Chicago   San Francisco   Athens   London   Madrid   Mexico City
Milan   New Delhi   San Juan   Seoul   Singapore   Sydney   Toronto

Medical Epidemiology: Population Health and Effective Health Care , Fifth Edition

1 2 3 4 5 6 7 8 9 0   DOC/DOC   21 20 19 18 17 16 15

ISBN 978-0-07-182272-5
MHID 0-07-182272-0
ISSN 1064-1025

Notice

Medicine is an ever-changing science. As new research and clinical experience broaden our knowledge, changes in treatment and drug therapy are required. The authors and the publisher of this work have checked with sources believed to be reliable in their efforts to provide information that is complete and generally in accord with the standards accepted at the time of publication. However, in view of the possibility of human error or changes in medical sciences, neither the authors nor the publisher nor any other party who has been involved in the preparation or publication of this work warrants that the information contained herein is in every respect accurate or complete, and they disclaim all responsibility for any errors or omissions or for the results obtained from use of the information contained in this work. Readers are encouraged to confirm the information contained herein with other sources. For example and in particular, readers are advised to check the product information sheet included in the package of each drug they plan to administer to be certain that the information contained in this work is accurate and that changes have not been made in the recommended dose or in the contraindications for administration. This recommendation is of particular importance in connection with new or infrequently used drugs.

This book was set in AGaramondPro, Regular, 10/10.5 pt by MPS Ltd.
The editor was Harriet Lebowitz.
The production supervisor was Richard Ruzycka.
Project management was provided by Asheesh Ratra of MPS Ltd.
The cover designer was Thomas De Pierro.
RR Donnelley was printer and binder.

To Leah, for her support and encouragement over many years and many editions.

Contents

Authors

David J. Ballard, MD, MSPH, PhD
Chief Quality Officer
Baylor Scott & White Health
President and Founder, STEEEP Global Institute
Dallas, Texas

Kathleen T. Brady, MD, PhD
Distinguished University Professor of Psychiatry and
    Behavioral Sciences
Associate Provost, Clinical and Translational Science
Medical University of South Carolina
and
Staff Physician, Ralph H. Johnson VA Medical
    Center
Charleston, South Carolina

Briget da Graca, JD, MS
Senior Medical Writer
Office of Chief Quality Officer
Baylor Scott & White Health
Dallas, Texas

Valerie L. Durkalski-Mauldin, MPH, PhD
Professor, Department of Public Health Sciences
Medical University of South Carolina
Charleston, South Carolina

Leonard E. Egede, MD, MS
Allen H. Johnson Endowed Chair & Professor
    of Medicine
Director, Center for Health Disparities Research
Medical University of South Carolina
Charleston, South Carolina
and
Director, Charleston VA
Health Equity and Rural Outreach Center
Ralph H. Johnson VA Medical Center
Charleston, South Carolina

Giovanni Filardo, PhD, MPH
Director, Epidemiology, Office of the Chief
    Quality Officer
Baylor Scott & White Health
and
Endowed Chair of Cardiovascular Epidemiology
Baylor University Medical Center
and
Research Associate Professor, Department of
    Statistical Science
Southern Methodist University
Dallas, Texas

Marvella E. Ford, PhD
Professor, Department of Public Health Sciences
Associate Director, Cancer Disparities, Hollings
    Cancer Center
Medical University of South Carolina
Charleston, South Carolina

Raymond S. Greenberg, MD, PhD
Executive Vice Chancellor for Health Affairs
The University of Texas System
Austin

Carolyn Jenkins, DrPH, APRN, RD, LD, FAAN
Professor and Ann Darlington Edwards Endowed
    Chair
College of Nursing
Medical University of South Carolina
Charleston, South Carolina

Daniel T. Lackland, DrPH
Professor, Department of Neurosciences
    and Neurology
Medical University of South Carolina
Charleston, South Carolina

Cathy L. Melvin, PhD, MPH
Associate Professor
Medical University of South Carolina
Charleston, South Carolina

David Nicewander, MS
Director, Analytics
Baylor Scott & White Health
Dallas, Texas

Annie N. Simpson, PhD
Assistant Professor
Department of Healthcare Leadership and
    Management
College of Health Professions
Medical University of South Carolina
Charleston, South Carolina

Kit N. Simpson, DrPH
Professor, Department of Healthcare Leadership
    and Management
College of Health Professions
and
Professor, Department of Public Health Sciences
College of Medicine
Medical University of South Carolina
Charleston, South Carolina

Michael D. Sweat, PhD
Professor and Director, Family Services Research
    Center
Department of Psychiatry and Behavioral Sciences
Medical University of South Carolina
Charleston, South Carolina

Joni L. Strom Williams, MD, MPH
Postdoctoral Fellow, Center for Health Disparities
    Research
Medical University of South Carolina
Charleston, South Carolina

Preface

It has been almost a quarter century since the first edition of ***Medical Epidemiology*** was written. That original text was developed out of the experience of teaching epidemiology to medical students at Emory University and the University of Cincinnati. Our goal was to present the field of epidemiology in an approachable manner, emphasizing how these methods can advance medical knowledge.

At the time, we could not have anticipated how widely the book would be used and read. Translation into multiple different languages has made ***Medical Epidemiology*** accessible to an international audience, and the publishers have been generous in their support of four subsequent editions to keep its contents current. Each successive edition provided an opportunity to revisit the examples that were used in a field that was evolving rapidly.

It has been a decade since the last iteration of this book appeared, and in the interim there have been transformative changes in the way epidemiologic methods are being used in health care. Some of these changes have been spurred on by the widespread adoption of electronic medical records, making clinical information much more accessible for research purposes. Also, the promotion of clinical and translational research by the National Institutes of Health has given additional focus to moving discoveries from the laboratory bench to the patient's bedside and ultimately to the community at large. Even as translational work has advanced, there has been a paucity of educational material to help prepare investigators for research careers in this area.

Major shifts also have occurred at the policy level, with a growing recognition that the quality of health care is uneven, that advances in medical knowledge often are slowly translated into clinical practice, and that many widely used treatments are poorly justified on the basis of patient-centered outcomes research. As increasing attention is being paid to reimbursement based on the quality and value of care, it will become incumbent upon practitioners to be able to interpret and use research on comparative effectiveness and quality improvement.

With all of these changes underway, we concluded that a fundamental rethinking was required about the contents of ***Medical Epidemiology***. As a consequence, this book has been rewritten in its entirety. In addition, new chapters have been added on many topics, including global health, social determinants of health, health inequalities, comparative effectiveness, quality of care, variations in care, and implementation science. We are not aware of any other existing book with such a broad range of topics, and we hope that the current work fills a void for students, as well as practitioners.

With such a broad range of topics, it was necessary to assemble a truly interdisciplinary team of authors. Gone are the days when a group of epidemiologists could write a textbook in isolation from investigators in other fields. In addition to our core epidemiologic expertise, the writing team for this book included, among others, experts in medical sociology, internal medicine, psychiatry, global health, health disparities, health economics, health services research, biostatistics, population sciences, community-based participatory research, database design, and translational science. If ever it took a village to write a book, this is a prime example.

We realize full well that with this breadth of material, some compromises had to be made in the level of detail provided. Accordingly, we view this book as a primer, and readers who wish to explore specific topics in greater depth are encouraged to pursue the cited work under Further Reading at the end of each chapter.

We have tried to keep this book grounded in medical care by introducing each chapter with a Health Scenario. We also encourage readers to assess their knowledge acquisition through Study Questions at the end of each chapter. Although any textbook on epidemiology is obliged to cover essential quantitative topics, we have attempted to keep this book accessible to a wide readership by limiting the methodological discussions to the most essential material. For those who are interested in more detail on the calculation of various epidemiologic measures, free, user-friendly resources are available, such as the Centers for Disease Control and Prevention's Epi Info (http://www.cdc.gov/epiinfo/).

Hopefully, this book will be a faithful heir to its four predecessors. At the same time, we have tried to expand on the original mission by highlighting the ways in which epidemiology can advance and be advanced by its sister sciences. There was never a time of greater need for appreciating how epidemiology can improve both the delivery of medical care and the health of populations. In some small measure, we hope that this book begins to fill that need.

Raymond S. Greenberg, MD, PhD
Austin, Texas
September 2014

Acknowledgments

The development of this book has been a team effort, with the participation of many colleagues at the Medical University of South Carolina in Charleston, South Carolina, and Baylor Scott & White Health in Dallas, Texas. We thank both institutions for their support and encouragement, as well as The University of Texas System, which served as the home institution for this collaboration.

We are grateful to the McGraw-Hill Education team who encouraged the preparation of this book and helped in all facets of its production. Particular thanks go to Harriet Lebowitz, the project development editor; Christine Diedrich and her successor, Sarah Henry, the associate editors of the Medical Publishing Division; and Jim Shanahan, the associate publisher of the Professional Group.

Deep gratitude is due to Dena Gregory at the Medical University of South Carolina and Trisha Meloncon at The University of Texas System for their patience and skill in preparing the manuscripts and serving as the glue to hold the entire project together.

Finally, and most important, we thank our families and loved ones for their support and encouragement, even when writing tasks stole precious time away from them. We hope that they find the final product justified their personal sacrifices to make it possible.

Raymond S. Greenberg, MD, PhD
Austin, Texas
September 2014

SECTION I
Population Health

Introduction to Epidemiology

Raymond S. Greenberg

HEALTH SCENARIO

A 53-year-old previously healthy man visited his physician with a chief complaint of a sore throat of 6 weeks' duration. The patient reported pain on swallowing but did not have a fever, cough, or congestion. He did not smoke and had an occasional glass of wine with dinner. A physical examination revealed a 3-cm mass on the left side of the posterior pharynx along with an ipsilateral 1-cm firm, immovable cervical lymph node. A referral was made to an otolaryngologist, who performed a biopsy yielding a diagnosis of squamous cell carcinoma of the posterior pharynx. The patient subsequently underwent a complete surgical resection of the primary tumor and a selective dissection of cervical lymph nodes, two of six of which had malignant cells present. Examination of the tumor specimen by situ hybridization was positive for human papillomavirus (HPV) type 16. The patient was treated additionally with external-beam radiation therapy, and there was no evidence of tumor recurrence within the initial 3 years after diagnosis.

CLINICAL BACKGROUND

Head and neck cancer most commonly arises as a squamous cell malignancy within the oral cavity, pharynx, or larynx. Worldwide, there are estimated to be more than half a million new head and neck cancers diagnosed each year and nearly one third of a million deaths annually from this disease. Head and neck cancer is the sixth most common type of cancer globally, ranking third highest among economically

emerging countries and eighth highest among high-income countries.

In the United States, the overall occurrence of head and neck cancer has been declining for several decades, with an average annual decrease of about 1.5% per year. When examined by anatomic site of the primary malignancy, however, differing patterns are observed, with decreases in the occurrence of lip, oral cavity, and laryngeal cancers and an increasing proportion of lesions arising in the oropharynx (base of the tongue, tonsils, and pharynx). Over this same time period, there was a progressive shift to more advanced oropharyngeal malignancies (disseminated to the adjacent tissue or spread remotely) at the time of diagnosis. With more extensive tumors, one might have anticipated declining survival rates for oropharyngeal cancers, but to the contrary, 5-year survival rates have risen, and most of the improvement has been observed among patients with nonlocalized disease.

Cigarette smoking is a well-established risk factor for head and neck cancer, increasing the risk by about 10-fold. It has been estimated that four out of five of these malignancies are attributable to tobacco use. Heavy alcohol consumption has been shown to increase the risk of developing head and neck cancer independently and even more dramatically when used in combination with tobacco use. The overall declining rate of new occurrences of head and neck cancer in the United States has been attributed to falling rates of cigarette smoking.

Human papillomavirus is a small virus containing double-strained circular DNA. More than 150 types of this virus have been identified, about a quarter of which are known to be sexually transmitted. In the United States, HPV infection is the most common form of sexually transmitted disease. It is spread by skin-to-skin contact, and more than half of all sexually active people are infected with the virus at some point during their lives. Typically, infection with HPV does not produce symptoms, and the host's immune system clears the virus within 1 to 2 years. About 10% of affected individuals will have persistent infections, with the virus persisting in host epithelial cells. HPV multiplies and produces proteins that interfere with normal mechanisms of regulatory cell growth and death in the host. It is estimated that half of persons with persistent infections will develop precancerous lesions that over time can evolve into malignancies.

Studies within the general population have revealed that HPV infection peaks among young adults in their 20s through early 30s and then again among older adults in their late 50s and early 60s. Infection is more common among persons of lower socioeconomic status and among African Americans. A number of aspects of sexual behavior are strongly associated with risk of HPV infection, including early age at onset of sexual activity, the lifetime number of sexual partners, and the number of sexual partners in the recent past.

The association of HPV with cancer was first demonstrated in the late 1970s and 1980s, when HPV particles were discovered first in genital warts and then in cancers of the uterine cervix. Subsequent studies revealed that there are more than a dozen types of HPV that are high risk for producing cervical cancer, among which types 16 and 18 are the most frequently occurring. It has been estimated that about two thirds of cervical cancers are related to HPV types 16 and 18.

In the 1980s, the identification of HPV structural proteins in oral squamous cell carcinomas raised the possibility that HPV may play a role in cancer causation in nongenital organs. At any point in time, about 7% of adults in the United States have an oral HPV infection, with type 16 being the most common variant. Men are more likely than women to have oral HPV infections, as are African Americans, smokers, and drinkers. HPV infections of the oral cavity are strongly correlated with ever having had sex and the total number of lifetime sexual partners.

Human papillomavirus DNA is detected in about one third of oropharyngeal cancers, with type 16 accounting for about 9 of 10 of these instances. Studies of HPV infection and oropharyngeal risk show strong associations, particularly when the measures are indicators of long-term infection (presence of an HPV 16 capsid protein) or impaired cellular control of growth and death (HPV 16 oncoproteins).

The proportion of oropharyngeal cancers that have evidence of HPV infection has risen dramatically, from about one in six cancers in the 1980s to almost three fourths in the early 2000s. These changes have been attributed in part to the decline of other risk factors, such as cigarette smoking, and in part to the rise of high-risk sexual practices, such as earlier onset of sexual activity and a larger number of sexual partners. HPV-related oropharyngeal cancers tend to occur at slightly younger ages and demonstrate weaker associations with alcohol and tobacco use. HPV-related oropharyngeal cancer tends to occur more than three times as often among men than women, which is consistent with about a threefold greater presence of oral HPV infection among men. The reasons for the male excess are unclear, perhaps reflecting higher transmission of HPV to men during oral sex and/or greater immunity to oral HPV among women because of prior genital infections.

The clinical behavior of HPV-related oropharyngeal cancers also differs from HPV-unrelated malignancies, with a greater tendency toward regional spread at the time of diagnosis. However, HPV-related cancers tend to have a more favorable prognosis, with lower risks of disease recurrence and death.

Two vaccines against HPV have been developed, both of which are targeted against the leading HPV types associated with cancer development. The vaccines were developed to prevent HPV genital infections and their consequences, including cervical cancer. The vaccines are delivered in three doses and contain noninfectious virus-like particles that incorporate a major protein found on the surface of the virus. The vaccinated host develops an immune response to the protein, thus protecting against infection with the wild virus. The vaccines have been shown to be safe and highly effective against the HPV types for which they were developed, as well as in preventing precancerous changes in the cervix. The protective effect is particularly strong among those who have not yet acquired natural infection; therefore, vaccination has been recommended for age groups before the onset of sexual activity. The first vaccine was licensed in the United States in 2006 for use among girls and young women (targeted at age 11–12 years, with catch-up to age 26 years). The second vaccine was licensed three years later, also for use among young women. Despite its clear benefit and recommendations, HPV vaccination has lagged behind the use of other recommended vaccines among adolescents. By 2010, only about one third of eligible adolescent girls had received the full three doses of HPV vaccine compared with more than 90% coverage for hepatitis B. Barriers to immunization include parental knowledge, attitudes, and belief, as well as cost and unsubstantiated concerns about safety. Wider immunization, including boys and young men, has been encouraged because of the recognition of the role of HPV in causing a broad range of cancers.

INTRODUCTION

Epidemiology is the study of the distribution and determinants of health and disease in human populations. By the distribution of a disease, we mean the pattern of its occurrence among people. Consider, for example, oral HPV infection as introduced in the **Health Scenario**. A basic question about this illness is how it is distributed within a population. To answer this question, a study was conducted on a sample of the population of the United States during 2009 and 2010. More than 5500 persons aged 14 to 69 years were included and samples of exfoliated oral cells were collected and analyzed for the presence of HPV. Overall, about 7% of examinees had HPV present in their oral cells. This summary measure provides a useful snapshot of the collective experience, and it is of value, therefore, as a general description. On the other hand, it may mask important underlying patterns of infection. By studying these underlying patterns, we may gain insight into how the virus is spread from person to person.

One of the most basic ways to begin to describe disease patterns is to characterize how they vary by age, race, and sex. In the instance of HPV oral infection, considerable variations in occurrence were seen by these demographic attributes. As shown in **Figure 1-1**,

the percentage of affected persons is lowest among adolescents. Infection appears to peak in two age groups, with the highest level among those in their late 50s and early 60s and a smaller peak among those in their late 20s and early 30s. Although this distribution by itself does not suggest a specific mode of transmission, it is noteworthy that the youngest age group has less than one third of the level of infection of those in their late teens and early 20s. At the other end of the age spectrum, a similar dramatic decline in infection is observed for those age 65 years or older.

When the study population was classified by race and ethnicity, variation was observed again, albeit not as great as the differences by age (**Figure 1-2**). The highest infection levels were found for non-Hispanic blacks followed by non-Mexican Hispanics. Intermediate percentages were detected for non-Hispanic whites and Mexican Americans, with the lowest rate among other races.

Further analysis by sex indicated that the infection was almost three times more common among men than women (**Figure 1-3**). Through these demographic patterns, we begin to see an emerging picture of who within the population is at greatest likelihood of being infected and who has the lowest likelihood of infection. The high infection groups include men, those in their late 50s and early 60s, and blacks. Those at comparatively low infection levels include young adolescents, women, and persons of other racial groups. Although these are fairly broad categories of occurrence and they may not be unique, the

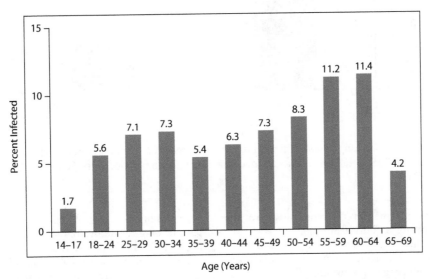

Figure 1-1. Percent of U.S. population with oral human papillomavirus infection, by age, 2009 to 2010. (Data from Gillison ML, Broutian T, Pickard RK, et al. Prevalence of oral HPV infection in the United States, 2009-2010. *JAMA.* 2012;307:693-703.)

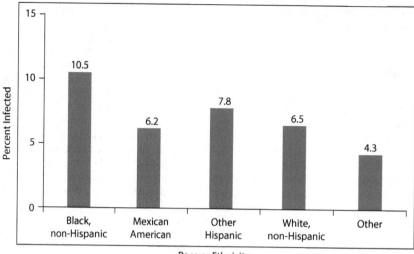

Figure 1-2. Percent of U.S. population with oral human papillomavirus infection, by race or ethnicity, 2009 to 2010. (Data from Gillison ML, Broutian T, Pickard RK, et al. Prevalence of oral HPV infection in the United States, 2009-2010. *JAMA.* 2012;307:693-703.)

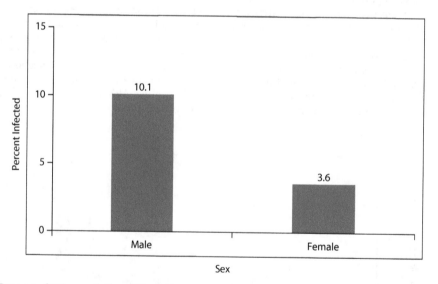

Figure 1-3. Percent of U.S. population with oral human papillomavirus infection, by sex, 2009 to 2010. (Data from Gillison ML, Broutian T, Pickard RK, et al. Prevalence of oral HPV infection in the United States, 2009-2010. *JAMA.* 2012;307:693-703.)

more we refine our analysis, the more distinctive the pattern becomes for oral HPV infection.

Observing these patterns, we begin to see the hallmark of one of the basic tenets of epidemiology: **diseases do not occur at random**. Within a population, some people are more likely than others to acquire a condition. These variations can occur because of differential exposure to a causative agent, greater susceptibility to it, or both. For example, the higher the level of oral HPV infection among men might reflect a greater level of exposure (e.g., more sexual partners), more frequent genital-to-oral transmission among men, or greater immunity to oral infection among women because of more frequent genital infections.

We characterize persons in groups with a higher likelihood of acquiring a disease as being at "high risk." It is important to recognize, however, that being in a high-risk group, such as men for oral HPV infection, does not mean that a particular individual within that group is likely to have the condition. Even though a man is three times more likely than a woman to be infected, 9 of 10 men are not infected at any particular moment in time.

The characterization of a disease pattern by demographic attributes such as age, race, and sex is one of the fundamental applications of epidemiology. It is what one might refer to as a **descriptive** use and serves a vital purpose in helping to identify high-risk individuals within the population. In some circumstances, such knowledge can lead to patient or public education for the purposes of prevention, early detection, or treatment strategies.

As a case in point, the same survey of oral HPV infection included questions about certain behavioral practices. As shown in **Figure 1-4**, those who were heavy cigarette smokers had almost a fourfold increased risk of oral HPV infection than persons who were either nonsmokers or never smokers. From this graph, one observes a progressive increase in infection risk with increasing level of cigarette smoking. Such a pattern could arise either because smokers are more likely to have other high-risk practices or because smoking adversely affects host immunity and thereby increases the likelihood of infection or its persistence. Similar, albeit not as strong, graded increases in risk of

oral HPV infection were seen with reported alcohol consumption and marijuana use.

Given that HPV is known to be sexually transmitted, further description of the population by sexual practices may shed light on the risk of oral infection. Persons who reported never having sex were one eighth as likely to have oral HPV infections as those who reported having sex. Among sexually active persons, sexual orientation was not related to oral HPV infection. A dramatic relationship was observed, however, for number of lifetime sex partners, as depicted in **Figure 1-5**. There was almost a 20-fold difference in likelihood of infection between those who reported never having sex and those who reported 21 or more sex partners during their lifetimes. A similar pattern was seen for number of lifetime vaginal sex partners.

The characterization of disease occurrence patterns across broad behavioral categories extends our understanding of oral HPV infection beyond the simple demographic patterns. From this descriptive epidemiology, we can appreciate that certain lifestyle practices increase the likelihood of acquiring infection. We can use these observations to be more targeted in providing educational and other interventions.

In addition to the descriptive role of epidemiology, we can identify a second broad area of application referred to as **analytic**. In this context, epidemiologic methods are used to understand the determinants, or causes, of disease. To illustrate this type of study,

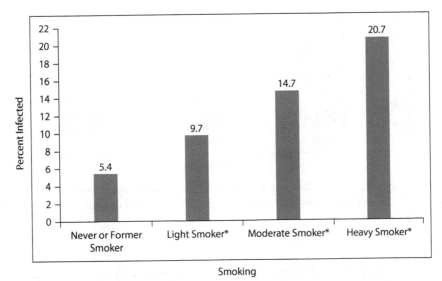

*Light, ≤10 cigarettes/day; Moderate, 11–20 cigarettes/day; Heavy, >20 cigarettes/day

Figure 1-4. Percent of U.S. population with oral human papillomavirus infection, by cigarette smoking status, 2009 to 2010. A light smoker smokes fewer than 10 cigarettes/day, a moderate smoker smokes 11 to 20 cigarettes/day, and a heavy smoker smokes more than 20 cigarettes/day. (Data from Gillison ML, Broutian T, Pickard RK, et al. Prevalence of oral HPV infection in the United States, 2009-2010. *JAMA.* 2012;307:693-703.)

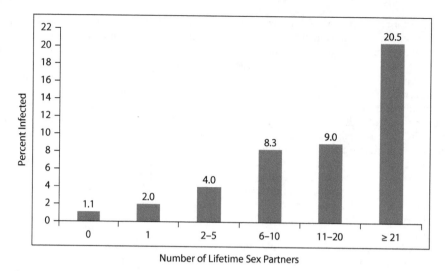

Figure 1-5. Percent of U.S. population with oral human papillomavirus infection, by number of lifetime sex partners, 2009-10. (Data from Gillison ML, Broutian T, Pickard RK, et al. Prevalence of oral HPV infection in the United States, 2009-2010. *JAMA*. 2012;307:693-703.)

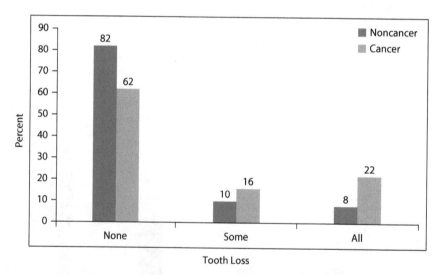

Figure 1-6. Percentages of patients with some or all tooth loss, by oropharyngeal cancer status. (Data from D'Souza G, Kreimer AR, Viscidi R, et al. Case-control study of human papillomavirus and oropharyngeal cancer. *N Engl J Med*. 2007;356:1944-1956.)

let us consider an investigation of 100 patients with newly diagnosed oropharyngeal cancer. These individuals were identified from an outpatient otolaryngology clinic between 2000 and 2005. For each cancer patient, two comparison subjects of the same sex and similar age who did not have cancer were identified. The cancer patients and the comparison subjects were then compared with regard to a wide range of characteristics.

As shown in **Figure 1-6**, patients with oropharyngeal cancer were more likely to have had a loss of some or all of their teeth. This suggests that poor oral hygiene is associated with oropharyngeal cancer. A series of other characteristics are depicted in **Figure 1-7**,

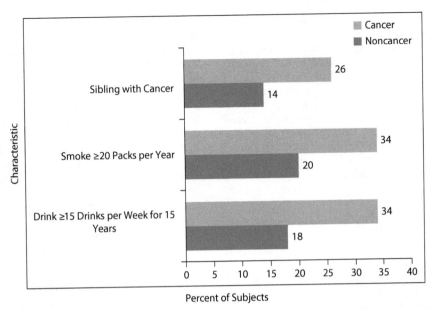

Figure 1-7. Percentages of patients with various characteristics, by oropharyngeal cancer status. (Data from D'Souza G, Kreimer AR, Viscidi R, et al. Case-control study of human papillomavirus and oropharyngeal cancer. *N Engl J Med*. 2007;356:1944-1956.)

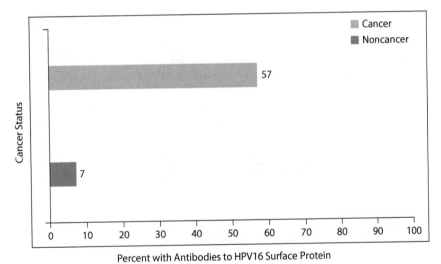

Figure 1-8. Percent of subjects seropositive for the L1 surface protein of human papillomavirus (HPV) 16, by oropharyngeal cancer status. (Data from D'Souza G, Kreimer AR, Viscidi R, et al. Case-control study of human papillomavirus and oropharyngeal cancer. *N Engl J Med*. 2007;356:1944-1956.)

indicating that the cancer patients were more likely to have had a family history of cancer, to smoke heavily, and to drink alcohol over a sustained period of time.

The relationship between lifetime exposure to HPV type 16 (as indicated by presence in the serum of antibodies to a type-specific viral surface protein) and oropharyngeal cancer is shown in **Figure 1-8**.

This relationship is very strong, that is to say, the differences between patients with and without cancer are extremely large. Differences in other characteristics (family history, alcohol and tobacco use, and oral hygiene) could not explain this intense association, thus suggesting a role for HPV type 16 in the development of oropharyngeal cancer.

Epidemiologic studies, whether descriptive or analytic in nature, can be conducted in a wide range of populations. At one extreme, one might attempt to characterize the worldwide situation and perform cross-national comparisons. More focused studies can be conducted within a single country or within its regions and cities. Beyond these general population investigations, one might undertake studies of special populations because they have distinctive (either high or low) patterns of disease occurrence. In the following sections, examples are presented of these various sampling strategies, with particular reference to HPV infection.

GLOBAL POPULATION

To describe patterns of HPV cervical infection around the world, the International Agency for Research on Cancer selected random samples of women in 11 countries. The countries were selected to represent areas with low, medium, and high risks of cervical cancer. In all, more than 15,000 sexually active women between the ages of 15 and 74 years were included. All subjects underwent a gynecologic examination with cervical specimens collected for HPV detection. Overall, 1429 women (9.2%) had evidence of cervical HPV infection.

The percentages of European women with cervical HPV infection varied widely by country (**Figure 1-9**), with a low level in Spain and a comparatively

high percentage in Italy and the Netherlands. The differences in infection rates were even more dramatic when compared across continents (**Figure 1-10**). The highest infection rates were observed in sub-Saharan Africa followed in turn by South America, Asia, and Europe. The distribution of types of HPV is varied by continent among women with cervical infections. Sub-Saharan women were less likely than others to have type 16 HPV but more likely to have other viral types. These international variations in HPV occurrences and subtype distributions could have important implications for vaccine effectiveness and immunization policies in differing parts of the world.

In general, global studies have great appeal because they cover a broad range of experience and can reveal similarities and differences across a range of populations. However, these investigations are relatively infrequent because they are expensive and logistically difficult to conduct. Working across national boundaries offers challenges in dealing with a variety of languages, cultures, and traditions. Standardizing protocols, training staff, adapting questionnaires, and coordinating data and specimen collection can be difficult, but rewarding, if executed successfully.

NATIONAL POPULATION

To study the relationship between HPV cervical infection and the subsequent risk of developing potentially precancerous changes of the cervix,

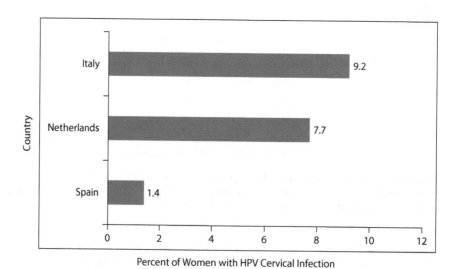

Figure 1-9. Percent of sexually active women with cervical human papillomavirus (HPV) infection, by country within Europe. (Data from Clifford GM, Gallus S, Herrero R, et al. Worldwide distribution of human papillomavirus types in cytologically normal women in the International Agency for Research on Cancer HPV prevalence surveys: a pooled analysis. *Lancet.* 2005;366:991-998.)

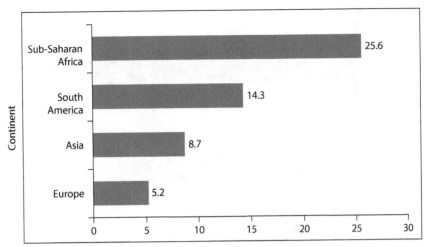

Figure 1-10. Percent of sexually active women with cervical human papillomavirus (HPV) infection, by continent. (Data from Clifford GM, Gallus S, Herrero R, et al. Worldwide distribution of human papillomavirus types in cytologically normal women in the International Agency for Research on Cancer HPV prevalence surveys: a pooled analysis. *Lancet*. 2005;366:991-998.)

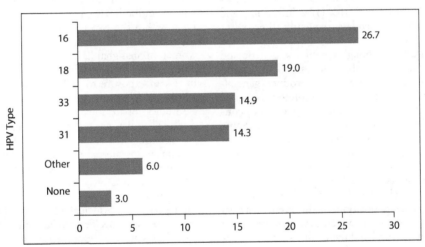

Figure 1-11. The risk of subsequently developing a potentially precancerous lesion of the cervix, by type of human papillomavirus (HPV) cervical infection, Denmark, 1991 to 2007. (Data from Kjaer SK, Frederiksen K, Munk C, Iftner T. Long-term absolute risk of cervical intraepithelial neoplasia grade 3 or worse following papillomavirus infection: role of persistence. *J Natl Cancer Inst*. 2010;102:1478-1488.)

investigators sampled more than 8000 women from the general population of Denmark. The women subjects underwent a series of gynecologic examinations and were followed for up to 13 years. The results are summarized in **Figure 1-11**. Those who had no evidence of HPV infection had a 3% chance of subsequently developing potentially precancerous cervical cells. In contrast, women who had HPV type 16 infection had a greater than one in four chance of developing potentially premalignant cellular abnormalities. Risks were also elevated for women with type 18 HPV and to lesser extents for those with types 33

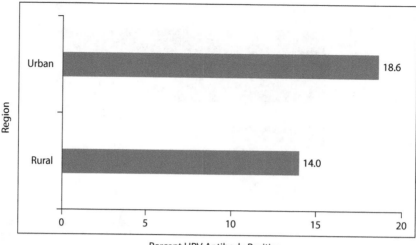

Figure 1-12. Percent of women with antibodies to human papillomavirus (HPV) in their blood, China, 2006 to 2007. (Data from Ji J, Sun HK, Smith JS, et al. Seroprevalence of human papillomavirus types 6, 11, 16 and 18 in Chinese women. *BMC Infect Dis.* 2012;12:137-147.)

or 31. These results help to define patient populations that should be more frequently screened for cervical cancer (those with high risk HPV infections) and those that can be screened less frequently (those without HPV infection).

National studies, although having less genetic and cultural diversity than global studies, still provide a broad base of experience and can produce generalized results at least to the country of interest. National studies also can be expensive and complicated to conduct, albeit less so than global investigations. Some settings are particularly suited for national studies, such as the one described here. Denmark has a national registration system, which facilitates both sampling of subjects and follow-up for medical outcomes. Denmark also has a stable, relatively homogeneous and small population, with excellent access to medical care. All of these factors contribute to the ease of identifying and following the study population. The ability to extrapolate results to other settings, however, may be limited by these distinctive characteristics.

REGIONAL POPULATION

To better characterize the patterns of HPV infection among Chinese women, samples were drawn at random from three rural and two urban areas. Nearly 5000 women completed a questionnaire and provided a sample of blood. Overall, the percentage of women with blood antibodies to HPV was much higher among women who reported being sexually active (15.8%) than among those who denied sexual activity (2.5%).

As illustrated in **Figure 1-12**, the women who resided in urban areas had a higher likelihood of having antibodies to HPV infection in their blood. Even within the two urban areas, there was noteworthy variation, with a higher proportion of infected women in Shanghai (22.1%) than in Beijing (15.3%). These patterns suggest that considerable heterogeneity in risk of exposure to HPV can occur across regions within a single country.

Studies of regional variation, such as the one described earlier, are logistically easier to conduct than global or national studies, but they lack the ability to extrapolate to external populations. For example, even within China, we cannot be certain whether the HPV infection patterns of other cities would be more similar to those of Beijing, Shanghai, or neither. Regional studies have two principal advantages. First, they allow greater focus on specific populations of interest, and second, they tend to be less expensive and logistically complicated to conduct. Ultimately, the decision to conduct a global, national, or regional study is governed by the goals of investigation, as well as by the fiscal, technical, and human resources available for the effort.

SPECIAL POPULATIONS

In each of the previous examples, the study populations were sampled from within a frame of reference related to place of residence. This is a common strategy and tends to allow extrapolation of results to the general population from which the subjects were selected. In certain circumstances, however, an investigator may choose to examine a population defined by other characteristics. Typically, the study of such a group is motivated because the subjects are recognized to have an unusual (either high or low) risk of developing the disease of interest. Several special populations with respect to HPV exposure are described in the following examples.

Because HPV is a sexually transmitted infection, it stands to reason that sex workers would have elevated risks of infection. A study was conducted in Alicante, Spain, of almost 550 female sex workers and more than 1000 women sampled from the general population. At baseline, about one third of sex workers, but only about 1 in 10 women in the general population had infections with high risk types of HPV (**Figure 1-13**). The women without infections were followed for the development of new infections. Even after taking into account other risk factors for HPV acquisition, female sex workers had about four times the likelihood of developing a new infection. Among those who had an initial infection, sex workers were about twice as likely as other women to have persistence of their infections.

Another group known to be at high risk of cervical cancer is incarcerated women. Accordingly, a group of more than 200 female prisoners was studied in Alicante, Spain, with regard to HPV infection. The proportion of women with cervical infections was greater than one in four, which was nearly the same as female sex workers and almost threefold greater than the general population. About 18% of prisoners had known infection with human immunodeficiency virus (HIV). As shown in **Figure 1-14**, women with HIV infection were more likely to have cervical HPV because of participating in higher risk behaviors, having reduced immunity, or both.

It should be noted that studies of prison populations have many logistical advantages given the captive nature of their confinement. At the same time, given the power imbalance of the situation, it is important to establish, as in the case of this study, that prisoners are fully informed about the risks and benefits of participating in the study. Protocols involving the study of prisoners involve a vulnerable population and therefore require even greater assurance than usual that participation is voluntary, refusal to participate has no adverse consequence, and withdrawal can occur without any jeopardy to the participant.

In the two examples of special populations cited thus far, the definition was based on occupational or social or behavioral considerations. In other circumstances, a special group might be selected for study because of a predisposing medical condition. One such circumstance relevant to HPV infection is patients who have undergone organ transplantation. Transplant recipients have their immune systems medically suppressed in order to reduce the risk of rejecting the transplanted organ. As a consequence, these patients are at increased risk of acquiring infections and having them persist. In addition, transplant recipients are known to be at increased risk of developing cancer.

A study of more than 400 recipients of organ transplants was conducted in five European countries.

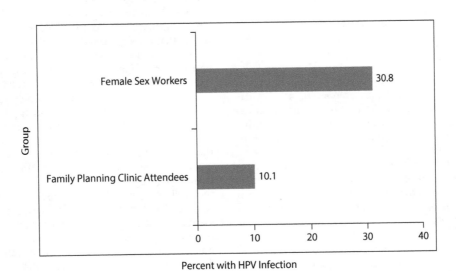

Figure 1-13. Percent of women with cervical human papillomavirus (HPV) infections, by group, Alicante, Spain, 2003 to 2006. (Data from Gonzalez C, Torres M, Canals J, et al. Higher incidence and persistence of high-risk human papillomavirus infection in female sex workers compared with women attending family planning. *Int J Infect Dis.* 2011;15:e688-94.)

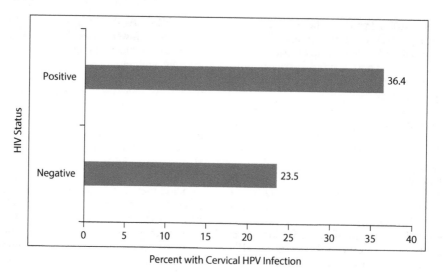

Figure 1-14. Percent of imprisoned women with cervical human papillomavirus (HPV) infections, by HIV status, Alicante, Spain, 2003 to 2006. (Data from Gonzalez C, Canals J, Ortiz M, et al. Prevalence and determinants of high-risk human papillomavirus (HPV) infection and cervical abnormalities in imprisoned women. *Epidemiol Infect.* 2008;136:215-221.)

After transplant, 8 of 10 patients had evidence of HPV infections, as indicated by antibodies to type-specific virus surface proteins. This level of infection is much greater than is observed in European general populations. Regular examinations over the 18 months after transplantation revealed little evidence of new antibodies, suggesting either few new infections or impaired ability to make antibodies to HPV. Nevertheless, the high level of HPV infections in this population means that they are at increased risk for cancers associated with this virus.

SUMMARY

In this chapter, we have introduced the field of epidemiology through the lens of research on a widespread infection, HPV, that has serious potential consequences. Epidemiology is the study of the distribution and determinants of health and disease in human populations. Epidemiologic research may be conducted for descriptive purposes in order to characterize the patterns of disease occurrence. A fundamental tenet of this type of investigation is that diseases do not occur at random. Some people are at increased risk of acquiring a particular disease, and others are at reduced risk. Characterizing these patterns of occurrence can give insight into strategies to prevent a disease, detect it early, or target treatment interventions. For HPV infection, we have observed a number of high-risk populations such as those residing in sub-Saharan Africa, female sex workers, prisoners, persons with HIV, and organ transplant recipients.

Another use of epidemiology, which may be termed **analytic**, is focused on ascertaining the determinants, or causes, of disease. We have seen, for example, that oropharyngeal cancer has been increasing in frequency, while other head and neck cancers have been declining. This suggests that different risk factors may be responsible for these cancers. The identification of HPV as a cause for cancers of the anogenital region led to speculation that sexual transmission of the virus might be responsible for oropharyngeal cancers. Indeed, there is now compelling evidence from epidemiologic and other studies that HPV is a cause of oropharyngeal cancer.

In this chapter, we also considered a range of human populations that might be sampled for epidemiologic studies. Global studies, involving multiple countries, can yield the most widely generalizable results but are infrequently conducted because they are expensive and complicated to undertake. Studies conducted at a single country level are more limited in the range of human biologic and social variation that can be examined but allow a more focused examination of the populations considered. Investigations at the local or regional level are the most constrained in terms of the ability to extrapolate results to other populations but are logistically and economically the easiest to conduct. Finally, special populations with either unusually high or low risk of the disease of interest can provide further insight into disease occurrence and determinants. These special populations may be characterized by social constructs, such as employment, or biologic ones, such as having a comorbid illness or having undergone a particular procedure.

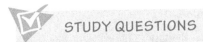

STUDY QUESTIONS

1. Which type of study would have the broadest generalizability to other populations?
   A. A study in 10 countries across five continents
   B. A study in a single country
   C. A study in a single region
   D. A study in a university hospital

2. Which type of study logistically would be the easiest to conduct?
   A. A study in 10 countries across five continents
   B. A study in a single country
   C. A study in a single region
   D. A study in a university hospital

3. Which of the following attributes is NOT associated with HPV infection?
   A. Age
   B. Race
   C. Sex
   D. None of the above

4. Which of the following studies is an example of descriptive epidemiology?
   A. A comparison of the number of lifetime sexual partners between persons with and without oropharyngeal cancer
   B. A study of the percent of persons with HPV infection in a prison population
   C. A study in which female sex workers are contrasted with women in the general population for risk of developing precancerous lesions of the cervix
   D. A trial in which HPV vaccine is administered by random assignment and subsequent development of precancerous lesions of the cervix is assessed

5. Which of the following conditions is likely to have a nonrandom pattern of occurrence within a population?
   A. Oropharyngeal cancer
   B. HPV infection
   C. Laryngeal cancer
   D. All of the above

6. The age group with the lowest risk of HPV infection is
   A. 0 to 10 years.
   B. 30 to 34 years.
   C. 45 to 49 years.
   D. 60 to 64 years.

7. Which of the following cancers have increased in occurrence in recent years?
   A. Cervix
   B. Larynx
   C. Oropharynx
   D. None of the above

8. Which of the following might be a special population of interest for a study of HPV infection?
   A. Female hospital workers
   B. Male truck drivers
   C. Men who have sex with men
   D. None of the above

9. A national study is logistically easier to conduct in Denmark than in the United States because of
   A. a national registration number that can be used to track health event.
   B. a relatively small geographic area.
   C. a relatively stable population.
   D. all of the above.

10. International variations in HPV infection are most likely related to differences in
    A. rates of organ transplantation.
    B. sexual practices.
    C. rates of incarceration.
    D. genetic variation.

FURTHER READING

Chaturvedi AK. Epidemiology and clinical aspects of HPV in head and neck cancers. *Head and Neck Pathol.* 2012;6:516-524.

Syrjänen S. Human papillomavirus (HPV) in head and neck cancer. *J Clin Virol. 2005;325*(suppl):S59-S66.

Zandberg DP, Bhargava R, Badin S, Cullen KJ. The role of human papillomavirus in nongenital cancers. *CA Cancer J Clin.* 2013;63:57-81.

REFERENCES

Clinical Background

Chaturvedi AK, Engels EA, Pfeiffer RM, et al. Human papillomavirus and rising oropharyngeal cancer incidence in the United States. *J Clin Oncol.* 2011;29:4294-4301.

Carvalho AL, Nishimoto IN, Califano JA, Kowalski LP. Trends in incidence and prognosis for head and neck cancer in the United States: a site-specific analysis of the SEER database. *Int J Cancer.* 2005;114:806-816.

Moscicki A-B. Human papillomavirus disease and vaccines in adolescents. *Adolesc Med State Art Rev.* 2010;21:347-363.

O'Rorke MA, Ellison MV, Murray LJ, Moran M, James J, Anderson LA. Human papillomavirus related head and neck cancer survival: a systematic review and meta-analysis. *Oral Oncol.* 2012;48:1191-1201.

Introduction

D'Souza G, Kreimer AR, Viscidi R, et al. Case-control study of human papillomavirus and oropharyngeal cancer. *N Engl J Med.* 2007;356:1944-1956.

Gillison ML, Broutian T, Pickard RK, et al. Prevalence of oral HPV infection in the United States, 2009-2010. *JAMA.* 2012;307:693-703.

Global Population

Clifford GM, Gallus S, Herrero R, et al; IARC HPV Prevalence Surveys Study Group. Worldwide distribution of human papillomavirus types in cytologically normal women in the International Agency for Research on Cancer HPV prevalence surveys: a pooled analysis. *Lancet.* 2005;366:991-998.

National Population

Kjaer SK, Frederiksen K, Munk C, Iftner T. Long-term absolute risk of cervical intraepithelial neoplasia grade 3 or worse following papillomavirus infection: role of persistence. *J Natl Cancer Inst.* 2010;102:1478-1488.

Regional Population

Ji J, Sun HK, Smith JS, et al. Seroprevalence of human papillomavirus types 6, 11, 16 and 18 in Chinese women. *BMC Infect Dis.* 2012;12:137-147.

Special Populations

Antonsson A, Waterboer T, Bouwes Bavinck JN, et al; EPI-HPV-UV-CA group. Longitudinal study of seroprevalence and serostability of 34 human papillomavirus types in European organ transplant recipients. *Virology.* 2013;436:91-99.

Gonzalez C, Canals J, Ortiz M, et al. Prevalence and determinants of high-risk human papillomavirus (HPV) infection and cervical abnormalities in imprisoned women. *Epidemiol Infect.* 2008;136:215-221.

Gonzalez C, Torres M, Canals J, et al. Higher incidence and persistence of high-risk human papillomavirus infection in female sex workers compared with women attending family planning. *Int J Infect Dis.* 2011;15:e688-94.

Epidemiologic Measures

Raymond S. Greenberg

HEALTH SCENARIO

Mr. W., a 73-year-old retired insurance executive, presented to the emergency department of his local hospital with a recent onset of shortness of breath and chest pain when breathing. The patient had undergone a total hip replacement (arthroplasty) 7 days earlier at the same hospital. He had been discharged on postoperative day 4 and was encouraged to ambulate as much as possible at home while recovering. His mobility was limited, however, because of pain on standing, and he had not yet begun a prescribed physical therapy regimen. Mr. W. was a 40-pack-year cigarette smoker and was morbidly obese.

Upon physical examination, the patient appeared anxious and was breathing rapidly (respiratory rate of 24 breaths/min) with shallow breaths. His heart rate was elevated at 92 beats/min, and his blood pressure was low (86/62 mm Hg). His temperature was slightly above normal (38.5° C). Upon auscultation, there were diffuse crackling sounds (rales) in his lung fields. No other abnormalities were observed on physical examination.

Further evaluation revealed a slight reduction in arterial oxygen pressure, evidence of a pleural effusion (fluid around the lungs) on chest radiograph, and indications of right ventricular strain on electrocardiography (ECG). Based on the history of sudden onset of respiratory distress 1 week after major orthopedic surgery and the findings on physical examination, the treating emergency physician suspected a possible pulmonary embolus (PE). To confirm this diagnosis, she ordered a rapid D-dimer blood test, and the result was positive. In addition, a multislice computed tomography study of the chest revealed blockages within multiple pulmonary arteries.

Mr. W. was started immediately on a so-called clot-busting drug, alteplase. The patient also was started on medications to improve cardiac contractions, as well as an anticoagulant. Mr. W. was admitted to the critical care unit, where his symptoms progressively resolved over the next 24 hours. Then he was transferred to a regular nursing care unit, where he was ambulated and was started on a regimen of oral anticoagulant medications and physical therapy along with instruction about preventing recurrence of venous thromboembolism (VTE). He was discharged 3 days later, remaining on oral anticoagulants for 3 months without any further complications.

CLINICAL BACKGROUND

The patient in the Health Scenario had a postoperative PE. A PE is the blockage of one or more pulmonary arteries by a blood clot. Typically, these clots arise in the deep veins of the leg, or less commonly, other parts of the body. Such a clot is referred to as deep vein thrombosis (DVT). Because PEs tend to occur in conjunction with DVTs, the two entities are aggregated together under the rubric VTE.

Trailing only myocardial infarction and stroke, VTE is the third most common life-threatening form of cardiovascular disease in the United States. More than a half million hospitalizations each year in this country are associated with a diagnosis of a VTE. Because many VTEs occur as an unintended consequence of medical care, groups dedicated to improving patient safety and health care quality have ranked VTE as the most common preventable cause of hospital death in this country.

An understanding of VTE begins with an appreciation of the factors that contribute to the formation of clots (thrombi) in deep veins. Classically, a triad of factors is associated with the genesis of thrombi: (1) diminished venous blood flow, (2) increased coagulability of blood, and (3) damage to the blood vessel wall.

A thrombus is a solid accumulation of platelets, fibrin, and trapped red and white blood cells that forms within and blocks a blood vessel. Fragments of the clot, referred to as emboli, may break off and get swept away into the circulation, eventually wedging themselves in the smaller blood vessels of the pulmonary vascular tree. The redistributed blood flow creates areas of low ventilation–perfusion within the lung, resulting in impaired gas exchange.

A number of factors may predispose a patient to experience a VTE. Some of these characteristics are related to an elevation in the risk of clotting. These traits include, among others, advanced age (older than 40 years), a prior history of VTE, cigarette smoking, the use of estrogens or birth control pills, cancer, and certain autoimmune diseases. Other predisposing factors are related to diminished blood flow. These conditions include, but are not limited to, a family history of VTE, obesity, recent surgery (particularly those involving the pelvis, hip, or knee), fracture of the pelvis or legs, bed rest, the postpartum period, and placement of a heart pacemaker through a catheter in the groin.

The symptoms of a DVT may include single-sided leg or thigh redness, warmth, pain, or swelling, but about half of DVTs have no associated symptoms. With PE, the onset of symptoms often is abrupt with shortness of breath and pain when breathing, sometimes associated with a cough or coughing up blood (hemoptysis). Complaints related to DVT may or may not be present. Upon examination, patients with PE often exhibit rapid breathing (tachypnea) accompanied by a rapid heart rate (tachycardia); low blood pressure (hypotension, and if extremely low, shock); fever; and if oxygenation is poor, a pale or bluish skin color.

The history and physical examination can produce a high level of suspicion of a VTE, but the definitive diagnosis requires further studies. For patients in respiratory distress, prompt measurement of arterial oxygenation is essential. A rapid test for D-dimer, a breakdown product of cross-linked fibrin is useful, but it can be elevated in other conditions, as well. An ECG is important to rule out a myocardial infarction but can also provide supporting evidence of right heart dysfunction, as can an echocardiography. Often, chest radiograph results are normal, but they may reveal changes in the pulmonary vascularity, or fluid between the lung and chest wall.

Computed tomography of the chest with injected contrast material may reveal a filling defect in the pulmonary vasculature. Other imaging studies, such as pulmonary angiography and ventilation–perfusion scans, also may be used. DVTs often can be detected by compression ultrasonography, with clots indicated by internal sound echoes and the inability to compress the vein.

An acute, massive PE is a medical emergency, with 3% of patients dying within 48 hours and 10% expiring during hospitalization. The clinical course is particularly ominous for patients who experience shock, respiratory failure, or both. Initial management, therefore, is focused on achieving hemodynamic stability and optimal oxygenation. Medications can be used to increase blood pressure and cardiac output, as necessary. Simultaneously, oxygenation can be enhanced by dissolving the embolus, if it is massive, using clot-busting drugs or by interventional mechanical removal. Further clot formation is prevented by the administration of intravenous anticoagulants followed by maintenance on injectable or oral anticoagulants for a minimum of 3 months. The use of graduated compression stockings and frequent ambulation also helps to reduce the risk of additional clots.

INTRODUCTION

Health care professionals often are confronted with life-threatening situations in which the benefits of a treatment must be weighed against the risks associated with it. In the Health Scenario, for example, the emergency physician must balance the benefits of breaking up the clots in the pulmonary arteries of the patient with the risk of inducing serious bleeding from the use of clot-busting drugs. Although this particular situation involves a relatively extreme comparison of risks and benefits, less dramatic appraisals are made routinely in patient care. In this chapter, we provide an overview of how epidemiologic measures can be used to characterize various outcomes and support evidence-based practice.

MEASURES OF DISEASE OCCURRENCE

Three measures are used to quantify the frequency of events that occur in health care. The first is **risk**, which relates to the likelihood that an event (e.g., disease development or death) will occur. The second is **prevalence**, which corresponds to the proportion of a population that is affected by a disease. Finally, **incidence rate** refers to the speed with which new instances of a disease are developing.

Risk

Risk, sometimes also referred to as cumulative incidence, is an indicator of the proportion of persons within a specified population who develop the outcome of interest (e.g., onset of disease or death), within a defined time period.

We can express this concept in the form of an equation:

$$R = \frac{\text{New cases}}{\text{Persons at risk}} = \frac{A}{N}$$

where R is the estimated risk; A is the number of new instances of the outcome of interest, often described as new cases; and N is the number of unaffected persons at the beginning of the observation period. It is important to emphasize that at the outset, all persons under consideration must be free of the outcome of interest. The risk of developing the outcome then can range anywhere between 0 (if no outcomes occur during the observation period) and 1 (if all unaffected persons become affected during the observation period). For simplicity, risk often is presented as a percentage by multiplying the proportion by 100. The following example illustrates the calculation of risk, and weighing risks and benefits.

Example 1. Vekeman and colleagues (2012) were interested in the risk of VTE after total hip or knee arthroplasty and whether the use of anticoagulants to prevent VTEs might induce an unacceptable number of episodes of serious bleeding. Through a large national database, the investigators were able to identify more than 820,000 inpatient hospital stays for adults age 18 years or older who underwent one of these procedures between 2000 and 2008. A total of 8042 VTEs were observed during these hospital stays. The risk of a VTE among total hip or knee replacement admissions, therefore, is:

$$R = \frac{8042}{820,197} = 0.0098 = 0.98\%$$

In other words, about 1 in 100 patients undergoing these particular orthopedic procedures experienced a VTE during their hospitalizations. Similarly, the risk of a major bleeding event was calculated as:

$$R = \frac{2740}{820,197} = 0.0033 = 0.33\%$$

This means that about 1 in 300 patients undergoing these particular orthopedic procedures experienced a major episode of bleeding during hospitalization. The risk of a clot, therefore, is about three times greater than the risk of a major bleeding episode during the immediate hospitalization. In reaching any definitive conclusion about the full risks and benefits of anticoagulation, however, one would need to consider the period beyond the immediate hospitalization, as well as the outcomes of the thrombotic and bleeding episodes.

Prevalence

The proportion of persons within a population who have the condition of interest is referred to as prevalence. Sometimes we designate this proportion further as relating to a specific point in time (point prevalence) or alternately, to a particular time period (period prevalence). The prevalence is calculated by dividing the number of affected persons (cases) by the number of persons in the source population. Mathematically, we calculate prevalence as:

$$P = \frac{C}{N}$$

where P is the prevalence, C is the number of cases, and N is the size of the source population. As with risk, prevalence can range from 0 (no persons with the condition of interest), to 1 (everybody in the source population is affected). We can also express prevalence as a percentage, by multiplying by 100. The following example illustrates the calculation of prevalence.

Example 2. Deitelzweig and colleagues (2011) were interested in estimating the prevalence of VTE in the United States. For that purpose, they accessed a database that combined commercial insurance claims with those of Medicare beneficiaries for the 5-year period 2002 to 2006. The source population of these databases included 12.7 million persons. Of these persons, 200,007 had a VTE, so the 5-year period prevalence was:

$$P = \frac{200,007}{12.7 \text{ million}} = 0.016 = 1.6\%$$

The investigators calculated the 5-year period prevalence separately for DVT (1.1%), PE (0.4%), and both DVT and PE (0.1%). The annual prevalence of VTE was observed to increase progressively over the 5-year study period, with a low of 0.32% in 2002, rising to a high of 0.42% in 2006. The investigators also demonstrated a strong predilection for VTE among persons aged 65 years and older.

Incidence Rate

The incidence rate measures the rapidity with which newly diagnosed cases of a disease develop. The faster the population is becoming affected, the higher the incidence rate. To estimate the incidence rate, one follows a source population of unaffected persons over time, counting the number of individuals who become newly affected (cases), and expresses it relative to person-time (PT), which is a combination of the size of the source population and the time period of observation.

The quantification of PT may seem a little confusing at first, so let us explore how it is calculated. The goal is to estimate the total amount of disease-free time that subjects in the source population are observed. For example, an individual who is followed for 1 year without developing the condition of interest contributes 1 year of observation. Another person may develop the condition of interest 6 months into the study. Although this individual may be followed for a full year, he or she only contributes a half year of disease-free observation to the study. In this manner, each individual contributes a specific amount of disease-free observation, which then can be summed over all persons in the source population, yielding a total PT of observation. Then, we can calculate the incidence rate as:

$$IR = \frac{A}{PT}$$

where IR is the incidence rate, A is the number of newly diagnosed occurrences of the condition of interest, and PT is the total amount of disease-free observation within the source population.

Example 3. To estimate the incidence rate of VTE in the Canadian province of Québec, Tagalakis and colleagues (2013) accessed health care administrative databases to identify all new cases of DVT or PE between 2000 and 2009. The overall incidence of VTE was found to be:

$$IR = \frac{91,761 \text{ cases}}{74,297,764 \text{ person-year}}$$

$$= 0.00124 \text{ cases/person-year}$$

To express the incidence rate with fewer decimal places, it is convenient to convert it to 1.24 cases/1000 person-years of observation. An equivalent expression would be 124 cases per 100,000 person-years of observation. In other words, among residents of the province of Québec during the decade of 2000 to 2009, the overall incidence rate of newly diagnosed VTEs was a little more than one 1000 persons followed for 1 year.

In a large population, such as that of the province of Québec, it would be difficult to enumerate the person-years of observation by summing the amount of observation for each individual person over the entire population. An approximation for the population time can be obtained by multiplying the average size of the population at risk (as estimated through a census) by the length of time the population is observed. The estimate will be reasonably accurate if the condition of interest is relatively infrequent in the general population (as is the case for VTE) and there are no major demographic shifts (e.g., in-migration or out-migration) during the period of observation.

It is important to note that the incidence rate relates to the first occurrence of the disease or condition of interest. VTE is a disorder that can recur, so if all episodes of VTE in a population (both initial and recurrent) are counted, the estimate of the VTE incidence rate will be inflated. To avoid this problem, the investigator must be able to exclude prior diagnoses of VTE when identifying incident cases.

DISTINCTIONS BETWEEN MEASURES OF DISEASE FREQUENCY

Risk, prevalence, and incidence rate are among the most commonly used measures in epidemiology and clinical medicine. Unfortunately, they also are often misunderstood and inappropriately used interchangeably. In reality, these terms relate to distinct concepts.

As an exercise in understanding the differences between these measures, it may be useful to consider the following illustration.

Example 4. Spencer and colleagues (2009) undertook a population-based study in Worcester, Massachusetts, to determine the incidence rates, clinical features, and outcomes of VTE. The patients were identified from hospital admissions, as well as from outpatient, emergency department, imaging, and laboratory facilities. First occurrences of VTEs were included for 3 years of diagnoses: 1999, 2001, and 2003. The patients were followed for about 3 years on average for determination of any recurrences.

In all, 1567 incident cases of VTE occurred, which corresponded to an incidence rate of 1.14 cases/1000 person-years, similar but slightly lower than the incidence rate previously noted for Québec province. As shown in **Figure 2-1**, the incidence rate for VTE was strongly age dependent, with the highest rates among elderly adults. Examination of incidence rates by gender (**Figure 2-2**) revealed higher rates among women than among men. Similarly, when incidence rates were examined over time, there was little suggestion of any increase (data not shown).

When the medical characteristics of these patients at the time of VTE diagnosis were considered, the prevalence of a recent (within 3 months) surgery was:

$$P = \frac{478 \text{ recent surgeries}}{1567 \text{ VTE patients}} = 0.305 = 30.5\%$$

Similarly, the prevalence of a recent (within 3 months) central venous catheterization was:

$$P = \frac{312 \text{ recent catheterizations}}{1567 \text{ VTE patients}} = 0.119 = 19.9\%$$

The risk of developing a recurrent VTE within an average follow-up period of about 3 years was:

$$R = \frac{260 \text{ recurrences}}{1567 \text{ VTE patients}} = 0.166 = 16.6\%$$

Over the same follow-up period, the risk of developing major bleeding on anticoagulant therapy was:

$$R = \frac{194 \text{ bleeding episodes}}{1567 \text{ VTE patients}} = 0.124 = 12.4\%$$

In this single study, the investigators have characterized aspects of VTE occurrence using all three types of measures of disease frequency. They used incidence rates to characterize the rapidity with which VTE was arising within the population of Worcester, Massachusetts. They further characterized patterns of occurrence by examining incidence rates by age, gender, and time period. They then described the clinical profile of the VTE-affected

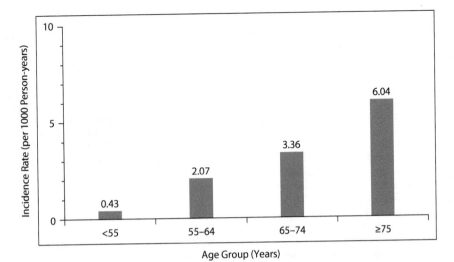

Figure 2-1. Incidence rates of venous thromboembolism, by age, Worcester, Massachusetts, 1999 to 2003. (Data from Emery C, Joffe SW, et al. Incidence rates, clinical profile, and outcomes of patients with venous thromboembolism. The Worcester VTE Study. *J Thromb Thrombolysis.* 2009;28:401-409.)

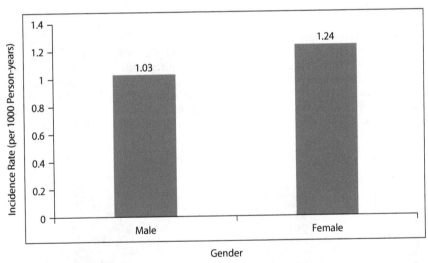

Figure 2-2. Incidence rates of venous thromboembolism, by gender, Worcester, Massachusetts, 1999 to 2003. (Data from Spencer FA, Emery C, Joffe SW, et al. Incidence rates, clinical profile, and outcomes of patients with venous thromboembolism. The Worcester VTE Study. *J Thromb Thrombolysis.* 2009;28:401-409.)

individuals at diagnosis by examining the prevalence of various risk factors of disease occurrence, such as recent surgery or central catheterization. Finally, they estimated the risk of subsequent adverse events, such as recurrent VTEs or bleeding, by following the patients over time to determine the percentage who experienced these complications. Each of these measures helps to complete the picture of the pattern of occurrence of VTE within the population.

SURVIVAL

For diseases, such as VTE, that can have serious impacts on an affected person's well-being, we may wish to characterize the likelihood of remaining alive, or survival, after a diagnosis. Mathematically, we would measure survival (S) as:

$$S = \frac{A - D}{A}$$

where A is the number of newly diagnosed patients with the condition of interest and D is the number of deaths. Survival is, therefore, a proportion that can range from 0 (when no patients survive) to 1 (when all patients survive). We can convert survival to a percentage by multiplying by 100. It is important to recognize that survival is a time-dependent phenomenon, therefore, it is essential to specify a time period for the measurement of survival, such as the 30-day survival, or the 1-year survival.

Example 5. In the previously cited study by Tagalakis and colleagues (2013) of VTE in Québec province, patients were followed for survival after their initial diagnosis. Among the 33,447 persons with a PE, there were 5654 deaths within the first 30 days after diagnosis. The 30-day survival, therefore, is calculated as:

$$S = \frac{33,447 - 5654}{33,447} = 0.83 = 83\%$$

Survival estimates provide a clear and meaningful way to characterize the prognosis of a condition. For example, in this same study population, among the 58,314 persons with a newly diagnosed DVT, the 30-day survival estimate was 93%. As shown in **Figure 2-3**, the near-term (30 day) prognosis after PE is worse (lower survival) than that for DVT. For both PE and DVT, the likelihood of surviving the first 30 days was highly related to the patient's age at diagnosis. The age-specific survival estimates are shown for PE in **Figure 2-4**. It can be seen from this graph that persons age 80 years or older have almost a one third

lower probability of surviving for 1 month after a PE than persons 40 years or younger. Thus, some basic information about the diagnosis and the personal characteristics of the patient can be helpful in predicting the clinical outcome.

It should be emphasized that although these likelihoods are derived from the experiences of a group of patients, they also represent our best predictions for an individual patient who fits within the corresponding group. In other words, the evidence from this investigation suggests that among a group of persons 80 years or older with a new PE, 71% will survive for at least 1 month after diagnosis. Similarly, our best estimate from these data of the 30-day survival rate for an individual 82-year-old patient with a new PE is 71%.

When the survival period of interest is relatively short, such as 30 days, the likelihood that one will be able to follow all patients to the end of the observation period is quite high. On the other hand, as the duration of the follow-up period increases, so does the likelihood that the investigator will not be able to track each and every subject for the full time period. For example, a patient may move away from the study area. In studies in which individual patients are being tracked for their outcomes, subjects may be lost to observation for a variety of reasons, such as relocation, changing names (through marriage or other circumstances), voluntarily withdrawing from participation, or because the study ends before the patient has completed the full observation period of interest. If such losses are substantial, excluding these patients with incomplete follow-up might introduce error

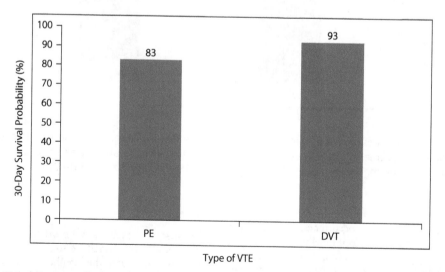

Figure 2-3. Thirty-day survival after a venous thromboembolism (VTE), by type (pulmonary embolus [PE] or deep vein thrombosis [DVT]), Québec province, 2000 to 2009. (Data from Tagalakis V, Patenaude V, Kahn SR, Suissa S. Incidence of and mortality from venous thromboembolism in a real-world population: the Q-VTE Study Cohort. *Am J Med.* 2013;126:832.e13-21.)

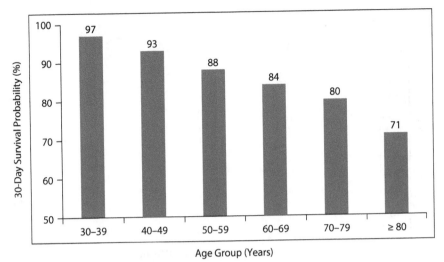

Figure 2-4. Thirty-day survival probabilities after a diagnosis of pulmonary embolus, by age at onset. (Data from Tagalakis V, Patenaude V, Kahn SR, Suissa S. Incidence of and mortality from venous thromboembolism in a real-world population: the Q-VTE Study Cohort. *Am J Med.* 2013;126:832.e13-21.)

in estimation, which we refer to as a bias. Consider for instance, that patients who move away have more favorable outcomes than those who remain. Excluding those subjects who relocate, therefore, would yield an erroneously low estimate of survival. Even if the outcomes do not differ, throwing out all information on patients who were lost to follow-up is wasteful in a statistical sense. By this, we mean that reducing the number of subjects under consideration is tantamount to reducing the sample size, and as a consequence, our survival estimates are not as precise as they might otherwise be if these individuals were included.

Fortunately, there are statistical techniques that allow an investigator to use all of the follow-up information that is available, even for patients who are lost to follow-up or for whom the study ends before they complete the full follow-up period. Two such techniques are life-table analysis and so-called Kaplan-Meier analysis. Although the methods for performing these calculations are beyond the scope of this discussion, readers who are interested in more detail may consult discussions of survival analysis in most biostatistics textbooks.

Survival results over time often are depicted in a graphical format, such as that shown in **Figure 2-5**. Here survival likelihood is shown for the first 2 years after a new VTE diagnosis among persons who also had cancer. On the horizontal axis, time since the first diagnosis of the VTE is depicted in months, with 0 time representing when the diagnosis was made. Over time, the percentage of persons surviving declines, with key observation periods every 6 months. It can

be seen that the most dramatic decrease in survival occurs in the first 6 months after a VTE, with smaller risk of death in subsequent observation periods.

Example 6. One might want to summarize the survival results with a single measure, such as the percentage of persons with cancer surviving for 2 years after a first VTE. To estimate this probability as shown in **Figure 2-6**, one first goes to the follow-up period of interest—in this case, 24 months—and draws a vertical line (A) to the survival curve. From the point at which line A intersects the survival curve, one draws a horizontal line (B) to the y axis. The point of intersection of line B with the y axis yields the survival probability—in this case, 35%.

Another useful measure to characterize the observed survival experience is the **median survival time**. This corresponds to the amount of time after diagnosis at which point half of the affected individuals remain alive. **Figure 2-7** shows how the median survival time is estimated. First, one draws a horizontal line from 50% survival on the y axis to the survival curve. From the point at which line A intersects the survival curve, one draws a vertical line (B) to the x axis. The point of intersection of line B with the x axis yields the median survival time—in this case, 12 months.

Case-Fatality

Another measure of prognosis after a diagnosis is the **case-fatality**. *This metric refers to the proportion (or percentage) of persons with a particular condition who die within a specified period of time.* Often, case-fatality is incorrectly referred to as a rate or a ratio, but it is

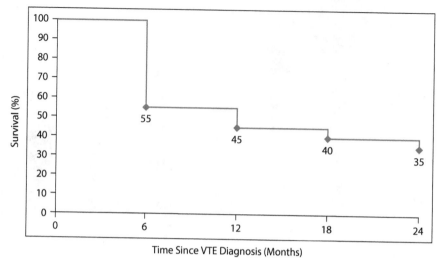

Figure 2-5. Survival curve from the time of an incident venous thromboembolism (VTE) diagnosis for persons with preexisting cancer.

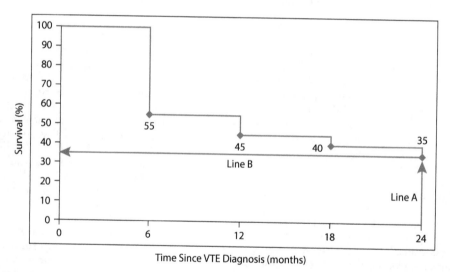

Figure 2-6. Approach to estimating the 2-year survival probability after a venous thromboembolism (VTE) diagnosis among persons with cancer.

more accurately described as a risk or probability. It is calculated mathematically as:

$$CF = \frac{\text{Number of deaths}}{\text{Number of diagnosed persons}} = \frac{D}{A}$$

where CF is case-fatality, D is the number of deaths, and A is the number of persons with the condition of interest. The case-fatality can range from 0 when there are no deaths observed during the specified timeframe to 1 when all affected persons with the condition of interest die during the specified timeframe. For simplicity, the case-fatality often is expressed as a percentage by multiplying by 100.

Example 7. The previously cited study of VTE in Québec province (Tagalakis et al, 2013) included information on case-fatality risks at 30 days and 1 year after diagnosis. The results are shown separately for DVTs and PEs in **Figure 2-8**. It can be seen that PEs have a much higher associated risk of death than do DVTs, with the excess appearing soon after the diagnosis and persisting through subsequent observation.

Because case-fatality reflects the probability of death within a defined period of time and survival relates to the

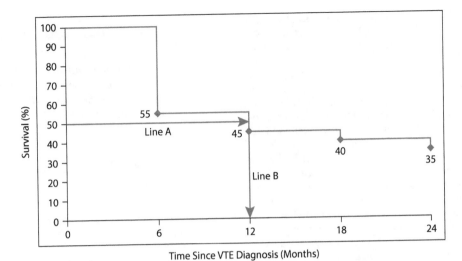

Figure 2-7. Approach to estimating the median survival time after a venous thromboembolism (VTE) diagnosis among persons with cancer.

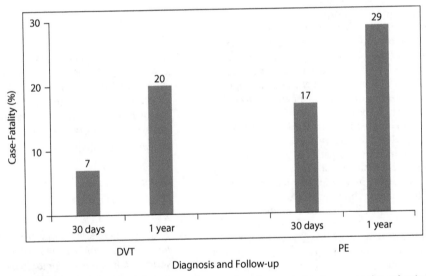

Figure 2-8. Case-fatality percentages at 30 days and 1 year after diagnosis for deep vein thrombosis (DVT) and pulmonary embolus (PE), Québec province, 2000 to 2009. (Data from Tagalakis V, Patenaude V, Kahn SR, Suissa S. Incidence of and mortality from venous thromboembolism in a real-world population: the Q-VTE Study Cohort. *Am J Med.* 2013;126:832.e13-21.)

probability of not dying in that defined period, the two measures may be thought of as inverse proportions—as one increases, the other, of necessity, decreases.

SUMMARY

In this chapter, we featured basic measures of disease frequency and prognosis. Each of these metrics is used commonly in epidemiology and clinical medicine.

Despite their routine appearance in the literature, the meaning and appropriate application of these measures often is misconstrued. To review, **risk** (also referred to as cumulative incidence) is the fraction of unaffected individuals within a defined population who newly develop the condition of interest during a specified time period. **Prevalence** also is defined as a proportion, but it refers to the fraction of persons within a population who have the condition of interest at any particular point or period of time. **Incidence rate** refers to the rapidity with which unaffected persons within a defined population develop the condition of interest. Risk, prevalence, and incidence rate are used typically to quantify the amount, sometimes called burden, of disease within a particular group of people.

Several measures are used to characterize the prognosis of a condition of interest after it has occurred. Risk can be used to characterize the likelihood that a particular outcome (favorable or unfavorable) will occur among newly affected persons with the condition of interest over a specified period of time. **Survival** is the probability of a particular outcome (remaining alive) during a specified period of time after diagnosis with the condition of interest. **Case-fatality** is the inverse of survival and represents the likelihood of a particular outcome (death) during a specified time period after diagnosis of the condition of interest.

We have seen how each of these measures can be used to help quantify aspects of VTE occurrence and prognosis. Specifically, we learned that whereas the risk of a VTE arising during the hospitalization for a total knee or hip replacement was about 1%, the risk of a major bleeding episode on routine anticoagulant therapy to prevent VTEs was one third as great. The 5-year period prevalence of VTE in the United States was shown to be between 1% and 2% of the general population. The incidence rate of VTE separately was found to be slightly more than one case for every 1000 person-years of observation. We learned that the incidence rate of VTE is highly related to age, with the highest rates among elderly adults. Among patients with a newly diagnosed VTE, the prevalence of recent surgery was almost one third, and the prevalence of a recent central venous catheterization was about one fifth.

In terms of prognosis, we learned that the risk of recurrence of a VTE over 3 years was about one in six patients, and the risk of a major bleeding episode was about one in eight patients. Finally, we learned that whereas a particularly serious form of VTE, PE, has a 30-day survival probability of only 83%, those diagnosed with a DVT had a 1-month survival probability of 93%. We also saw that survival probability was strongly related to age, with 30-day survival from PE much more likely among young adults. Finally, we found that the case-fatality percentage at 1 year after diagnosis of a PE was much higher (29%) than the corresponding 1-year case-fatality for DVT (20%).

Together, these measures have painted a very clear picture of VTE in the general population. This is a common condition, with particularly high risk among persons undergoing invasive medical procedures. The prognosis is strongly related to the type of VTE and the age of the patient at diagnosis, with significant loss of life in the first month after diagnosis.

STUDY QUESTIONS

1. To characterize the burden of diabetes mellitus on a population, an investigator conducts a household survey of residents. The most appropriate measure in this context is
   A. risk.
   B. prevalence.
   C. incidence rate.
   D. survival.
   E. case-fatality.

2. To assess prognosis after a diagnosis of diabetic coma, an investigator collects information on deaths within 30 days. The most appropriate measure in this context is
   A. cumulative incidence.
   B. prevalence.
   C. incidence rate.
   D. attributable risk.
   E. case-fatality.

3. To assess the likelihood of women developing diabetes during pregnancy, an investigator follows 10,000 nondiabetic women from inception to completion of pregnancy and determines the percentage of them who develop gestational diabetes. The most appropriate measure in this context is
   A. cumulative incidence.
   B. prevalence.
   C. incidence rate.
   D. attributable risk.
   E. case-fatality.

4. To assess the rapidity with which diabetes mellitus develops among a cohort of morbidly obese young adults, an investigator follows each nondiabetic obese student for the development of newly diagnosed diabetes mellitus from matriculation at a university through graduation. The most appropriate measure in this context is
   A. cumulative incidence.
   B. prevalence.
   C. incidence rate.
   D. attributable risk.
   E. case-fatality.

5. Which of the following measures may be thought of as the inverse of case-fatality?
   A. Cumulative incidence
   B. Prevalence

C. *Incidence rate*

D. *Survival*

E. *Attributable risk*

Questions 6 to 10. To better understand the epidemiology and clinical outcomes of diabetes mellitus, an investigator screens the workforce of 1500 adult employees at a large retail business. Of the workers screened, 500 have diabetes mellitus. Among the remaining workers, check-ups are performed each year for 1 decade, and 100 new cases of diabetes are diagnosed. For the diabetic patients, follow-up is continued for 10 years after diagnosis, yielding 10 cases of diabetic retinopathy and 1 death.

6. *The prevalence (%) of diabetes in the workforce at the outset was*

    A. *1.*

    B. *10.*

    C. *33.*

    D. *100.*

    E. *500.*

7. *The incidence rate (cases/person-year) was*

    A. *0.01.*

    B. *0.1.*

    C. *1.0.*

    D. *10.0.*

    E. *100.0.*

8. *The 10-year cumulative incidence (%) of diabetes was*

    A. *0.01.*

    B. *0.1.*

    C. *1.0.*

    D. *10.0.*

    E. *100.0.*

9. *The 10-year case-fatality (%) was*

    A. *0.01.*

    B. *0.1.*

    C. *1.0.*

    D. *10.0.*

    E. *100.0.*

10. *The 10-year risk (%) of diabetic retinopathy was*

    A. *0.01.*

    B. *0.1.*

    C. *1.0.*

    D. *10.0.*

    E. *100.0.*

FURTHER READING

Heit JA. The epidemiology of venous thromboembolism in the community. *Arterioscler Thromb Vasc Biol.* 2008;28:370-372.

Wong P, Baglin T. Epidemiology, risk factors and sequelae of venous thromboembolism. *Phlebology.* 2012;27(suppl 2):2-11.

REFERENCES

Clinical Background

Pollak AW, McBane RD. Succinct review of the new VTE prevention and management guidelines. *Mayo Clin Proc. 2014;89*:394-408.

Wells PS, Forgie MA, Rodger MA. Treatment of venous thromboembolism. *JAMA.* 2014;311:717-728.

Risk

Vekeman F, LaMori JC, Laliberté F, et al. In-hospital risk of venous thromboembolism and bleeding and associated costs for patients undergoing total hip or knee arthroplasty. *J Med Econ.* 2012;15:644-653.

Prevalence

Deitelzweig SB, Johnson BH, Lin J, Schulman KL. Prevalence of clinical venous thromboembolism in the USA: current trends and future projections. *Am J Hematol.* 2011;86:217-220.

Incidence

Tagalakis V, Patenaude V, Kahn SR, Suissa S. Incidence of and mortality from venous thromboembolism in a real-world population: the Q-VTE Study Cohort. *Am J Med.* 2013;126(832):e13-21.

Distinctions Between Measures of Disease Frequency

Spencer FA, Emery C, Joffe SW, et al. Incidence rates, clinical profile, and outcomes of patients with venous thromboembolism. The Worcester VTE Study. *J Thromb Thrombolysis.* 2009; 28:401-409.

Survival

Tagalakis V, Patenaude V, Kahn SR, Suissa S. Incidence of and mortality from venous thromboembolism in a real-world population: the Q-VTE Study Cohort. *Am J Med.* 2013;126(832):e13-21.

Case-Fatality

Tagalakis V, Patenaude V, Kahn SR, Suissa S. Incidence of and mortality from venous thromboembolism in a real-world population: the Q-VTE Study Cohort. *Am J Med.* 2013;126(832):e13-21.

Patterns of Occurrence

3

Raymond S. Greenberg

HEALTH SCENARIO

A 62-year-old healthy female office manager with fair skin visited her dermatologist for the evaluation of a recently appearing itchy black mole on her left thigh. Upon examination, the mole was approximately 8 mm in diameter with an asymmetrical shape, irregular borders, black and brown coloration, and a flat surface. An excisional biopsy with 1-cm surgical margins was performed revealing a superficial spreading melanoma of 0.6-mm thickness without ulceration or evidence of rapid cell division. There was no disease spread beyond the primary anatomic site, and the patient was followed with regular examinations, which revealed no recurrence or spread during the following 5 years.

CLINICAL BACKGROUND

Melanoma is a malignancy of pigment-producing cells (melanocytes) principally found in the skin. It is the fifth most common form of cancer in the United States, with more than 75,000 cases diagnosed each year. Although fewer than 5% of skin cancers are melanomas, four out of five deaths from skin cancer are related to melanoma.

Melanomas typically present, as in the patient described, as nonuniform pigmented skin lesions that have changed over time. The lesions may have shades of brown, black, red, or blue discoloration. The appearance usually is asymmetrical, and the boundaries are often indistinct or irregular. At diagnosis, the size usually exceeds a half centimeter.

Melanoma occurs much more frequently among whites than among those of other races. It tends to arise more frequently in older persons but can occur as early as the second or third decades of life. Fair-skinned persons, as in the patient described earlier, are at increased risk as are those with light hair color, blue eyes, and a predisposition to freckling.

Persons with a family history of melanoma are at increased risk, and a number of genes have been associated with a predisposition to developing this disease. Persons who have had a previous melanoma are at greatly elevated risk of developing a second melanoma. By far, the strongest environmental risk factor for this disease is exposure to ultraviolet (UV) radiation. This can occur through sunlight exposure, as demonstrated by cumulative indices of exposure, as well as frequency of sunburn events. The use of tanning beds also has been linked to melanoma risk, especially among young adults who are regular users.

A diagnosis of melanoma is confirmed by a surgical biopsy that removes some or all of the lesion for microscopic examination by a pathologist. There are five subtypes of melanoma, with about two thirds classified as the superficial spreading type. These cancers begin as a proliferation of melanocytes in the basal layer of the skin and tend to grow by radial (outward) expansion followed eventually by vertical (upward) expansion.

Several microscopic features have been shown to be related to the prognosis of melanomas. One of the most important attributes is the vertical penetration of the lesion, with tumors divided into thin (<1 mm), intermediate (1–4 mm), and thick (>4 mm) levels. Patients with thinner melanomas tend to have better clinical outcomes. Other attributes that affect prognosis are ulceration (loss of the overlying epithelium), which is associated with worse prognosis, and mitotic activity, with higher levels of cell reproduction being linked to poorer outcomes.

The primary treatment for cutaneous melanoma is surgical removal. It is important that the entire malignancy be removed, as evidenced by margins that lack cancer cells. The recommended width of the clear margins depends on the size of the tumor. For the majority of patients with thin, nonulcerated, low mitotic rate tumors, as in our example, no further evaluation generally is required. For those with adverse prognosis factors, however, imaging studies or sampling of lymph nodes (or both) may be indicated to determine whether the cancer has spread to regional lymph nodes or beyond. For patients with high-risk or advanced disease, interferon is the only treatment shown to slow the spread of disease and improve overall survival. Interferon is a glycoprotein that binds to a specific membrane receptor, leading to the activation of genes that produce substances that interfere with cancer growth by inhibiting cell proliferation and preventing the growth of new blood vessels to nourish the tumor. Other systemic treatments for disseminated melanoma are under evaluation.

DESCRIPTIVE EPIDEMIOLOGY

In Chapter 1, we learned that one of the primary uses of epidemiology is **descriptive**, by which we mean evaluation of the distribution of a disease within a population. We contrasted this application with **analytic** epidemiology, which focuses on the study of potential causes of a disease.

These two types of epidemiology each serve essential purposes and may be seen as complementary in nature. Descriptive studies often lead to speculation about underlying patterns of occurrence and why some population groups appear to be at higher (or lower) risk of becoming affected. These theories could be tested in a subsequent analytic study. Similarly, analytic studies may shed light on reasons for variation in disease occurrence within populations, leading to more focused surveillance strategies.

In this chapter, we focus on descriptive epidemiology, using malignant melanoma as the illustrative example. For this purpose, we will use the tools of measurement that were introduced in Chapter 2. We are guided in this effort by three basic questions of descriptive epidemiology:

1. **Who** develops the disease (melanoma)?
2. **Where** does the disease (melanoma) tend to occur?
3. **When** does the disease (melanoma) tend to occur?

In answering these questions, we characterize the distribution of melanoma by **person**, **place**, and **time**. We can think of these three dimensions as helping us to map out the population distribution of melanoma, as depicted schematically in **Figure 3-1**.

PERSON

As noted in Chapter 1, one of the fundamental tenets of epidemiology is that diseases do not occur at random. In other words, some people, by virtue of their personal characteristics, have a heightened risk of developing the disease. Other persons, by virtue of their own attributes, have a lowered risk of the disease. The job of the epidemiologist is to ascertain which of these personal attributes is most highly associated with risk.

The most basic place to begin with is demographic characteristics such as age, race, and sex. This information is available routinely from clinical and other sources of information on the affected individuals, as well as on the population from which they arose.

The incidence of melanoma in the United States is shown by age in **Figure 3-2**. Incidence data are available for cancer in the United States through a variety of mechanisms. One is the Surveillance, Epidemiology and End Results (SEER) Program of the National Cancer Institute. The SEER Program, created in 1973, involves a network of cancer registries that collectively cover more than one quarter of the U.S. population. A disease registry is an organized system for collecting information on

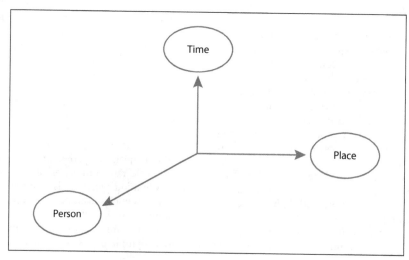

Figure 3-1. Schematic representation of the standard dimensions used to characterize disease occurrence.

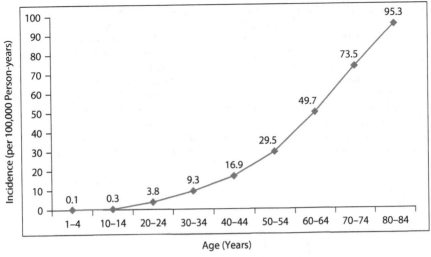

Figure 3-2. Incidence rates for melanoma, by age, United States, 2006 to 2010. (Data from Howlader N, et al. *SEER Cancer Statistics Review, 1975-2010*. Bethesda, MD: National Cancer Institute; 2013.)

persons with a disease of interest. Registries can be hospital based, meaning that they focus on patients treated at a specific health care facility or group of facilities. Other registries are population based, meaning that an attempt is made to collect information on all affected persons who reside within a particular area. The SEER registry system is population based and involves 20 areas selected to be broadly representative of the United States.

A second population-based cancer registration system in the United States is the National Program of Cancer Registries, first organized in 1992 and coordinated by the Centers for Disease Control and Prevention (CDC). Today, this program includes data from 45 states and territories, which correspond to 96% of the U.S. population.

The data presented in **Figure 3-2** were derived from the SEER Program. We can see that melanoma is a strongly age-dependent condition, with a dramatic rise in incidence with age. In general, cancer is a disease that tends to predominate at older ages.

The incidence of melanoma is depicted by race and ethnicity in **Figure 3-3**. There is a dramatic differential,

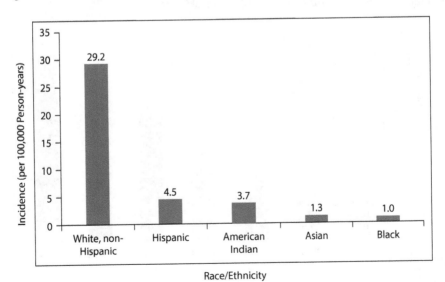

Figure 3-3. Incidence rates of melanoma, by race/ethnicity, in the United States, 2006 to 2010. (Data from Howlader N, et al. *SEER Cancer Statistics Review, 1975-2010*. Bethesda, MD: National Cancer Institute; 2013.)

with the highest risk among non-Hispanic whites and the lowest risks among Asians and blacks. Twenty- to 30-fold difference in risk across race/ethnic groups is highly unusual and is therefore an important clue to the underlying risk factors. One possible explanation for this pattern is that darker, more pigmented skin tends to protect against the damage caused by UV radiation. Other factors related to European ancestry may be involved as well, including genetic susceptibility.

The incidence of melanoma by sex is illustrated in **Figure 3-4**. Here we see a 60% excess of disease among males. These summary results are heavily reflective of the pattern among non-Hispanic whites because that particular race/ethnic group so dominates the overall occurrence patterns. A male excess is seen in some, but not all, race/ethnic groups in the United States and elsewhere, so there may be factors related to sunlight exposure patterns or other risk factors that explain this disparity.

It is also worth noting that the male excess of melanoma in the United States appears principally at older ages. As illustrated in **Figure 3-5**, there is a progressive increase in the male-to-female ratio of melanoma

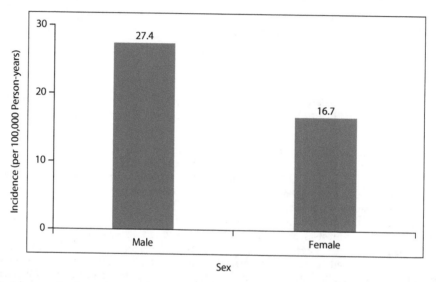

Figure 3-4. Incidence rates for melanoma, by sex, United States, 2006 to 2010. (Data from Howlader N, et al. *SEER Cancer Statistics Review, 1975-2010*. Bethesda, MD: National Cancer Institute; 2013.)

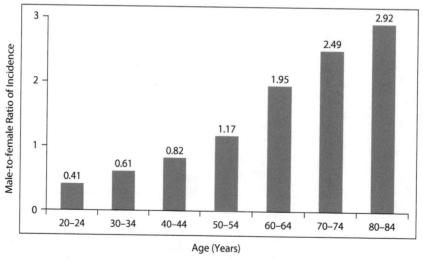

Figure 3-5. Male-to-female ratio of melanoma incidence among whites, by age, United States, 2008 to 2010. (Data from Howlader N, et al. *SEER Cancer Statistics Review, 1975-2010*. Bethesda, MD: National Cancer Institute; 2013.)

incidence with age. Before age 50 years, females exhibit excesses of the disease, with male excesses occurring over age 50 years. It has been speculated that the high risk among young women may relate to more frequent UV radiation exposure by sunlight, use of tanning beds, or both.

PLACE

Variation in disease occurrence by place of residence can be examined across countries or within them. In

Figure 3-6, incidence rates for melanoma among men are shown for representative countries of residence. Tremendous variation is seen, with the highest rates in the Oceanic region (Australia and New Zealand) and the lowest rates in Asia. (African countries were not included here because of extremely low rates and poor registration systems.) North American and Northern European countries tend to have moderately high rates, with lower rates in Southern Europe and South America. The corresponding incidence patterns for females are shown in **Figure 3-7**, with

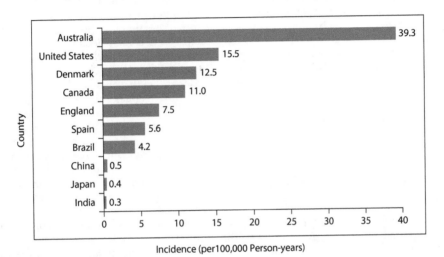

Figure 3-6. Incidence rates for melanoma, by country, for males, 2000 to 2002. (Data from Erdman F et al. International trends in the incidence of malignant melanoma 1953-2008: are recent generations at higher or lower risk? *Int J Cancer.* 2013;132:385-400.)

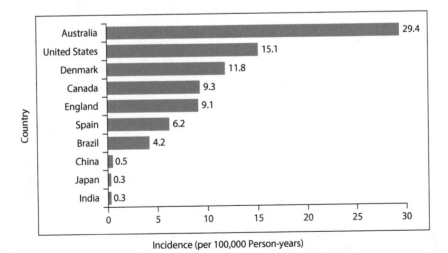

Figure 3-7. Incidence rates for melanoma, by country, for females, 2000 to 2002. (Data from Erdman F et al. International trends in the incidence of malignant melanoma 1953-2008: are recent generations at higher or lower risk? *Int J Cancer.* 2013;132:385-400.)

similar rankings, except for Denmark replacing the United States with the second highest rates.

These patterns of international variation in melanoma incidence tend to support the general notion of elevated rates among fair-skinned populations (Northern Europe, North America, and Oceania). Within Europe, the gradient of increasing rates with rising latitude is consistent with a gradient in skin pigmentation. The combination of fair skin and heavy sunlight exposure, as occurs in Oceania, results in the highest overall risk of melanoma.

Variation in disease occurrence also can be examined by place of residence within a single country. One such analysis was performed in Norway, a country with a homogeneous, fair-skinned population. Overall, Norway is located at high latitude, but it extends across a considerable geographic range (57–72° N), allowing a comparison of incidence in the northern and southern parts of the country. The rates in the south of Norway are twice the corresponding rates in the north of the country, consistent with the greater sunlight exposure in the south.

CORRELATIONS WITH DISEASE OCCURRENCE

The variation of disease occurrence patterns across population groups can be used to generate hypotheses about the reasons for this variation. Such a study may be useful for suggesting potential risk factors

for the disease because it is relatively quick, inexpensive, and easy to perform. This type of investigation is referred to as an **ecologic study** because it examines the pattern of risk at the group or population level rather than on a person-by-person basis. Such a study might also be referred to as a **correlation study** because it results in a measure of how strongly disease occurrence is related to some potentially predictive characteristics.

To illustrate an ecologic study, data are presented in **Figure 3-8** on the mortality rate of melanoma in relation to the annual number of days of very high UV index, a measure of intensity of UV radiation from the sun. For this analysis, eight Midwestern states were chosen because they have stable populations and are relatively homogeneous with respect to race and ethnicity. The states included were North Dakota, South Dakota, Minnesota, Iowa, Nebraska, Missouri, Kansas, and Oklahoma. Mortality rates were used here rather than incidence rates because the former was readily available for all states. The UV index data were from a period more than a decade before the mortality experience, thereby accounting for a lag in time from exposure to the development of disease and subsequent clinical course. An even longer lag period might have been justified given the presumed length of exposure required for melanoma to develop, but earlier measures of UV index were not universally available.

The scatterplot in **Figure 3-8** reveals a generally positive relationship between days of very high UV index

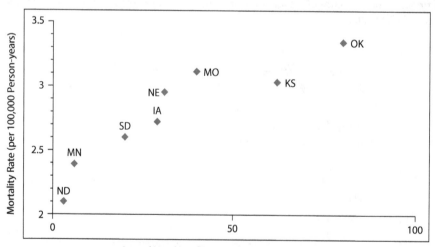

Figure 3-8. Scatterplot of mortality rate of melanoma (2006–2010) in relation to annual days of very high ultraviolet index (1995) for eight selected states in the Midwestern United States. (Melanoma data from Howlader N, et al. *SEER Cancer Statistics Review, 1975-2010.* Bethesda, MD: National Cancer Institute; 2013. UV index data from Climate Prediction Center, National Weather Service, National Oceanic and Atmospheric Administration: *UV Index: Annual Time Series.* College Park, MD; 2013.)

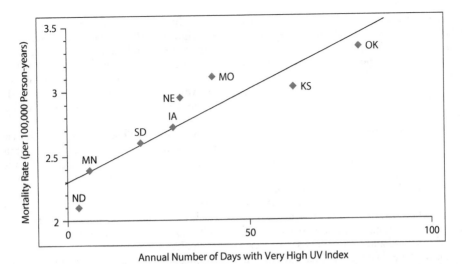

Figure 3-9. Regression line for regression of mortality from melanoma (2006–2010) on annual days of very high ultraviolet index (1995). (Melanoma data from Howlader N, et al. *SEER Cancer Statistics Review, 1975-2010.* Bethesda, MD: National Cancer Institute; 2013. UV index data from Climate Prediction Center, National Weather Service, National Oceanic and Atmospheric Administration: *UV Index: Annual Time Series.* College Park, MD; 2013.)

and mortality from melanoma, with states with more days of intense sunlight exposure (e.g., Oklahoma and Kansas) experiencing higher rates of death from melanoma. In contrast, states with fewer days of intense solar radiation (e.g., North Dakota and Minnesota) had lower rates of death from melanoma.

To assess the strengths of relationships between days of very high UV index and death rate from melanoma, a correlation analysis was performed on these data. If very high UV index and melanoma mortality were maximally correlated, the **correlation coefficient** would be 1.0. If there was no relationship at all, then the correlation coefficient would be zero. If there was a maximally inverse relationship (i.e., melanoma deaths tended to occur more frequently in areas with lower UV index), the correlation coefficient would be -1.0. The calculated correlation coefficient was 0.91, which confirms the visual impression that the measure of intense solar radiation and melanoma death rates are strongly and positively linked.

The square of the correlation coefficient is 0.83, and this is referred to as the **coefficient of determination**. An interpretation of this finding is that more than four fifths of the variation observed in melanoma mortality rates can be accounted for by the number of days of very high UV index.

A linear regression analysis of these data revealed the following equation:

$$\text{Mortality} = 2.30 + 0.014(\text{Days UV index})$$

A graph of this regression line is shown in **Figure 3-9**. This relationship is highly statistically significant, meaning that it is very unlikely that the observed relationship could have occurred by chance alone. The regression line can be used to predict melanoma mortality. For instance, in the absence of any days of very high UV index, the predicted mortality from melanoma would be 2.30 deaths per 100,000 person-years. For every 10 days of very high UV index, the death rate increases 0.14 deaths per 100,000 person-years.

As shown visually and by regression analysis, the relationship between intense solar UV radiation and risk of melanoma death is very strong, raising the question of whether intense solar UV radiation might be a cause of melanoma. Unfortunately, this type of ecologic study cannot prove whether an association arises from a causal link. The observations are at the group (state) level of experience, so we do not know what is happening at the individual person level. Although the overall group risk of melanoma death is higher for populations living in areas with more intense sun exposure, the persons who developed melanoma in these communities may have less solar exposure because they have fair skin and burn easily. Epidemiologists refer to this type of inconsistency as an **ecologic fallacy**. That is to say, at the group level, a risk factor and a disease appear to be tightly linked, but at the personal level, there is no such association.

Given the potential for an ecologic fallacy, one might wonder why such a study would be undertaken in the first place. The motivation for conducting an ecologic study is that it relies on easily accessible already collected data. It is quick and inexpensive, therefore, to conduct such an investigation compared with the more definitive types of study on individual subjects. This type of "quick and dirty" study might be used to develop clues or hypotheses about disease causation. We refer to such an investigation as a **hypothesis-generating** study because its purpose is to develop a theory about disease causation that can be tested subsequently in a more definitive study. These more definitive investigations are more time consuming, complicated, and expensive to conduct, as we will see in later chapters. We refer to these investigations of individual exposure and disease risk as **hypothesis-testing** studies. Many hypothesis-testing studies have been conducted on personal exposure to solar (and other types of UV) radiation and the risk of melanoma. In general, these investigations have found the most compelling evidence for risk associated with recurrent sunburns in childhood and adolescence.

TIME

The incidence of a disease also can be tracked over time. As shown in **Figure 3-10**, in the United States, melanoma occurrence has been rising steadily over the years between 1975 and 2010. During this 35-year period of time, the incidence tripled. In recent years, the annual increase has averaged about 2.6%. This pattern is at odds with the experience for cancer of all types, which experienced rising incidence rates until 1992 followed by a progressive decline of about 0.5% per year on average thereafter.

It should be noted that the time trend depicted in **Figure 3-10**, although representing the experience of the population of the United States, does not correspond to a single, fixed group of people. Over a span of 35 years, the composition of the population evolves as new persons are added by birth and immigration, and other persons are removed by emigration or death.

A slightly different picture might emerge if we were to track the disease occurrence among a group of people born in a particular year or time period (a **birth cohort**) as they aged through life. For this purpose, it is helpful to have many years of observation, so that multiple successive birth cohorts can be tracked through their lifespans. On a national level, collection of data on cancer occurrence did not start in the United States until the 1970s, but the State of Connecticut has been collecting data on cancer incidence since the 1930s. Data from the Connecticut Tumor Registry are shown in **Figure 3-11**. For simplicity, age-specific incidence rates are presented for males only and for two time periods. It is clear that there has been a dramatic increase in the occurrence of melanoma between these two data collection periods 30 years apart. The disparity is particularly strong at the age groups above 50 years.

A somewhat different picture emerges if we examine the incidence not by age and time period but rather by age and birth cohort (**Figure 3-12**). For each successive birth cohort, beginning in 1910 and continuing through 1940, there was a progressively higher incidence of melanoma at each age group. The most recent birth cohort, men born in 1950,

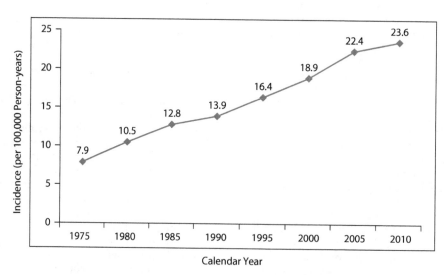

Figure 3-10. Incidence of melanoma, by year, in the United States, 1975 to 2010. (Data from Howlader N, et al. *SEER Cancer Statistics Review, 1975-2010.* Bethesda, MD: National Cancer Institute; 2013.)

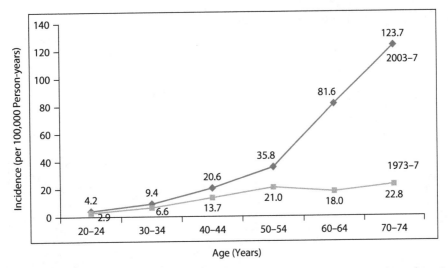

Figure 3-11. Incidence of melanoma among males, by age and time period, Connecticut. (Data from Geller AC, Clapp RW, Sober AJ, et al. Melanoma epidemic: an analysis of six decades of data from the Connecticut Tumor Registry. *J Clin Oncol.* 2013;33:4172-4178.)

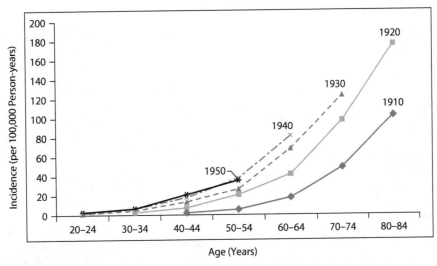

Figure 3-12. Incidence of melanoma among males, by age and birth cohort, Connecticut. (Data from Geller AC, Clapp RW, Sober AJ, et al. Melanoma epidemic: an analysis of six decades of data from the Connecticut Tumor Registry. *J Clin Oncol.* 2013;33:4172-4178.)

however, had age-specific incidence rates that were similar to men born in 1940. Of course, not enough time has elapsed for the men born in 1950 to reach the highest risk years for melanoma. It is possible, therefore, that there may be greater separation of the 1940 and 1950 birth cohorts with regard to melanoma risk at older ages. Nevertheless, from the data available, it appears that there may be a leveling off of melanoma risk for the later birth cohorts of men,

suggesting a generational stabilization of exposure to UV radiation.

It should be noted that the Connecticut data reveal a different pattern for women, with a continued rise in age-specific incidence rates for successive birth cohorts, with no evidence of a plateau (**Figure 3-13**). These observations tend to support a continuing generational increase in exposure to UV radiation among females through sunlight, tanning devices, or both.

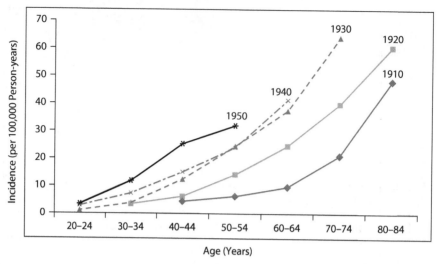

Figure 3-13. Incidence of melanoma among females, by age and birth cohort, Connecticut. (Data from Geller AC, Clapp RW, Sober AJ, et al. Melanoma epidemic: an analysis of six decades of data from the Connecticut Tumor Registry. *J Clin Oncol.* 2013;33:4172-4178.)

MIGRATION AND DISEASE OCCURRENCES

Another technique available in descriptive epidemiology is to examine whether migration affects the rate of disease occurrence. Such a study may help to establish the extent to which a disease is determined by genetic factors, environmental exposures, or both. Consider, for example, a study in which persons from a country known to be at low risk for a particular disease migrate to a country known to be at high risk for that same disease. If the disease risk among migrants remains low, we might conclude that a change in environment did not affect risk, so that disease susceptibility is either established by heredity or premigration environmental exposure. If we follow disease risk into the next generation, and children of migrants born and raised in the adopted country continue to have a low risk, the reduced risk is transferable across generations and suggests a hereditary basis for the disease.

If, in contrast, migrants from a low-risk country move to a high-risk nation and experience a higher rate of disease than those who did not migrate, we might conclude that environmental exposures do affect risk. In the next generation, as the children of immigrants assimilate into the cultural patterns of the new home country and have a full lifetime of exposure, we would expect disease rates to closely parallel those of native-born persons for conditions that are determined mostly by environmental causes.

A number of migrant studies have been conducted in relation to risk of melanoma. One setting that is especially suited for this type of investigation is Israel, where there are large numbers of immigrants coming from a variety of settings. Investigators in Israel studied melanoma risk among Israeli men of European descent according to when they arrived in Israel. In general, the European countries of origin have much lower incidence rates for melanoma than does Israel. As shown in **Figure 3-14**, the migrants from Europe who arrived in Israel at 10 years of age or younger experienced risk of melanoma virtually identical to those who were born in Israel. However, migrants from Europe who arrived in Israel at ages older than 10 years had a 40% lower risk of developing melanoma. In other words, environmental exposures early in life appear to be important determinants of risk of malignant melanoma. If one spends the first decade of life in a low-risk setting and then moves to a higher risk country, the relative protection of the low-risk childhood environment appears to persist. The protective effect is lost if one migrates during the first decade of life.

This observation does not establish early childhood sun exposure as a definitive cause of melanoma, but it is consistent with that hypothesis. One cannot exclude other early childhood exposures or hereditary factors from playing some role in causation. Indeed, a number of other lines of investigation support a contribution from genetics to risk of developing melanoma. Nevertheless, it appears that early life experience is important in determining a person's subsequent risk of melanoma.

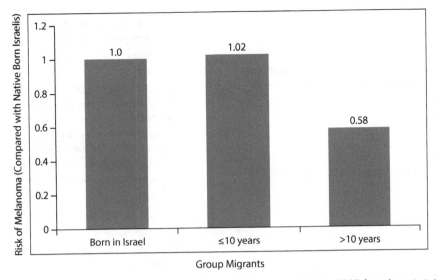

Figure 3-14. Risk of melanoma among Israeli men of European descent, 1967 to 2005, by migrant status and age at migration. (Data from Levine H, Afek A, Shamiss A, et al. Country of origin, age at migration and risk of cutaneous melanoma: a migrant cohort study of 1,100,000 Israeli men. *Int J Cancer.* 2013;133:486-494.)

SUMMARY

In this chapter, the methods of descriptive epidemiology were illustrated with data on the occurrence of melanoma. Fundamental to descriptive epidemiology is the premise that diseases do not occur at random. Some persons, by virtue of their personal characteristics, are at increased risk of the disease, and other persons are at reduced risk of being affected. These patterns often are revealed by answers to three basic questions:

1. **Who** gets the disease?
2. **Where** does the disease occur?
3. **When** does the disease occur?

These features of disease occurrence relate respectively to **person**, **place**, and **time**.

The standard approach to characterizing who gets the disease begins with demographic attributes such as age, race, and sex. For melanoma, we observed that the disease occurs with increased frequency in older persons, white non-Hispanics, and males.

The place of occurrence can be evaluated on the international, national, or regional levels. For melanoma, the greatest incidence rates tend to occur in Oceania followed by North America and northern Europe. Within some countries, gradients of risk by geographic latitude also are observed.

Unlike cancer overall in developed countries, the incidence of melanoma is increasing over time, with more than a 2% per year increase in the United States. When 6 decades of data from Connecticut were examined by birth cohort, that is, by groups born in the same year or period, increasing incidence appears to apply to successive birth years for both males and females up until 1950. Thereafter, a leveling off was observed among males, and continuing generational increases were seen for females.

Ecologic studies can be conducted to correlate the group level exposure to a putative causative agent with the occurrence of disease. We illustrated this approach with data from eight states in the Midwestern United States concerning annual number of days with very high UV index and subsequent mortality rates for melanoma. Although a strong correlation was demonstrated, the absence of data at the individual subject level prevents one from concluding that heavily UV-exposed persons bear an increased risk of melanoma. An **ecologic fallacy** exists when an exposure and disease appear to be linked at the population level but not within specific individuals.

Finally, we considered how investigation of migrant populations can help to distinguish whether a disease is primarily determined by inherited traits or is more greatly influenced by environmental exposures. An illustrative study was cited in which migrants from Europe to Israel had incident rates of melanoma similar to native-born Israelis if they migrated within the first decade of life. If they migrated later, however, they tended to retain risks of melanoma that were more similar to those of their European countries of origin. These findings tend to support the notion that environmental exposures early in life are particularly critical in determining the risk of melanoma later in life.

STUDY QUESTIONS

1. Which of the following attributes is NOT typically used to characterize who gets a disease?
   A. Sex
   B. HLA type
   C. Race
   D. Age

2. Persons born in the same year are referred to as
   A. a birth cohort.
   B. gestational peers.
   C. conception cohort.
   D. none of the above.

3. For a genetic disease, when persons from a high-risk country migrate to a low-risk country, we expect their risk of disease to
   A. decrease.
   B. increase.
   C. remain unchanged.
   D. vary based on age at migration.

4. For an environmentally determined disease, when persons migrate from a high-risk country to a low-risk country, we expect their risk of disease to
   A. decrease.
   B. increase.
   C. remain unchanged.
   D. be similar to their children's risk.

5. In an ecologic study of cell phone use and incidence of brain cancer, the coefficient of determination is found to be 0.3. This suggests that
   A. cell phone use accounts for most of the variation in risk of brain cancer.
   B. cell phone use is a cause of brain cancer.
   C. cell phone use has no association with risk of brain cancer.
   D. cell phone use accounts for about a third of the variation in brain cancer risk.

6. In an ecologic study of dietary folate intake and risk of neural tube defects, the correlation coefficient was -0.86. This means that
   A. high dietary folate intake is associated with a higher risk of neural tube defects.
   B. high dietary folate intake is associated with a lower risk of neural tube defects.

C. there is no association between dietary folate intake and neural tube defects.
   D. dietary folate intake causes neural tube defects.

7. In a correlation study, the prevalence of obesity is associated at the population level with the incidence of prostate cancer. When examined on a person-by-person basis, however, obese individuals do not have an increased risk of developing prostate cancer. This is an example of
   A. the Hawthorne effect.
   B. a selection bias.
   C. an ecologic fallacy.
   D. regression to the mean.

8. A registry for Alzheimer's disease is described as population-based. This means that
   A. only persons born within a specific population are considered for registration.
   B. an attempt is made to assemble a population of Alzheimer's disease patients from specialized treatment centers.
   C. only data from population surveys are used to find persons with Alzheimer's disease.
   D. an attempt is made to identify all Alzheimer's disease patients from a population defined within geographic boundaries.

9. Human papillomavirus (HPV) is known to be the principal cause of uterine cervical cancer. If an ecologic study was performed, one would expect the following correlation coefficient between incidence of HPV cervical infection and incidence of cervical cancer to be closest to
   A. -1.
   B. 0.
   C. 1.
   D. 100.

10. Which of the following is NOT a descriptive epidemiology study?
    A. A study of trends over time in the mortality from diabetes
    B. A study of variation in stroke incidence by race and sex
    C. A study of the risk of stomach cancer among migrants
    D. A study of the risk of suicide among veterans as compared with nonveterans

FURTHER READING

Gabe C, Leiter U. Melanoma epidemiology and trends. *Clin Dermatol.* 2009;27:3-9.

Little EG, Eide MJ. Update on the current state of melanoma incidence. *Dermatol Clin.* 2012;30:355-361.

REFERENCES

Clinical Background

Dunki-Jacobs EM, Callender GG, McMasters KM. Current management of melanoma. *Curr Probl Surg.* 2013;50:351-382.

Descriptive Epidemiology

Person

Howlader N, et al. *SEER Cancer Statistics Review, 1975-2010.* Bethesda, MD: National Cancer Institute; 2013.

Place

Cicarma E, Juzeniene A, Porojnicu AC, Bruland ØS, Moan J. Latitude gradient for melanoma incidence by anatomic site and gender in Norway, 1966-2007. *J Photochem Photobiol B.* 2010;101:174-178.

Erdmann F, Lortet-Tieulent J, Schüz J, et al. International trends in the incidence of malignant melanoma, 1953-2008: are recent generations at higher or lower risk? *Int J Cancer.* 2013;132:385-400.

Correlations with Disease Occurrence

Climate Prediction Center, National Weather Service, National Oceanic and Atmospheric Administration: *UV Index: Annual Time Series.* College Park, MD: Author; 2013.

Howlader N, et al. *SEER Cancer Statistics Review, 1975-2010.* Bethesda, MD: National Cancer Institute; 2013.

Time

Geller AC, Clapp RW, Sober AJ, et al. Melanoma epidemic: an analysis of six decades of data from the Connecticut Tumor Registry. *J Clin Oncol.* 2013;33:4172-4178.

Howlader N, et al. *SEER Cancer Statistics Review, 1975-2010.* Bethesda, MD: National Cancer Institute; 2013.

Migration and Disease Occurrence

Levine H, Afek A, Shamiss A, et al. Country of origin, age at migration, and risk of cutaneous melanoma: a migrant cohort study of 1,100,000 Israeli men. *Int J Cancer.* 2013;133:486-494.

Global Burden of Disease

Raymond S. Greenberg

4

HEALTH SCENARIO

At 4:53 PM on Tuesday, January 12, 2010, an earthquake measuring 7.0 on the Richter scale hit Haiti. The earthquake was the most powerful to strike the island in more than 200 years, and it was centered near the capital city, Port-au-Prince, where a quarter of the nation's nearly 10 million citizens lived.

The devastation caused by the earthquake was severe, with an estimated 250,000 residences and 30,000 commercial buildings either collapsed or severely damaged. The exact number of fatalities was uncertain, but the death toll was estimated to be 200,000 to 300,000, with another 300,000 nonfatal injuries. The number of displaced persons was estimated to be 1.3 million, with nearly 400,000 still residing in temporary shelters a year and a half after the earthquake.

The catastrophic dimensions of the earthquake can be attributed to a number of factors. Haiti is a very poor country, with 80% of its citizens living under the poverty level. As a consequence of the economic conditions, buildings there are poorly designed, constructed, and inspected. Construction materials are of inferior quality, and many buildings are sited on hillsides without adequate structural support. Moreover, the earthquake was centered in a densely populated area, increasing the number of people affected.

The tragedy of the earthquake was compounded by the logistical challenges of getting relief workers and supplies into the country. In addition, nearly two thirds of Haiti's hospitals were destroyed by the earthquake, adversely impacting the speed and capacity of the medical response.

The devastation caused by the earthquake was followed 10 months later by an outbreak of cholera. This epidemic began in a region about 100 km north of Port-au-Prince, with the source presumed to be drinking water drawn from a contaminated river. Because three out of four Haitian households lack running water and sanitation conditions are poor, the disease was easily transmitted from person to person. Within 10 weeks, the disease had spread throughout the country, ultimately affecting 6% of all Haitians. Hundreds of thousands of persons were hospitalized, and more than 3000 deaths were reported within 2 months. New cases were still arising years after the outbreak, with peaks occurring during the rainy season and after hurricanes.

The earthquake and ensuing cholera epidemic in Haiti demonstrate dramatically that death and disability from natural disasters and communicable diseases still burden substantial human populations, particularly those in economically challenged parts of the world. In this chapter, we will examine general patterns of health and disease throughout the world, with a focus on variations across person, place, and time.

GLOBAL BURDEN OF DISEASE STUDY

Imagine an effort to characterize the distribution and determinants of human health and disease around the world. Such an undertaking would require a large number of data sources; a highly collaborative, interdisciplinary team of investigators; extensive computational resources; complicated protocols and analyses; and substantial financial investment. All of these elements were brought together in a monumental effort referred to as the Global Burden of Disease Study 2010 (GBD 2010). The purpose of the GBD 2010 was to measure the relative amounts of health loss resulting from diseases, injuries, and risk factors, with assessment of trends over time, place, and personal attributes. After being assembled, this information can be applied for the following purposes:

1. To better understand the leading contributors to losses in human health and to describe how these contributions vary by person, place, and time

2. To help set priorities for initiatives to promote human health

3. To measure progress in addressing the leading health problems worldwide

4. To identify gaps in information on human health in order to improve the quality and quantity of data available

The GBD 2010, by virtue of its size, scale, rigor, and complexity, has set a new standard for descriptive epidemiology at the international level.

Study Design

The GBD 2010 followed three earlier versions in 1990, 1999 to 2002, and 2004. GBD 2010 greatly expanded the prior studies by including more diseases, more risk factors, more age groups, and multiple time periods. GBD 2010 was undertaken as a partnership between seven primary institutions: the University of Washington, Harvard University, Johns Hopkins University, the University of Queensland, Imperial College of London, the University of Tokyo, and the World Health Organization. The collaborative team of investigators included 486 scientists from 302 institutions in 50 counties.

The study was initiated in 2007 and was completed 5 years later. About 100,000 sources of data were identified by a systematic search for potential use in deriving estimates of the burden of disease. The resulting database contained information on 800 million deaths between 1950 and 2010. A major challenge in assembling the database was the fact that vital registration systems that include medical certification are not established in many countries, particularly those in the developing world. For example, in a recent year, only 36% of all deaths occurred in countries using physician certification. Even when medical input is required, comparisons across countries may be affected by varying skills of physicians, variability in information available at the time the death certificate is completed, differing practices in assigning underlying causes of death, and other legal and procedural issues.

For deaths that are not medically certified, a variety of other sources of information were used, including, among others, surveillance systems, disease registries, demographic surveys, and police reports. The diversity of data origins and potential errors associated with them contribute to uncertainty in the resulting death rates. Ranges of uncertainty were presented for estimated measures in the results. Because the emphasis of the present summary is to capture the major patterns and trends, only the best estimates are reported here. GBD 2010 used a list of 291 diseases and injuries and 1160 sequelae of these conditions, the latter being defined as the direct consequences of disease or injury that were not otherwise captured. In addition, 67 risk factors for disease were estimated. Separate estimates of outcomes were made for 187 individual countries. These countries were also grouped into 21 regions based on demographic similarity and geographic proximity, and outcomes were estimated for these regions.

The computational requirements for GBD 2010 were enormous. Using a network of more than 100 computers, the amount of data stored after a modeling process could exceed 3 terabytes of information. The human effort of summarizing and interpreting these results was similarly demanding.

Mortality

There were 52.8 million deaths in the world in 2010. This represents an increase of 6.3 million deaths (13.5%) compared with the number of death in 1990. The rise in the number of deaths does not imply that human health declined during this 20-year period. In reality, age-standardized death rates declined by 21.5% during this interval.

The seemingly paradoxical rise in the number of deaths occurred because the population grew and aged between 1990 and 2010. As shown in **Figure 4-1**, if the population size and age composition had remained unchanged and the 1990 death rates had continued in 2010, an extra 8.5 million deaths would have occurred. A further 9 million deaths would have occurred in 2010 if the 1990 death rates applied to the larger and older world population in 2010.

The 10 leading causes of death in 2010 are shown in **Table 4-1** along with the respective age-standardized mortality rates. Collectively, these leading causes of death account for more than half of all deaths and more than half of the overall age-standardized mortality rate. Six of the top 10 causes of death, including the top three, are noncommunicable diseases or injuries. Compared with the corresponding ranking 2 decades earlier, the most dramatic increases were the rise of HIV/AIDS (rank 35 to 6), diabetes (rank 15 to 9), lung cancer (rank 8 to 5), and road injuries (rank 10 to 8). The largest declines in ranking during this 20-year interval were seen for preterm birth complications (rank 7 to 15), tuberculosis (rank 6 to 10), diarrhea (rank 5 to 7), and lower respiratory infections (rank 3 to 4).

To the extent that declining age-standardized mortality rates reflect progress in controlling diseases, some of the more dramatic success stories are shown in **Figure 4-2**. It is noteworthy that four of the top five cause-specific declines in mortality are related to the control of infectious diseases. These changes reflect the so-called **epidemiologic transition** in which improvements in nutrition, sanitation, immunization, and medical care in developing nations led to a reduction in mortality from infectious diseases, with consequent growth and aging of the population and a rise in degenerative and human-made diseases.

The list of causes of death with increasing age-adjusted death rates between 1990 and 2010 is far more limited (data not shown). By far, the most dramatic rise in mortality was for HIV/AIDS, with the death rate climbing nearly 260% during this 2-decade

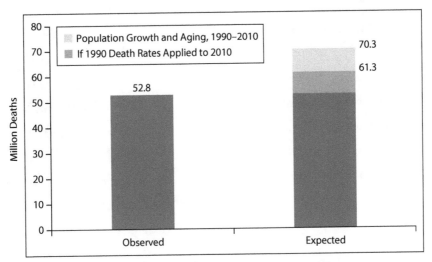

Figure 4-1. Observed numbers of deaths in the world, 2010. Expected numbers were calculated using the 1990 death rates and separately accounting for the aging and growth of the population between 1990 and 2010. (Data from Lozano R, Pourmalek F, Raju M, et al. Global and regional mortality from 235 causes of death for 20 age groups in 1990 and 2010: a systematic analysis for the Global Burden of Disease Study 2010. *Lancet*. 2012;380:2095-2128.)

Table 4-1. The 10 leading causes of death in 2010 along with the age-standardized mortality rates.

Cause	Age-Standardized Mortality Rate[a]
1. Ischemic heart disease	105.7
2. Stroke	88.4
3. Chronic obstructive pulmonary disease	43.8
4. Lower respiratory infections	41.0
5. Lung cancer	23.4
6. HIV/AIDS	21.4
7. Diarrheal disease	20.9
8. Road injuries	19.5
9. Diabetes	19.5
10. Tuberculosis	18.0

[a]Per 100,000 persons.
Data from Lozano R, et al. Lozano R, Pourmalek F, Raju M, et al. Global and regional mortality from 235 causes of death for 20 age groups in 1990 and 2010: a systematic analysis for the Global Burden of Disease Study 2010. *Lancet*. 2012;380:2095-2128.

period. More modest elevations also were seen for neurologic disorders (38%) and diabetes (20%).

The epidemiologic transition is associated with declines in childhood deaths principally because of the fall of fatal infectious diseases, with a concomitant rise in deaths among adults, attributable primarily to increases in degenerative and human-made diseases. This pattern was observed in GBD 2010, as shown in **Figure 4-3**.

Life Expectancy

Estimated age-specific death rates were used to estimate likelihoods of surviving each age period, and ultimately the number of years a person is expected to live from a particular baseline age. For simplicity, life expectancy at birth was used as a summary measure. In 2010, the life expectancy at birth was 67.5 years for males and 73.3 years for females. During the 20-year interval between 1990 and 2010, the life expectancy at birth increased 4.7 years for males and 5.2 years for females.

In 2010, there was considerable variation in life expectancy across different regions of the world. Among females, the region with the greatest life expectancy at birth (High Income Pacific) had an almost 27-year advantage over the region with the lowest life expectancy at birth (Central sub-Saharan Africa). For males, the range of life expectancies between the highest region (Australasia) and the lowest region (central sub-Saharan Africa) was more than 25 years. **Table 4-2** shows the four countries with the highest and the four countries with the lowest life expectancies at birth in 2010 by sex. The countries with the longest lived populations are the same for males and females, although the rankings differ slightly. All of these countries are located in the high-income regions of Asia and Western Europe.

The counties with the shortest life expectancies at birth and their rank order are the same for males and females (**Table 4-2**). These countries are located in the low-income regions of the Caribbean and sub-Saharan Africa. The low life expectancies in sub-Saharan African countries reflect the severe impact of

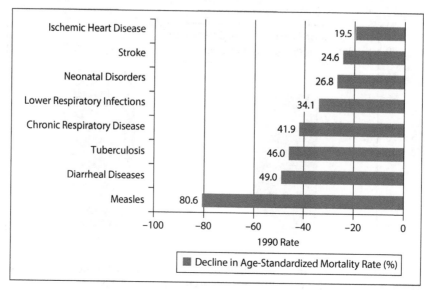

Figure 4-2. Percent declines in age-standardized mortality rates, 1990 to 2010, for selected causes of death. (Data from Lozano R, Pourmalek F, Raju M, et al. Global and regional mortality from 235 causes of death for 20 age groups in 1990 and 2010: a systematic analysis for the Global Burden of Disease Study 2010. *Lancet.* 2012;380:2095-2128.)

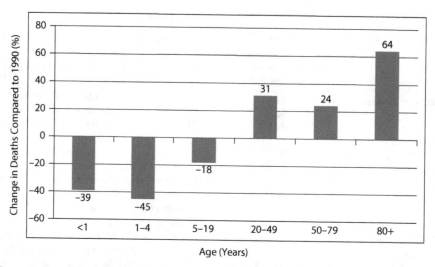

Figure 4-3. Percent change in numbers of deaths by age group, 2010 versus 1990. (Data from Wang H, Dwyer-Lindgren L, Lofgren KT, et al. Age-specific and sex-specific mortality in 187 countries, 1970-2010: a systematic analysis for the Global Burden of Disease Study 2010. *Lancet.* 2012;380:2071-2094.)

HIV/AIDS in these populations. The low life expectancy in Haiti is attributable to the earthquake that ravaged the country in 2010.

Healthy Life Expectancy

As noted already, progress has been made in virtually all countries toward reducing death rates, with concomitant increases in life expectancy for both males and females. The aging of the population is accompanied by a rise in degenerative and human-made diseases, many of which have considerable morbidities. A reasonable question, therefore, is what proportion of the additional years of life are characterized by good health (i.e., a lack of disability and functional limitations)? In GBD 2010, an attempt was made to address this question by calculation of **healthy life expectancy**. This measure corresponds to the number

Table 4-2. The four countries with the highest and lowest life expectancies at birth, 2010, by sex.

Males		Females	
Highest Life Expectancies			
Iceland	80.0	Japan	85.9
Andorra	79.8	Andorra	85.2
Switzerland	79.7	Switzerland	84.5
Japan	79.3	Iceland	84.4
Lowest Life Expectancies			
Swaziland	47.4	Swaziland	51.4
Lesotho	44.1	Lesotho	50.7
Central African Republic	43.6	Central African Republic	49.3
Haiti	32.5	Haiti	43.6

Data from Wang H, Dwyer-Lindgren L, Lofgren KT, et al. Age-specific and sex-specific mortality in 187 countries, 1970-2010: a systematic analysis for the Global Burden of Disease Study 2010. *Lancet.* 2012;380:2071-2094.

of years a person can be anticipated to live in good health beyond some baseline age. To calculate healthy life expectancy, one needs to account for age-specific death rates, morbidity, and limitations in functional status.

A particularly challenging aspect of this analysis was to calculate the years lived with disability. To make the best possible determinations, the investigators calculated the prevalence of 1160 sequelae of disease by age, sex, country, and year. More than 100,000 data sources were used to help derive these estimates. The GBD 2010 study had many strengths,

such as the use of a wide range of data, and when possible, the incorporation of biomarkers and functional measurement as well as the assessment of severity of impairment. Nevertheless, it must be appreciated that there is considerable uncertainty involved in the estimates of years lived with disability.

Figure 4-4 depicts the total and healthy life expectancies at birth in 2010 for the world by sex. For males, the life expectancy of 67.5 years includes 59.0 years (87.4%) of healthy life. For females, the expected life span of 73.3 years includes 63.2 years (86.2%) of healthy life. Between 1990 and 2010, 4.2 of the 4.7 years gained in life expectancy for males were healthy years. Of the 5.2 years of additional life for females, 4.5 were healthy years.

As with life expectancy, considerable variation existed in the distribution of healthy life expectancies (**Table 4-3**). The highest levels were seen in Japan for both males and females, with the leading nations coming from the high-income Pacific and Western European regions. Haiti again had the lowest levels for both males and females, with the same three sub-Saharan African nations that trailed in life expectancy at birth also having low levels of healthy life. The most extreme contrast of experience between the highest and lowest ranking nations revealed about a 4-decade longer healthy life expectancy at birth for natives of Japan compared with Haitians.

In all but two of the 21 regions of the world, healthy life expectancy at birth increased between 1990 and 2010. The two regions that experienced declines were the Caribbean because of the 2010 earthquake in Haiti and Southern sub-Saharan Africa because of HIV/AIDS. Most of the loss of healthy

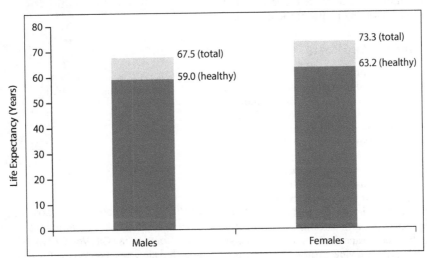

Figure 4-4. Life expectancy at birth and healthy life expectancy at birth (dark shaded) in the world, 2010. (Data from Salomon JA, Wang H, Freeman MK, et al. Healthy life expectancy for 187 countries, 1990-2010: a systematic analysis for the Global Burden of Disease Study 2010. *Lancet.* 2012;380:2144-2162.)

Table 4-3. The four countries with the highest and lowest healthy life expectancies at birth, 2010, by sex.

Males		Females	
Highest Healthy Life Expectancies			
Japan	70.6	Japan	75.5
Singapore	69.6	Spain	73.0
Switzerland	69.1	South Korea	72.6
Spain	68.8	Singapore	72.6
Lowest Healthy Life Expectancies			
Swaziland	40.4	Swaziland	43.3
Lesotho	37.7	Lesotho	42.6
Central African Republic	37.7	Central African Republic	41.7
Haiti	27.8	Haiti	37.1

Data from Salomon JA, Wang H, Freeman MK, et al. Healthy life expectancy for 187 countries, 1990-2010: a systematic analysis for the Global Burden of Disease Study 2010. *Lancet.* 2012;380:2144-2162.

life expectancy of about 6 years in both of these two regions was attributable to increased deaths in persons age 5 years or older. In Eastern Europe, a small decrease in deaths among children younger than 5 years of age was offset by an increase in mortality among older persons, resulting in minimal change in healthy life expectancy. For the remaining 18 regions, gains in healthy life expectancy ranged from 2 to more than 6 years, with improvements driven by reductions in mortality in the first 5 years of life, among older persons, or a combination of both. There was little contribution to improved healthy life expectancy as a result of diminished disability in any of these regions.

Disability-Adjusted Life Years

Healthy life expectancy provides a convenient summary measure of a population's health status. Disability-adjusted life years (DALYs) provide another way of characterizing the burden of disease within a population. The concept of DALYs was developed initially by the investigators of the first GBD Study in 1990. In brief, DALYs combine information on two components: years of life lost because of premature death and years lived with disability. The years of life lost are determined against the most favorable life expectancy, which is derived by applying the lowest observed age-specific death rates in the world. By summing together lost years of life and years lived with disability, DALYs provide a summary measure of the absolute loss of health due to death or nonfatal illness and are influenced, therefore, by the size and demographic features of the population.

In 2010, there were 2.49 billion DALYs in the world. Premature mortality accounted for more than two thirds (69%) of the loss of healthy life, with the reminder (31%) related to disabilities. The proportion of DALYs related to disabilities has increased over time, reflecting a gradual shift in the burden of disease from rapidly fatal causes to more chronic conditions. As depicted in **Figure 4-5**, more than half of all DALYs were attributable to noncommunicable diseases; another third coming from communicable, maternal, infant, and nutritional diseases; and the remainder attributable to injuries.

Some of the leading noncommunicable diseases contributing to DALYs are shown in **Figure 4-6**. The top three diseases—cancer, heart disease, and stroke—were all major causes of death and therefore were responsible for premature loss of life. This contrasts with two of the other leading noncommunicable disease contributors to DALYs—low back pain and depression—which impacted the population primarily as sources of disability.

The DALYs for the five leading communicable diseases are shown in **Figure 4-7**. These same five diseases were the top causes of death, but the relative lethality varies: HIV/AIDS is ranked second as a cause of death given that it is more likely to be fatal than either malaria or diarrheal disease. Beyond the infectious diseases and the chronic degenerative conditions, other leading contributors to DALYs include preterm birth complications (77.0 million DALYs) and road injuries (75.5 million DALYs).

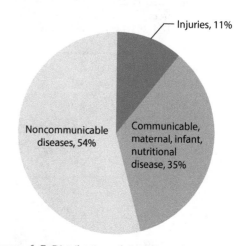

Figure 4-5. Distribution of disability-adjusted life years according to broad groupings of causes, 2010. (Data from Murray CJL, Vos T, Lozano R, et al. Disability-adjusted life years (DALYs) for 291 diseases and injuries in 21 regions, 1990-2010: a systematic analysis for the Global Burden of Disease Study 2010. *Lancet.* 2012;380:2197-2223.)

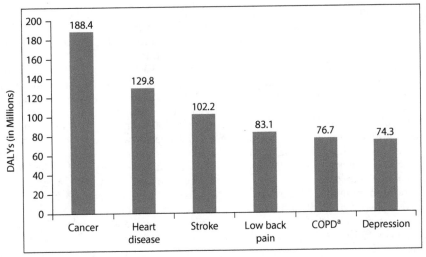

ªCOPD—Chronic obstructive pulmonary disease

Figure 4-6. Disability-adjusted life years (DALYs) related to leading noncommunicable diseases, 2010. (Data from Murray CJL, Vos T, Lozano R, et al. Disability-adjusted life years (DALYs) for 291 diseases and injuries in 21 regions, 1990-2010: a systematic analysis for the Global Burden of Disease Study 2010. *Lancet.* 2012;380:2197-2223.)

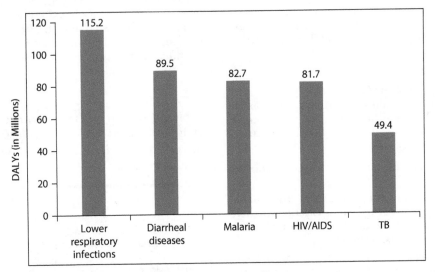

Figure 4-7. Disability-adjusted life years (DALYs) related to leading communicable diseases, 2010. TB, tuberculosis. (Data from Murray CJL, Vos T, Lozano R, et al. Disability-adjusted life years (DALYs) for 291 diseases and injuries in 21 regions, 1990-2010: a systematic analysis for the Global Burden of Disease Study 2010. *Lancet.* 2012;380:2197-2223.)

Over time, the burden of disease has shifted from the youngest age groups to older persons. For example, in 1990, children younger than 5 years of age accounted for 41% of DALYs. By 2010, the corresponding percentage had dropped to 25%. This dramatic decline in DALYs among children was driven by reductions over time in the two leading causes of DALYs in 1990, lower respiratory infections

(44% fall by 2010) and diarrheal diseases (51%). Because four fifths of these illnesses occur in children younger than 5 years of age, the proportion of DALYs incurred during childhood fell accordingly. A smaller, but still noteworthy decrease (27%) in DALYs was observed for preterm birth complications, further lowering the DALYs among children.

Other success stories between 1990 and 2010 with respect to the control of leading communicable diseases included measles (80% decline), meningitis (22% decrease), and tuberculosis (19% fall). Malaria was an exception to this pattern, with a 20% increase in DALYs between 1990 and 2010.

The rise of noncommunicable diseases as contributors to DALYs between 1990 and 2010 was particularly striking for diabetes (69%), low back pain (43%), depression (38%), ischemic heart disease (29%), and stroke (19%).

Regional differences in the composition of DALYs in 2010 were substantial, with about half of the totals in the high income regions of Asia, Western Europe, Australasia, and North America related to disabilities compared with only about one fifth of the DALYs in the low-income region of sub-Saharan Africa. The underlying causes differed strikingly as well: in the high-income regions, communicable, maternal, neonatal, and nutritional disorders contributed 7% of DALYs, but these same conditions constituted more than two thirds of all DALYs in sub-Saharan Africa.

Risk Factors

The investigators of the GBD 2010 study attempted to characterize the underlying risk factors contributing to the burden of disease globally. The process of estimating the impact of an individual risk factor required multiple elements:

1. Locating data on population exposure to the risk factor
2. Obtaining sufficient prior research that could be used to define strengths of associations between the risk factors and disease outcomes, as well as support for casual inferences
3. Determining that the relationships observed between the risk factor and outcome were generalizable to populations other than the ones in which the associations were established

The disease burden contributions of individual risk factors were assessed against a baseline level; no exposure when possible (i.e., tobacco smoking) or when not possible (i.e., systolic blood pressure), against a minimum risk of exposure level that was supported by epidemiologic evidence and was theoretically possible in a population. The investigators quantified the burden of disease in terms of deaths and separately in

DALYs. For simplicity, only the analyses in relation to DALYs are summarized here. A total of 67 individual risk factors and clusters of risk factors were considered in this study.

The 10 leading factors in terms of contributions to DALYs in 2010 are shown in **Table 4-4**. Elevated blood pressure had the greatest impact on burden of disease followed by tobacco smoking and household pollution from the use of solid fuels. Childhood underweight was the only one of the top 10 risk factors that did not relate to the risk of chronic, degenerative disease. The global decline in the burden from communicable, maternal, neonatal, and nutritional diseases was associated with a corresponding fall in contribution of the risk factors for these conditions. In 1990, childhood underweight was the risk factor with the greatest global disease burden, but it fell to number 8 by 2010. Similarly, suboptimal breastfeeding fell from the fifth highest risk factor contribution in 1990 to 14th in 2010. Other risk factors that declined appreciably in impact on disease burden over those two decades were sanitation (15th to 26th), vitamin A deficiency (17th to 29th), zinc deficiency (19th to 31st), and unimproved water (22nd to 34th). The risk factors that gained the most in terms of contribution to global burden of disease during this time interval were high blood pressure (4th position to 1st), low fruit consumption (7th to 4th), alcohol use (8th to 5th), high body mass index (BMI) (10th to 6th), and drug use (25th to 19th).

Table 4-4. Burden of disease contributions of the 10 leading risk factors, as measured by percentage of global disability-adjusted life years (DALYs) in 2010.

Risk Factor	Percent of DALYs
High blood pressure	7.0
Tobacco smoking	6.3
Household air pollution from solid fuels	4.3
Diet low in fruits	4.2
Alcohol use	3.9
High body mass index	3.8
High fasting plasma glucose	3.6
Childhood underweight	3.1
Ambient particulate air pollution	3.1
Physical inactivity	2.8

Data from Lim SS, Vos T, Flaxman AD, et al. A comparative risk assessment of burden of disease and injury attributable to 67 risk factor clusters in 21 regions, 1990-2010: a systematic analysis for the Global Burden of Disease Study 2010. *Lancet.* 2012;380:2224-2260.

There were many parallels between males and females for leading risk factors, with a few key differences. Tobacco smoking was the leading risk factor for males, accounting for 8.4% of DALYs. Among females, however, tobacco smoking was ranked fourth and was responsible for only 3.7% of DALYs. Alcohol use was the third highest risk factor among males, corresponding to 5.4% of DALYs. In contrast, for females, alcohol use was the 12th highest risk factor, accounting for only 2% of DALYs. In contrast, iron deficiency ranked 10th among risk factors for females and contributed to more than 2% of DALYs. For males, iron deficiency ranked 18th and was responsible for less than 1% of DALYs. Similarly, intimate partner violence was ranked 16th for females at 1.5% of DALYs but was not quantified for males.

Not surprisingly, considerable differences were observed across regions in the relative contributions of various risk factors. For example, childhood underweight, household air pollution from solid fuels, suboptimal breastfeeding, and iron deficiency were the top four risk factors in Eastern, Central, and Western sub-Saharan Africa. Alcohol use was the leading risk factor in three regions: Eastern Europe, Andean Latin America, and Southern sub-Saharan Africa. High BMI was the leading risk factor in Australasia, Southern and Central Latin America, whereas it made a comparatively smaller contribution in Asia and sub-Saharan Africa. Physical inactivity played a greater role in the high-income regions of Asia, Western Europe, Australasia, and North America than in most other parts of the world.

SUMMARY

In this chapter, we have reported key findings about global health from one of the most comprehensive assessments ever undertaken, the GBD Study of 2010. Key results included:

1. An estimated 52.8 million deaths occurred in 2010.
2. Compared with 1990, a greater number of deaths occurred in 2010 despite lower age-specific death rates because the world's population had grown and aged in the interim.
3. The leading cause of death worldwide was ischemic heart disease, and the three top causes of death all were noncommunicable diseases.
4. The greatest declines in age-standardized mortality rates were for three communicable diseases, measles, diarrheal diseases, and tuberculosis.
5. The observed decline of mortality from infectious disease in developing countries resulting from improved sanitation, nutrition, immunization, and medical care with consequent rises in noncommunicable diseases and growth and aging of the population is referred to as the **epidemiologic transition**.
6. Between 1990 and 2010, the global life expectancy at birth grew almost 5 years to 67.5 in males and more than 5 years to 73.3 in females.
7. In 2010, the shortest life expectancies were observed in Haiti, largely driven by the devastating earthquake there, and in sub-Saharan Africa because of HIV/AIDS.
8. In 2010, the longest life expectancies were found in the high-income regions of Asia and Western Europe.
9. In 2010, the global healthy life expectancy was 59.0 years for males and 63.2 years for females.
10. DALYs were used as a global measure of disease burden, combining information on both premature deaths and years lived with disability.
11. In 2010, there were 2.5 billion DALYs calculated for the world, with premature deaths accounting for about two thirds of the disease burden, although a shift over time to a greater contribution from disabilities was observed.
12. In 2010, more than half of all global DALYs related to noncommunicable diseases, with another third associated with communicable, maternal, neonatal, and nutritional deficiency conditions and the remainder attributable to injuries.
13. Cancer, heart disease, and lower respiratory infections were the three leading causes of loss of healthy life in 2010.
14. Over time, the global burden of disease has shifted from children younger than 5 years of age, although in sub-Saharan Africa, communicable, maternal, neonatal, and nutritional deficiency diseases still account for two thirds of loss of healthy life.
15. The top three risk factors contributing to premature death and disability globally in 2010 were elevated blood pressure, tobacco smoking, and household air pollution from the use of solid fuels.

STUDY QUESTIONS

1. *Which of the following is NOT associated with the epidemiologic transition?*

   A. *Aging of the population*

   B. *A decline in infectious diseases*

   C. *Growth of the population*

   D. *A decline in noncommunicable diseases*

2. Worldwide, the leading cause of death in 2010 was

A. HIV/AIDS.

B. ischemic heart disease.

C. diarrheal disease.

D. stroke.

3. In 2010, which one of the following countries had the highest life expectancy among females?

A. United States

B. Germany

C. Japan

D. Sweden

4. From a global perspective, which one of the following risk factors contributes to the greatest burden of disease?

A. High blood pressure

B. Obesity

C. Underweight children

D. Unsafe sexual practices

5. Between 1990 and 2010, the greatest percentage decline in age-standardized mortality rates was found from which disease?

A. Ischemic heart disease

B. Stroke

C. Measles

D. HIV/AIDS

6. Between 1990 and 2010, the age group with the greatest percentage reduction in numbers of deaths was

A. less than 5 years.

B. 5 to 19 years.

C. 20 to 49 years.

D. 80+ years.

7. The greatest percentage contribution to global burden of disease in 2010, as measured by DALYs, relates to which of the following?

A. Communicable diseases

B. Noncommunicable diseases

C. Injuries

D. Neonatal diseases

8. The noncommunicable disease with the greatest contribution to global burden of disease in 2010, as measured by DALYs is

A. heart disease.

B. depression.

C. low back pain.

D. cancer.

9. The communicable disease with the greatest contribution to global burden of disease in 2010 is

A. lower respiratory infections.

B. malaria.

C. HIV/AIDS.

D. tuberculosis.

10. DALYs include consideration of the impact from which of the following?

A. Premature mortality

B. Disability

C. Both premature mortality and disability

D. Neither premature mortality nor disability

FURTHER READING

Are C, Rajaram S, Are M, et al. A review of global cancer burden: trends, challenges, strategies, and a role for surgeons. *J Surg Oncol.* 2013;107:221-226.

Eaton J, McCay L, Semrau M, et al. Scale up of services for mental health in low-income and middle-income countries. *Lancet.* 2011;378:1592-1603.

Friel S, Bowen K, Campbell-Lendrum D, Frumkin H, McMichael AJ, Rasanathan K. Climate change, noncommunicable disease, and development: the relationships and common policy opportunities. *Annu Rev Public Health.* 2011;32:133-147.

Gaziano TA, Bitton A, Anand S, Abrahams-Gessel S, Murphy A. Growing epidemic of coronary heart disease in low- and middle-income countries. *Curr Probl Cardiol.* 2010;35:72-115.

Harper K, Armelagos G. The changing disease-scape in the Third Epidemiological Transition. *Int J Environ Res Public Health.* 2010;7:675-697.

Kohl HW 3rd, Craig CL, Lambert EV, et al. Lancet Physical Activity Series Working Group.The pandemic of physical inactivity: global action for public health. *Lancet.* 2012;380:294-305.

Malik VS, Willett WC, Hu FB. Global obesity: trends, risk factors and policy implications. *Nat Rev Endocrinol.* 2013;9:12-27.

Walker CL, Rudan I, Liu L, et al. Global burden of childhood pneumonia and diarrhea. *Lancet.* 2013;381:1405-1416.

REFERENCES

GBD 2010

Das P, Samarasekera U. The story of GBD 2010: a "super-human" effort. *Lancet.* 2012;380:2067-2012.

Murray CJL, Ezzati M, Flaxman AD, et al. GBD 2010: design, definitions, and metrics. *Lancet.* 2012;380:2063-2066.

Mortality

Lozano R, Pourmalek F, Raju M, et al. Global and regional mortality from 235 causes of death for 20 age groups in 1990 and 2010: a systematic analysis for the Global Burden of Disease Study 2010. *Lancet.* 2012;380:2095-2128.

Life Expectancy

Wang H, Dwyer-Lindgren L, Lofgren KT, et al. Age-specific and sex-specific mortality in 187 countries, 1970-2010: a systematic analysis for the Global Burden of Disease Study 2010. *Lancet.* 2012;380:2071-2094.

Healthy Life Expectancy

Salomon JA, Wang H, Freeman MK, et al. Healthy life expectancy for 187 countries, 1990-2010: a systematic analysis for the Global Burden of Disease Study 2010. *Lancet.* 2012; 380:2144-2162.

Disability-Adjusted Life Years

Murray CJL, Vos T, Lozano R, et al. Disability-adjusted life years (DALYs) for 291 diseases and injuries in 21 regions, 1990-2010: a systematic analysis for the Global Burden of Disease Study 2010. *Lancet.* 2012;380:2197-2223.

Risk Factors

Lim SS, Vos T, Flaxman AD, et al. A comparative risk assessment of burden of disease and injury attributable to 67 risk factor clusters in 21 regions, 1990-2010: a systematic analysis for the Global Burden of Disease Study 2010. *Lancet.* 2012;380:2224-2260.

Social Determinants of Health

5

Michael D. Sweat and Kathleen T. Brady

HEALTH SCENARIO

A series of studies beginning in 1967 in the United Kingdom conducted by Sir Michael Marmot, known as the "Whitehall" studies, followed 17,530 men working as government employees and discovered dramatically different health outcomes over time based mostly on the employee's type of job. Men in jobs classified as "higher grade," such as administrators and executives, had significantly better health over time than men in "lower grade" positions, such as clerical workers and unskilled manual laborers. A careful analysis of these data showed that differences in health status were only partially associated with known risk factors. Moreover, when risk factors were controlled for, there were still large and statistically significant differences in health status attributed to the employee's relative position in the work hierarchy. These differences persisted among the men followed for more than 20 years, and these strong effects of job status on health were later replicated among both male and female government workers.

Perhaps not unexpectedly, participants in the Whitehall study had markedly different risk factors identified at the start of the study across job grades. Compared with administrators and executives, men who were in the lowest job grade were approximately twice as likely to smoke cigarettes, were less likely to have active leisure activities, had more weight anomalies (very heavy or very thin), were significantly shorter in height, and had higher blood pressure. Only plasma cholesterol was higher for those in higher status job grades. What was surprising was that baseline differences in risk factors for health problems were not the best predictors of the incidence of serious health problems and death.

After following the government workers enrolled in the Whitehall study for 7.5 years, striking differences in the health of participants were found across employment grades. Interestingly, even when the baseline effects of age, blood pressure, cholesterol, smoking, and height were adjusted through statistical analysis,

it still was found that compared with the most senior employees (administrators), there was a strong linear relationship between job grade and mortality from coronary heart disease, with twice the mortality for professional executives, three times more for clerical workers, and four times more for the lowest grade workers (**Figure 5-1**). Remarkably, more than 60% of these large differences in mortality from coronary heart disease were attributable to job grade differences, and only 40% of the effect could be explained by traditional risk factors.

This seminal study identified the profound effects of social factors, such as job status, in the production of health and ushered in an era of evolving research highlighting the compelling and complex relationship between health and societal forces. In this chapter, we will explore the relationship between social factors and health outcomes; review emerging themes in this area, including a life-course perspective on the social determinants of health; and suggest intervention strategies that reflect the profound causal relationships identified by the Whitehall studies.

OVERVIEW

There is growing recognition that the health of individuals and populations is strongly influenced by factors beyond biomedical and behavioral risk factors. In recent years, the term "social determinants of health" has been used to capture these wide-ranging factors. This term grew out of research focused on identifying the mechanisms by which members of differing socioeconomic groups came to experience varying degrees of health and wellness. There are a variety of approaches to characterizing the social determinants of health, but all focus on the organization and distribution of economic and social resources. As shown in **Table 5-1**, wide ranges of economic and social resources have been examined in the study of social determinants of health. A World Health Organization (WHO) workgroup in 2003 charged with the task of

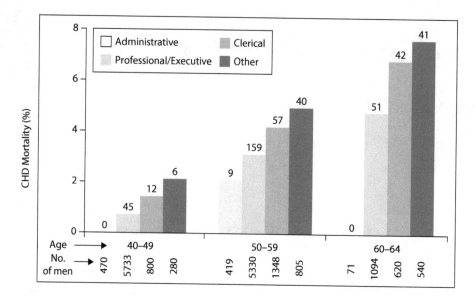

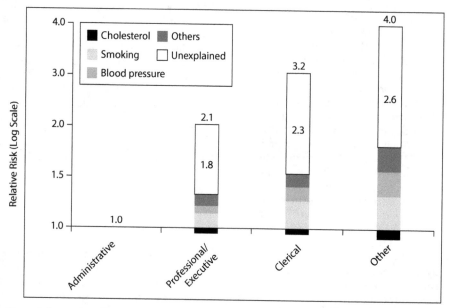

Figure 5-1. Linear relationship between job grade and mortality. CHD, congestive heart disease. (Reproduced with permission from Marmot MG, Rose G, Shipley M, Hamilton PJ. Employment grade and coronary heart disease in British civil servants. *J Epidemiol Community Health.* 1978;32(4):244-249.)

identifying the social determinants of health included social gradient, stress, early life, social exclusion, work, unemployment, social support, addiction, food, and transportation. In 2005, the Centers for Disease Control and Prevention highlighted socioeconomic status, transportation, housing, access to services, discrimination by social grouping, and social or environmental stressors in their listing.

Support for the importance of social determinants of health can be found in several lines of research, including the classic Whitehall study described earlier. Studies of causes of the profound improvement

Table 5-1. Economic and social resources assessed as social determinants of health.

Canadian Institute of Advanced Research	World Health Organization	US Centers for Disease Control and Prevention	Systematic Review of Empiric Studies
• Income and Social Status • Social Support Networks • Education • Employment and Working Conditions • Physical and Social Environments • Biology and Genetic Endowment • Personal Health Practices and Coping Skills • Healthy Child Development • Health Services	• Social Class Health Gradient, Stress, Early Life • Social Exclusion • Work • Unemployment • Social Support • Addiction • Food • Transport	• Socioeconomic Status • Transportation • Housing • Access To Services • Discrimination By Social Grouping (e.g., Race, Gender, or Class) • Social or Environmental Stressors	• Aboriginal Status • Early Life • Education • Employment and Working • Conditions • Food Security • Health Care Services • Housing • Income and its Distribution • Social Safety Net • Social Exclusion • Unemployment and Employment Security

Data from Canadian Institute of Advanced Research: Evans RG, Barer ML, Marmor TR. *Why are Some People Healthy and Others Not? The Determinants of Health Of Populations.* New York: A. de Gruyter; 1994. World Health Organization: Wilkinson RG, Marmot M. *Social Determinants of Health: The Solid Facts.* Copenhagen: The World Health Organization, European Office; 2003. U.S. Centers for Disease Control and Prevention: Centers for Disease Control and Prevention. *Social Determinants of Health Working Group.* Atlanta; 2005. Systematic Review of Empiric Studies: Raphael D, ed. *Social Determinants of Health: Canadian Perspectives.* Toronto: Canadian Scholars' Press; 2004.

in health status in individuals living in developed nations over the past 100 years emphasize the importance of social determinants in population health. Although advances in health care are clearly responsible for some increased longevity over the past 100 years, most analyses conclude that improvement in conditions of everyday life related to early life, education, food processing and availability, housing, and social services are responsible for a large percentage of the health status improvement. The importance of social determinants of health is also supported by the vast health differences observed among populations within the same nation and the differences in population health seen between different countries with similar levels of development and socioeconomic status.

The operational relationships between the various factors that constitute the social determinants of health are overlapping and complex. Clearly, poverty is an underlying issue of importance in determining access to health care, food, transportation, and adequate housing. Childhood (younger than age 5 years) mortality is the health outcome most sensitive to poverty. In **Figure 5-2**, mortality rates for children younger than age 5 years by socioeconomic status across four countries are displayed. As can be seen, although child mortality varies widely among countries, within any one country, there is a consistent social gradient with the highest child mortality rates in the poorest households. There are a number

of examples of countries with similar incomes, but strikingly different health records, however. Greece, for example, with a per capita gross national product (GNP) of just more than $17,000, has a life expectancy of 78.1 years, but the United States, with a per capita GNP of more than $34,000, has a life expectancy of 76.9 years. Costa Rica and Cuba both have per capita GNPs less than $10,000 and yet have life expectancies of 77.9 years and 76.5 years, respectively. A recent Institute of Medicine study found that the United States ranks poorly in terms of both prevalence and mortality for multiple diseases, risk factors, and injuries compared with 16 comparable high income or "peer" countries. This U.S. health disadvantage is not limited to socioeconomically disadvantaged groups, but even the most advantaged Americans are in worse health than their counterparts in other "peer" countries as shown in a report by the Institute of Medicine in 2013.

Where material deprivation is severe, a social gradient in mortality is more likely to be a function of the degree of absolute deprivation. In rich countries with relatively low levels of material deprivation, the focus changes from absolute to relative deprivation. With respect to relative deprivation, consideration of the impact of a broader approach to human needs is critical. This means considering the importance of both material and physical needs and capability as well as spiritual or psychosocial needs on human

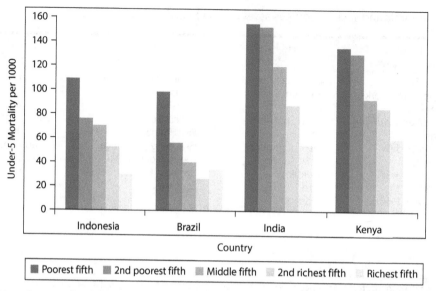

Figure 5-2. Mortality rates for children younger than age 5 years by socioeconomic status across four countries. (Reproduced with permission from Victora CG, Wagstaff A, Schellenberg JA. Applying an equity lens to child health and mortality: more of the same is not enough. *Lancet.* 2003 Jul 19;362(9379):233-241.)

health. Consistent with this approach toward the relationship between the level of material deprivation and social determinants of health, in Africa the major contributor to premature death is communicable disease, while in every other region of the world, noncommunicable disease makes the largest contribution to premature mortality. Analysis of the global burden of disease in developed countries has emphasized the importance of risk factors, such as being overweight, smoking, alcohol, and poor diet, a different set of social determinants than those that dominate in countries with higher indices of poverty (see Chapter 4).

EMERGING THEMES IN SOCIAL DETERMINANTS

An overarching theme that cuts across the various disciplines and theories addressing social determinants of health is that social factors, independent of behaviors and biologic causes, strongly influence population-level health. The idea that societal factors are strong precursors to health outcomes is not a new concept. In the 19th century, a host of theorists described political, economic, and social correlates of disease and mortality. Although there is widespread acceptance that the distribution of social and economic resources is highly correlated with health, there is also a wide range of theoretical approaches regarding the causal mechanisms for these effects. Empiric data show that

since the beginning of the 20th century, there have been large-scale improvements in human health. It is widely assumed that this is the byproduct of the development of technological advancements of industrial societies that allow them to deliver more effective and high-quality health care and that human behavior has changed in ways that lead to longer, more healthy lives. Yet multiple scientific studies have shown that only about 10% to 15% of the improvement in longevity since 1900 can be accounted for by improved health care, and health behaviors themselves are highly correlated with the material conditions of everyday life. These findings imply that there is something more fundamental than access to health care and individual behaviors actually driving health outcomes. One key factor that emerges across theories is that societal inequality is a major driving force behind social determinants of health. Three major theoretical perspectives have been advanced in this regard: materialist, neo-materialist, and comparative psychosocial theories.

Materialist theories of the social determinants of health are the earliest theories that emerged, and they persist to this day. The materialist approach argues that access to resources is the most basic driving force in determining the quality of health of both individuals and populations. Those with greater income, wealth, and the associated material possessions that income and wealth generate are posited to have the best health and longest lives. Empirical data well justify this assertion. For example, the overall wealth of a nation is a very strong predictor of the quality of health of its population. Within nations, wealth is well documented to be associated with health such that individuals with a better socioeconomic position are more likely to have better health and longer lives. As noted by Raphael (2006), "Material conditions predict likelihood of physical (infections, malnutrition, chronic disease and injuries), developmental (delayed or impaired cognition, personality, and social development), educational (learning disabilities, poor learning, early school leaving), and social (socialization, preparation for work and family life) problems." Poverty also is associated with increased stress, which itself is highly associated with poor health outcomes, both physical and psychiatric. In addition, unhealthy behaviors such as smoking and substance abuse sometimes have been associated with poverty, perhaps as a strategy to cope with stress and deprivation.

Neo-materialist theories have a slightly different perspective on the role of wealth as a primary social determinant of health. These theorists argue that the production of health is not related to just the absolute level of material resources available but also to the relative distribution of resources. For example, although a nation may be wealthy overall, health will be affected negatively if there are wide gaps in how resources are distributed across population groups or geographic areas. In essence, neo-materials posit that

health is not just a function of how wealthy a nation is but also how equal the population is within the nation. A host of research has shown that indeed there is a relationship between the level of inequality in a society and health, and this relationship is independent of the overall level of wealth. An example can be found in **Figure 5-3**, which shows the relationship between the Gini coefficient (high values represent higher levels of inequality) and various measures of health status. The graphic shows that poor individuals have fewer healthy days, and this effect is amplified with greater levels of inequality across members of a community.

Finally, the neo-materialist perspective has been elaborated on with regard to causal mechanisms related to psychosocial comparisons that emerge from inequality. In this theoretical perspective, the degree of perceived hierarchy and social distance that occurs in a society is thought to be correlated with health outcomes. The primary tenet of the psychosocial comparison perspective is that one key mechanism by which health is produced in the psychological self-perception that members of society have with regard to their standing in the social hierarchy. There are two primary mechanisms that drive these effects: (1) through the stress derived from feeling unequal and (2) from the reduction in communal "social capital" that results from inequality. In the first instance,

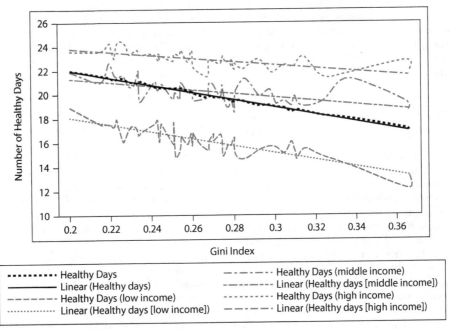

Figure 5-3. The relationship among wealth, inequality, and health. (Reproduced with permission from Frieden TR. Forward: CDC Health Disparities and Inequalities Report—United States, 2011. *MMWR Surveill Summ.* 2011;60(suppl):1-2.)

societal inequality is thought to directly promote stress among individuals, and as discussed earlier, stress is associated with poor health. The second mechanism, reduction in social capital driven by inequality, is a process by which the ties that bind people together in communities (also known as "social capital") are eroded by inequality, and this results in a diminution of health through distrust of others, a lack of social support, and smaller social networks, which can disadvantage people in navigating complex health care systems. These theorists argue that social cohesiveness promotes better population health.

One challenge when exploring the relationships between health and its social determinants is that the myriad relationships between health and such factors as access to material resources, inequality, self-perceptions of equity, communal ties, and social capital are linked in complex ways. Although there are strong empirical correlations between these variables and health outcomes, as has been described earlier, the pathways and mechanisms by which social forces impact health are difficult to tease apart. One emerging discipline that has attempted to do this is social epidemiology, a branch of epidemiology that concerns itself with the relationship between social forces and disease, with an emphasis on bringing rigorous epidemiologic methods to the study of these relationships. These scientists have focused on both what are known as "horizontal structures" (proximal variables experienced by an individual, such as the family structure and work environment) and "vertical structures" (distal variables, such as larger scale political and economic forces), as well as how these two interact. This is a rich area of inquiry that has provided insight into the specific causes and pathways for the influence of social variables on health.

THE LIFE-COURSE PERSPECTIVE ON SOCIAL DETERMINANTS OF HEALTH

Although traditional approaches to health and prevention efforts emphasize addressing biomedical risk factors and unhealthy behaviors in a contemporaneous manner, life-course approaches, which emphasize the accumulated impact of experiences across the lifespan on health, may make more sense in addressing the social determinants of health. In particular, investment during the early years of life has great potential in reducing health inequities. For example, brain development is highly sensitive to external influences such as good nutrition (including in utero), nurturing, and psychosocial stimulation. There is accumulating evidence to support the fact that early nutrition and experiences impact the risk of developing obesity, heart disease, mental health problems, and criminality

in later life. Early childhood experiences also have long-lasting impact on subsequent health and quality of life through skills development, education, and occupational opportunities.

Hertzman (1999) describes three classes of health effects that are relevant to a life-course perspective. Latent effects refer to biologic or developmental early life experiences that impact health later in life. The association between low birth weight and adult-onset diabetes and cardiovascular disease is one example of a latent effect. Recent studies demonstrate that adolescent cannabis use is associated with neuropsychological decline across multiple domains of function that is not fully restored with abstinence. This is likely associated with the poorer education achievement, lower earning potential, increased social welfare dependence, and decreased life satisfaction seen in individuals who were heavy cannabis users in adolescence.

Pathway effects refer to experiences that set individuals onto trajectories that influence health and well-being over the course of a lifetime. For example, entering school with delayed cognitive development can lead to lower education expectations, poorer employment opportunities, and a greater likelihood of illness across the lifespan. Cumulative effects refer to the accumulation of advantage or disadvantage over time, which manifests in health status. Cumulative effects can operate through latent or pathway effects. The life-course perspective allows for consideration of how social determinants of health operate at every level of development to immediately influence health and to provide the basis for health and illness later in life. As an example, the Australian National Public Health Partnership conceptualized the risk of tobacco use with a social determinants perspective that also considered the specificity of effects over the lifespan, as shown in **Figure 5-4**.

RECOMMENDATIONS

In 2005, the WHO established a Commission on the Social Determinants of Health, led by Marmot and colleagues, to foster attention on the role of social determinants of health and make recommendations for interventions. The Commission's analysis and recommendations are codified in a final report published in 2008. This report highlighted three key areas for interventions: (1) improving daily living conditions; (2) reducing the inequitable distribution of power, money, and resources; and (3) measuring and understanding social determinants of health to better plan interventions. This seminal report articulates well the key opportunities for interventions and stresses the role of government policy and international cooperation in maximizing human health through interventions

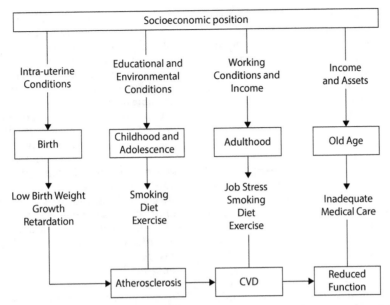

Figure 5-4. Socioeconomic influence on cardiovascular disease (CVD) from a life-course perspective. (Reproduced with permission from The National Public Health Partnership. National Public Health Partnership. Preventing Chronic Disease: A Strategic Framework. Background Paper. http://www.nphp.gov.au/publications/strategies/chrondis-bgpaper.pdf. Accessed November 19, 2014.)

whose primary focus is to improve health by addressing its social determinants. In this section, we summarize many of the core intervention recommendations highlighted in the report.

To improve daily living conditions, a fundamental strategy is to first improve life chances by enhancing early childhood development, including physical, cognitive, linguistic, social, and emotional development. Major strategies to achieve these goals include enhancing prenatal care, child nutrition, support to families for safe and supportive living environments for children, and access to quality preschool education. There is also potential to improve daily living conditions by improving the physical environment in which people live. Urbanization is dramatically increasing globally, and this is leading to an associated increase in population health problems dominated by noncommunicable diseases, accidents, and violent injuries. A large proportion of such risks can be mitigated through improved housing and shelter, improved access to clean water and sanitation, land use policies that minimize dependence on cars for transportation, automobile safety enhancements, and urban planning that supports healthy and safe behaviors. In rural settings, there are special needs with regard to access to services, poverty reduction, access to land, and links to transportation.

Another key component of improving daily living conditions is fair employment and decent work. Work is considered a fundamental social determinant of health because it consumes a large amount of life's efforts, subjects people to risks, is a major determinant of social status, affects self-esteem, and provides necessary income. Temporary workers also have much higher mortality rates than permanent workers, and unstable employment is associated with poor mental health. Poor working conditions, especially prevalent in low-income countries, expose workers to health hazards, especially among poorly paid employees. It is notable that occupations in which workers have little control over their work result in significantly greater health problems, such as was described in the Whitehall study earlier, an effect consistently identified in numerous other studies. Interventions to improve access to decent and fair work include provision of a living wage, strong protective health and safety standards in the workplace, a reasonable balance between work and life and home and life, and giving workers a voice in operational decision making, especially those that affect the worker's direct work activities.

Another major intervention area highlighted by the Commission on the Social Determinants of Health is the need for social protection to ensure that unexpected events in a person's life do not lead to impoverishment. In all countries, rich and poor, virtually everyone will need assistance during vulnerable periods of their lives such as during periods of illness, unemployment, and disability. There is strong evidence that government policies such as social welfare and social security insurance programs have an enormous impact on mitigation of the dire effects of vulnerability and the associated negative impacts on health. Moreover, there is also evidence that countries with strong systems and policies of social protection have significantly lower rates of poverty and healthier people, and they have more resilient economies better able to rebound in periods of economic recession. Examples of such effective policies include setting minimum living standards, financial support and job retraining during periods of unemployment, and systems that guarantee basic pensions in old age.

Finally, one of the most important social determinants of health identified by the Commission on the Social Determinants of Health is the need for universal access to health care. Health care in virtually all countries in the world, both rich and poor, is considered a basic human right, and the vast majority of countries worldwide have systems of government-financed universal health care. Some countries finance their systems through taxation and others through mandatory universal insurance, and the degree to which the state or private sector provides care also varies widely. Regardless of whether health care is financed and provided through public or private means, equitable access to health care as a basic human right is a principle that has striking impacts on the quality and length of life. It is estimated that upward of 100 million people annually are impoverished due to health care costs caused by catastrophic illness.

The second major recommendation of the Commission on the Social Determinants of Health is to reduce the inequitable distribution of power, money, and resources by setting coherent and coordinated policies, both public and private, that maximize health. The Commission stressed the importance of policy coherence to promote societal health. For example, public health policy that stresses good nutrition should not be undercut by trade policies that encourage the production, trade, and consumption of a poor-quality diet. Some policies that could have a major impact on improving health include progressive taxation systems that assure government resources to provide for social welfare programs, increased development aid for the poorest nations, and coordination of foreign development aid that is transparent and evidence based with regard to impact on improving the health and well-being of recipients. In addition, the Commission also strongly recommended that economic

markets be regulated to minimize "economic inequalities, resources depletion, environmental pollution, unhealthy working conditions, and the circulation of dangerous and unhealthy goods" and that health and health care not be treated as a commodity to be traded but rather to be considered as a human right accessible to all based on need.

Other polices recommended by the Commission on the Social Determinants of Health include those that foster gender equity, political empowerment, and improved global governance. The Commission notes that although the status of women has improved substantially over the past century, there remain significant challenges for girls and women because they continue to have poor education and employment opportunities globally compared with men. This can be mitigated by, for example, legislation that outlaws gender discrimination; increasing educational opportunities for girls and women; increased funding for sexual and reproductive health; and accounting for housework, care work, and voluntary work. Political empowerment also is pointed to as an important social determinant of health and one that is especially needed globally for indigenous populations, ethnic minorities, the poor, those with disabilities, and members of the LGBT (lesbian, gay, bisexual, and transgender) community. Interventions include state support for comprehensive human rights and the right to social and political inclusion and support and growth of civil society groups that give voice to the underrepresented. In a related vein, there are stark inequalities cross-nationally, and the Commission's 2008 report stressed the importance of global governance that stresses a multilateral system "in which all countries, rich and poor, engage with an equitable voice."

This review of possible interventions to address social determinants of health elucidates the far-reaching and complex nature of the topic. One final recommendation in the report from the Commission on the Social Determinants of Health was that we need to know more about social determinants in order to better craft and generate sustained support for interventions to improve health. Therefore, a strong recommendation was made to support the collection of more standardized and complete data on social determinants of health to allow for better analysis of these complex relationships. Without solid and rigorously collected data, it is impossible to unearth the casual forces at play, and it is difficult to generate policy support for intervention strategies. In addition, evaluation data on the efficacy of interventions are a powerful tool to both improve programs and generate societal and policy support for intervening on what has been demonstrably shown to be major causes of morbidity and mortality throughout the world.

CHALLENGES

Despite growing recognition of the importance of social determinants of health, a number of challenges are limiting action and implementation of policies based on this knowledge. As mentioned earlier, one clear need is in the area of basic data systems and mechanisms to ensure that the data can be disseminated and understood. Many countries do not even have basic systems to register all births and deaths, and countries with the worst health problems have the poorest data. Without basic data on mortality and morbidity stratified by socioeconomic indicators, countries will continue to have difficulties moving forward on health equity issues. Good evidence on levels of health and its distribution is essential to understand the scale of the problem, recommend actions to be taken, and monitor the impact of policy and other changes in social determinants that might be affecting public health.

In addition, the evidence base on health inequities and how they can be improved needs further strengthening. Unfortunately, most health research funding remains focused on a clinically oriented, individual patient approach to disease. In addition, research grants often are funded to deal with specific diseases and support researchers working in programs that focus on a particular disease state or risk factors. This emphasis produces a group of disease experts and expertise-driven intervention programs rather than programs that focus on fundamental issues impacting health in daily lives. In addition, traditional hierarchies of evidence that value randomized controlled trials and laboratory experiments above other types of evidence generally do not work for research on the social determinants of health. As such, we need new models for gathering and determining the quality of scientific evidence as it applies to population health and social determinants. Routine monitoring systems for health equity and the social determinants of health are needed. Such systems will enable generation and sharing of new evidence on the ways in which social determinants influence population health and health equity and on the effectiveness of measures to reduce inequities through action on social determinants.

Evidence alone does not ensure changes in the factors impacting social determinants of health, however. Education is necessary so that practitioners, policymakers, and the general public can understand the importance of these social factors. There is little evidence of penetration of concepts related to social determinants of health into either public health discourse or government policymaking. The emphasis on the market as the arbiter of societal functioning in many capitalistic countries conflicts with a social determinants of health approach that requires commitment to equitable income distribution and support of public social infrastructure that provides adequate housing, food security, and strong public health and social services.

Another challenge is the fact that both studying and addressing the social determinants of health is a complex, multilevel process that requires an interdisciplinary approach. If we take, for example, the incredible decline in cigarette smoking rates in the United States over the past 20 years, it is clear that numerous forces in operation at various levels influenced this decline. Knowledge about smoking addiction and treatments from basic and clinical research was applied in developing and using evidence-based treatments for smokers. In addition, there was a great deal of public information about the health risks of smoking, the price of cigarettes was increased, and access to cigarette machines was limited. In addition, severe limitations on advertising and smoking in public places were imposed. In other words, the partnerships and policies that helped to change the prevalence and health consequences of smoking went far beyond the narrow confines of the health care and biomedical research fields.

CONCLUSIONS

The social determinants of health approach offers a window into the processes by which social influences can impact health or illness and an opportunity to consider the processes by which power relationships and political ideology can ultimately influence the health of a population. However, there is much work to be done in gathering the data needed to explicate these social influences and to explore approaches to using social determinants to improve health and quality of life. In particular, bridging the gap between knowledge about social determinants and enacting coherent policies to address critical areas is an enormous challenge that will require breaking out of disciplinary silos with well-coordinated efforts operating at multiple levels.

SUMMARY

Social determinants of health refer to societal factors that contribute to health and well-being or the loss thereof. Variations in health status within human populations according to social class have been recognized since at least the 19th century. The landmark Whitehall Study, however, launched in the United Kingdom 50 years ago, brought great focus to the fact that persons of lower social status had worse health measures even after adjusting for baseline differences in known biomedical and behavioral risk factors.

The economic and social attributes classified under the umbrella of social determinants of health vary by context but typically include some or all of the following: income, education, employment, housing, transportation, food security, social connections and support, and access to health care. Improvements in these conditions over the past century have driven most of the gains in the quality and duration of life during this period. In contrast, technical breakthroughs in health care services account for a comparatively small part of the general progress in health outcomes.

The manner in which social factors have an impact on health is complex. Economic resources are critical to determining access to and quality of many services and therefore have an important impact upon health. This is certainly evident in comparing health outcomes across countries with widely varying economic resources. Even within wealthy countries, however, varying levels of deprivation can be seen and correlated with gradients in health status. Those with fewer resources are likely to experience higher stress and reduced social cohesion, as manifest by greater levels of distrust and inadequate social support and networks. Individually and collectively, these characteristics can adversely affect health and interaction with the health care system. Investigators in the field of social epidemiology focus on understanding the mechanisms by which these attributes interrelate and affect health.

Social factors can impact health along the entire human lifespan, with particular susceptibility during the early years of life when growth and development are most active. Some of these effects may not be observed for years, in part because of multistep processes or the cumulative impact of repeated exposures.

Although there are many gaps in our understanding of the mechanisms by which social factors impact health, the highly reproducible effects have led bodies such as the WHO to make recommendations for reducing these gaps in health. The main thrusts of these proposals are to (1) improve living conditions, (2) assure as equitable distribution of essential resources as possible, and (3) improve the measurement and understanding of how social determinants influence health.

STUDY QUESTIONS

1. What landmark investigation helped to focus attention on the role of social factors in determining health status?
   A. The Framingham Study
   B. The Whitehall Study
   C. The British Doctors Study
   D. The Nurses' Health Study

2. Which of the following aspects of poverty is likely to contribute to health status?
   A. Food security
   B. Transportation
   C. Adequate housing
   D. All of the above

3. Population level health status has improved during the past century principally because of
   A. a decline in cigarette smoking.
   B. advances in pharmaceutical treatments.
   C. enhanced social and economic resources.
   D. improved management of acute care hospitalizations.

4. Psychological self-perception is thought to impact health through
   A. stress from perceived inequalities.
   B. loss of trust and social connections.
   C. both A and B.
   D. neither A nor B.

5. Social inequities during which of the following phases of life have the greatest impact on health outcomes?
   A. The early childhood years
   B. The adolescent years
   C. The young adult years
   D. The older adult years

6. What aspects of employment likely contribute to health status?
   A. Poor working conditions
   B. Temporary work
   C. Lack of worker control
   D. All of the above

7. Which of the following is NOT typically considered a social determinant of health?
   A. Education
   B. Social drinking
   C. Transportation
   D. Housing

8. Which of the following groups of workers is likely to have the lowest mortality rate?
   A. Senior executives
   B. Support staff
   C. Skilled workers
   D. Semi-skilled laborers

9. Which of the following countries has the highest levels of both income and health inequity?

A. Japan

B. United States

C. Canada

D. United Kingdom

10. Which of the following programs is likely to have the greatest impact on social determinants of health?

A. A physical fitness campaign

B. A healthy nutrition program

C. Early childhood education

D. Smoking cessation

FURTHER READING

Friel S, Marmot MG. Action on the social determinants of health and health inequities goes global. *Annu Rev Public Health.* 2011;32:225-236.

Galea S, Tracy M, Hoggatt KJ, Dimaggio C, Karpati A. Estimated deaths attributable to social factors in the United States. *Am J Public Health.* 2011;101:1456-1465.

Muennig P, Fiscella K, Tancredi D, Franks P. The relative health burden of selected social and behavioral risk factors in the United States: implications for policy. *Am J Public Health.* 2010;100:1758-1764.

REFERENCES

Health Scenario

Marmot MG, Rose G, Shipley M, Hamilton PJ. Employment grade and coronary heart disease in British civil servants. *J Epidemiol Community Health.* 1978;32(4):244-249.

Marmot M. Social determinants of health inequalities. *Lancet.* 2005;365(9464):1099-1104.

Marmot M, Ryff CD, Bumpass LL, Shipley M, Marks NF. Social inequalities in health: next questions and converging evidence. *Soc Sci Med.* 1997;44(6):901-910.

Marmot MG. Tackling health inequalities since the Acheson inquiry. *J Epidemiol Community Health.* 2004;58(4):262-263.

Marmot MG, Smith GD, Stansfeld S, et al. Health inequalities among British civil servants: the Whitehall II study. *Lancet.* 1991;337(8754):1387-1393.

Overview

Centers for Disease Control and Prevention. *Social Determinants of Health Working Group.* Atlanta: Author; 2005.

Davey Smith G, Dorling D, Shaw M. *Poverty, Inequality and Health in Britain: 1800-2000: A Reader.* Bristol, UK: Policy Press; 2001.

Evans RD. *Interpreting and Addressing Inequalities in Health: From Black to Acheson to Blair to ...?: 7th Annual Lecture.* London: Office of Health Economics; 2002.

Fogel RW. *The Fourth Great Awakening and the Future of Egalitarianism.* Chicago: University of Chicago Press; 2000.

Institute of Medicine. *US Health in International Perspective: Shorter Lives, Poorer Health.* http://www.iom.edu/~/media/Files/Report%20Files/2013/US-Health-International-Perspective/USHealth_Intl_PerspectiveRB.pdf. Accessed January 15, 2013.

Marmot M. *Status Syndrome.* London: Bloomsbury; 2004.

Sen A. *Development as Freedom.* Oxford: Oxford University Press; 1999.

United Nations Development Programme. *Human Development Report.* New York: Oxford University Press; 2003.

Victora CG, Wagstaff A, Schellenberg JA, Gwatkin D, Claeson M, Habicht JP. Applying an equity lens to child health and mortality: more of the same is not enough. *Lancet.* 2003;362(9379):233-241.

World Health Organization. *Reducing Risks, Promoting Healthy Life.* Geneva: Author; 2002.

World Health Organization. *The World Health Report 2004.* Geneva: Author; 2004.

Wilkinson RG, Marmot M. *Social Determinants of Health: The Solid Facts.* Copenhagen: The World Health Organization, European Office; 2003.

Wilkinson RG. *The Impact of Inequality: How to Make Sick Societies Healthier.* London: Routledge; 2005.

Emerging Themes

Benzeval M, Judge K. Income and health: the time dimension. *Soc Sci Med.* 2001;52(9):1371-1390.

Berkman LF, Kawachi Io. *Social Epidemiology.* New York: Oxford University Press; 2000.

Berkman LF. Seeing the forest and the trees: new visions in social epidemiology. *Am J Epidemiol.* 2004;160(1):1-2.

Blakely TA, Lochner K, Kawachi I. Metropolitan area income inequality and self-rated health—a multi-level study. *Soc Sci Med.* 2002;54(1):65-77.

Bloom DE, Canning D. Policy forum: public health. The health and wealth of nations. *Science.* 2000;287(5456):1207, 1209.

Brady KT, Sonne SC. The role of stress in alcohol use, alcoholism treatment, and relapse. *Alcohol Res Health.* 1999;23(4):263-271.

Evans GW, English K. The environment of poverty: multiple stressor exposure, psychophysiological stress, and socioemotional adjustment. *Child Dev.* 2002;73(4):1238-1248.

Frieden TR. Forward: CDC Health Disparities and Inequalities Report—United States, 2011. *MMWR Surveill Summ.* 2011;60(suppl):1-2.

Horton R. The health (and wealth) of nations. *Lancet.* 2002;359(9311):993-994.

Karriker-Jaffe KJ, Roberts SC, Bond J. Income inequality, alcohol use, and alcohol-related problems. *Am J Public Health.* 2013;103(4):649-656.

Karriker-Jaffe KJ, Zemore SE, Mulia N, Jones-Webb R, Bond J, Greenfield TK. Neighborhood disadvantage and adult alcohol outcomes: differential risk by race and gender. *J Stud Alcohol Drugs.* 2012;73(6):865-873.

Kawachi I, Kennedy BP. Health and social cohesion: why care about income inequality? *BMJ.* 1997;314(7086):1037-1040.

Kawachi I, Kennedy BP. Income inequality and health: pathways and mechanisms. *Health Serv Res.* 1999;34(1 Pt 2):215-227.

Kennedy BP, Kawachi I, Prothrow-Stith D. Income distribution and mortality: cross sectional ecological study of the Robin Hood index in the United States. *BMJ*. 1996;312(7037):1004-1007.

Kivimaki M, Nyberg ST, Batty GD, et al. Job strain as a risk factor for coronary heart disease: a collaborative meta-analysis of individual participant data. *Lancet*. 2012;380(9852):1491-1497.

Kondo N, van Dam RM, Sembajwe G, Subramanian SV, Kawachi I, Yamagata Z. Income inequality and health: the role of population size, inequality threshold, period effects and lag effects. *J Epidemiol Community Health*. 2012;66(6):e11.

Malik P. Wealth of nations is health of nations. *Can J Cardiol*. 2007;23(7):516.

O'Campo P, Dunn JR. *Rethinking Social Epidemiology : Towards a Science of Change*. New York: Springer; 2012.

Pickett KE, Wilkinson RG. Greater equality and better health. *BMJ*. 2009;339:b4320.

Raphael D. Social determinants of health: present status, unanswered questions, and future directions. *Int J Health Serv*. 2006;36(4):651-677.

Subramanian SV, Kawachi I. The association between state income inequality and worse health is not confounded by race. *Int J Epidemiol*. 2003;32(6):1022-1028.

Wilkinson RG. *Unhealthy societies : the afflictions of inequality*. New York: Routledge; 1996.

The Life Course

Ellickson PL, Martino SC, Collins RL. Cannabis use from adolescence to young adulthood: multiple developmental trajectories and their associated outcomes. *Health Psychology*. 2004; 23(3):299-307.

Felitti VJ, RF. A. The relationship of adverse childhood experiences to adult health, well-being, social function, and health care. In: Lanius R, Vermetten E, Pain C, eds. *The Effects of Early Life Trauma on Health and Disease: The Hidden Epidemic*. Cambridge: Cambridge University Press; 2010.

Fergusson DM, Boden JM. Cannabis use and later life outcomes. *Addiction*. 2008;103(6):969-976; discussion 977-968.

Hertzman C. Population health and human development. In: Keating DP, Hertzman C, eds. *Developmental Health and the Wealth of Nations: Social, Biological and Educational Dynamics*. New York: Guilford Press; 1999.

Lynch J, Kaplan GA. Socioeconomic position. In: Beckman LF, Kawachi I, eds. *Social Epidemiology*. New York; 2000.

Macleod J, Oakes R, Copello A, et al. Psychological and social sequelae of cannabis and other illicit drug use by young people: a systematic review of longitudinal, general population studies. *Lancet*. 2004;363(9421):1579-1588.

Marmot M, Friel S, Bell R, Houweling TA, Taylor S. Closing the gap in a generation: health equity through action on the social determinants of health. *Lancet*. 2008;372(9650):1661-1669.

Murray C, Michaud C, McKenna M, Marks J. *US patterns of mortality by county and race: 1965-94*. Cambridge: Harvard Center for Population and Development Studies; 1998.

The National Public Health Partnership. *National Public Health Partnership. Preventing Chronic Disease: A Strategic Framework. Background Paper*. http://www.nphp.gov.au/publications/strategies/chrondis-bgpaper.pdf. Accessed November 19, 2014.

Challenges

Artazcoz L, Benach J, Borrell C, Cortes I. Social inequalities in the impact of flexible employment on different domains of psychosocial health. *J Epidemiol Community Health*. 2005;59(9):761-767.

Kivimaki M, Vahtera J, Virtanen M, Elovainio M, Pentti J, Ferrie JE. Temporary employment and risk of overall and cause-specific mortality. *Am J Epidemiol*. 2003;158(7):663-668.

Marmot M, Friel S, Bell R, Houweling TA, Taylor S. Closing the gap in a generation: health equity through action on the social determinants of health. *Lancet*. 2008;372(9650):1661-1669.

UNICEF. State of the World's Children 2007: Women and Children: The Double Dividend of Gender Equity. http://www.unicef.org/publications/files/The_State_of_the_Worlds__Children__2007_e.pdf. Accessed November 19, 2014.

Health Disparities

6

Leonard E. Egede, Marvella E. Ford, and Joni L. Strom Williams

HEALTH SCENARIO

Two male coworkers were referred by their supervisor to the same primary care physician for annual physical examinations. One patient was a 55-year-old African American man; the other was a 55-year-old European American man. Both men worked at the same job for nearly 30 years and had the same insurance coverage. Both patients were previously diagnosed with diabetes, which was managed by taking oral medications. An indicator of long-term blood glucose levels, the glycosylated hemoglobin A1c (HbA1c), for the African American and European American men, were 10.9% and 8.2%, respectively, which are both elevated. The African American patient had a positive family history of diabetes, with several first-degree relatives having amputations secondary to poor glycemic control. Amputations are performed because of recurrent severe infections of skin ulcerations that cannot be controlled otherwise.

During the visits, physical examinations were completed on each patient, and blood samples for appropriate laboratory tests were obtained. After examinations of his feet for evidence of ulceration, the European American patient was offered the influenza vaccination and received counseling on preventive services, such as annual dental and eye examinations. Despite a personal and extensive family history of risk factors for diabetes, the African American patient did not receive recommendations for preventive care services, including getting his feet examined. Months later, the African American patient developed septicemia (a blood infection arising from the infected foot ulcers), was hospitalized and treated with intravenous antibiotics, and ultimately underwent a lower limb amputation as a result.

CLINICAL BACKGROUND

Despite significant advances in the diagnosis and treatment of most chronic diseases, there is evidence that (1) racial and ethnic minorities tend to receive lower quality of care, including preventive care, than nonminorities and (2) patients of minority ethnicity experience greater morbidity and mortality from various chronic diseases than nonminorities. In 2002, the Institute of Medicine (IOM) published a report on unequal treatment, concluding that "racial and ethnic disparities in healthcare exist and, because they are associated with worse outcomes in many cases, are unacceptable." The IOM report defined disparities in health care as "racial or ethnic differences in the quality of health care that are not due to access-related factors or clinical needs, preferences, and appropriateness of intervention." Since the publication of the IOM report, there has been renewed interest in understanding the sources of disparities, identifying contributing factors, and designing and evaluating effective interventions to reduce or eliminate racial and ethnic disparities in health care.

Racial variations in health might be assumed to arise from genetic factors. Under this model, race is considered in biologic terms, genes that differ between races are linked with the genes that determine health, and the health of a population is determined predominantly by biologic factors. Recent studies have shown, however, that there is more genetic variation within races than between races and that race is more of a social construct than a biologic construct. Therefore, the concept of race, although useful from a social and cultural perspective, is of limited biologic relevance. In addition to the limitations of race as a biologic construct, there are problems with the validity and reliability of race as measured in most research studies. Methods for collecting data on race include self-report, direct observation, proxy report, and extraction from records. In general, self-reported race is most reliable and is the preferred method. With the increase in the number of people who belong to multiple racial categories, however, it is increasingly difficult to classify individuals into discrete racial categories, which further complicates the interpretation of effects associated with race in health care, as well as research studies.

Diabetes is one of the most prevalent and fastest growing chronic illnesses, affecting more than 346 million people worldwide. It is emerging as a global epidemic because of the rapid rise of obesity and decline in physical activity. The combined impacts of poor awareness, insufficient access, limited services, and inadequate resources make diabetes the leading cause of blindness, amputation, and kidney failure worldwide. Additionally, for type 2 diabetes (T2DM), in which the physiologic responses to insulin are diminished, patients have greater comorbidity and complications, including cardiovascular disease (CVD), renal disease, nerve damage, and retinal eye disease.

In conjunction with these population shifts, the number of racial/ethnic minorities developing diabetes also is growing continuously. Men and minorities—non-Hispanic blacks (NHBs), Hispanics (Mexican Americans, Puerto Ricans, and Cubans), and American Indians/Native Americans/Pacific Islanders—are affected more often than women and non-Hispanic whites (NHWs), respectively. Studies have shown consistently that NHBs are twice as likely to be diagnosed with and die as a result of diabetes compared with NHWs. This racial and ethnic disparity has existed over the past 20 years and continues to persist. Additionally, NHBs are two to four times more likely to experience diabetes-related complications than NHWs.

Although preventable, T2DM accounts for 90% of all cases of diabetes observed worldwide. Evidence shows that at least 30 minutes of moderate exercise once daily 5 days a week along with healthy eating habits aids in preventing and managing diabetes and diabetes-related outcomes. These behaviors, in addition to other self-care activities such as home blood glucose monitoring, taking medications as prescribed, obtaining preventive services, and limiting alcohol intake and tobacco use, make living and adjusting to a life with diabetes more manageable.

INTRODUCTION

The term "health disparities" is used widely in health outcomes research. The purpose of this chapter is to define health disparities, address measurement issues in health disparities research, describe health disparities in the United States, identify some of the causes of health disparities, and discuss potential solutions to health disparities.

The IOM defines disparities in health care as racial or ethnic differences that are not a result of access-related factors, clinical needs, preferences, or appropriateness of treatment intervention (**Figure 6-1**). These differences may be attributed to a lack of health insurance coverage and other barriers to care, such as lack of geographic access to clinicians, high copayments, and lack of transportation to health care sites. Disparities in health care are associated with disparities in health outcomes, which are widespread and persistent. Health disparities are differences in health outcomes that are attributable to the inequitable distribution of resources. The National Institutes of Health (NIH) defines health disparities as differences in the incidence, prevalence, mortality, and burden of diseases and other health conditions that exist among specific population groups.

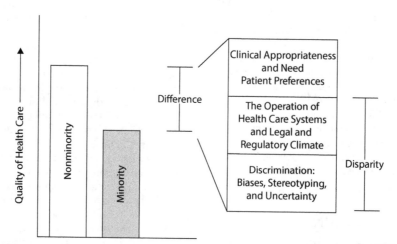

Figure 6-1. Definition of health disparities in health care. (Reproduced with permission from Smedley BD, Stith AY, Nelson AR, eds. *Unequal Treatment: Confronting Racial and Ethnic Disparities in Healthcare.* Washington, DC: Institute of Medicine; 2003.)

As will be discussed later in greater detail, for almost every category of disease, including CVD, diabetes, cancer, and renal disease, African Americans have poorer health, and other racial and ethnic minorities have poorer health outcomes than European Americans. For example, mortality rates due to hypertension are about 15 deaths per 100,000 people for European men and women, about 40 per 100,000 for African American women, and more than 50 per 100,000 for African American men. Moreover, an estimated 13.2% of African Americans and 11.9% of Hispanics have diabetes compared with 7.1% of European Americans. Prostate cancer death rates, although decreasing in men of all racial/ethnic groups, remain twice as high among African Americans as any other group. Overall, the death rate for cancer among African American men is 27% higher than for European American men, and the death rate for cancer among African American women is 11% higher than for European American women. For HIV/AIDS, in 1987, African Americans' mortality rate was three times higher than for European Americans; in 2011, African Americans' HIV/AIDS mortality rate was 1.9 times greater than that for European Americans. In 2011, 28% of African Americans and 25% of Hispanics/Latinos lived below the poverty line compared with 10% of European Americans. In Chapter 5, we learned that social determinants, such as income, are strong predictors of health outcomes. Even when socioeconomic status (SES) is taken into account, however, racial and ethnic disparities often persist.

The interface between social and economic health status determinants and the presence of racial and ethnic disparities in health outcomes is well documented. Race is associated with societal prejudices, which in turn produce increased susceptibility to disease; reduced access to health care; and subsequent health disparities in disease incidence, prevalence, morbidity, and mortality. From this perspective, race interacts with social and environmental factors, such as lack of access to grocery stores that provide healthy foods or access to safe areas in which to engage in physical activity. These social inequities in turn lead to increased susceptibility to disease. Socioeconomic factors such as employment and lack of health insurance negatively impact access to health care. The model in **Figure 6-2** depicts these relationships. Together, the factors in this model have significant contributions to observed health disparities.

Slightly more complex models are shown in **Figures 6-3 and 6-4**, which suggest that structural life inequalities based on access to high-quality education, good nutrition, well-paying jobs, safe living

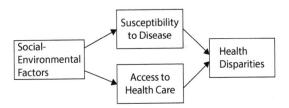

Figure 6-2. Impact of social determinants of health on health disparities. (Reproduced with permission from Baker TA, Whitfield KE. *Handbook of Minority Aging.* New York: Springer; 2013.)

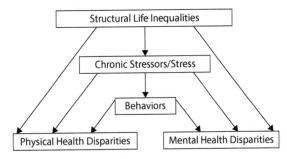

Figure 6-3. Impact of social determinants of health on health disparities. (Data from Williams DR, Mohammed SA. Racism and health II: a needed research agenda for effective interventions. *Am Behav Sci.* 2013;57(8):1200-1226.)

environments, reliable transportation, adequate health insurance coverage, and culturally competent health care are chronic stressors for people who face these inequalities on a daily basis. Facing these chronic stressors results in chronic activation of the hypothalamic–pituitary–adrenal axis system and subsequent downregulation of the immune system. Therefore, in response to chronic stressors, people tend to engage in activities that make them feel good and bring a temporary relief from the stressors, such as eating comfort food, smoking, and overusing drugs and alcohol. Others may develop health-damaging psychological responses to the structural life inequalities, such as internalized racism or feelings of self-blame for poor living conditions. It has been noted that engaging in these activities initially reduces activation of the stress-response network. The unfortunate consequence lies in the fact that the very activities that people use to temporarily reduce their levels of stress eventually lead to increased risk of disease and to poor health outcomes, contributing ultimately to further long-term stress.

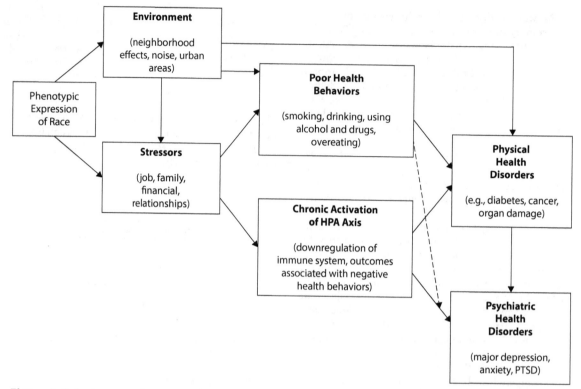

Figure 6-4. Environmental stressors, physiologic stress responses, negative behavioral coping strategies, and subsequent physical and psychiatric health disorders. HPA, hypothalamic–pituitary–adrenal; PTSD, posttraumatic stress disorder. (Data from Baker TA, Whitfield KE. *Handbook of Minority Aging.* New York: Springer; 2013.)

MEASUREMENT ISSUES IN HEALTH DISPARITIES RESEARCH

As noted earlier, race and ethnicity interface with social determinants of health to produce health disparities. Before these disparities can be accurately evaluated and described, however, race and ethnicity first must be accurately defined and conceptualized.

By the year 2050, racial and ethnic minorities will comprise 47.5% of the total U.S. population. In 2010, African Americans made up 12.6% of the U.S. population, an increase from 12.3% in 2000. In 2010, Hispanics/Latinos comprised 16.3% of the total U.S. population, almost half again as high as it was a decade earlier.

Race and ethnicity are complex and multidimensional constructs. For racial and ethnic categorizations to be most meaningful, they should lead to consistent data over time, allow data from populations and surveys to be compared, and use terms that are understood by the people who complete the surveys (Sawyer, 1998).

What Is Race?

Despite the use of phenotypic expressions of racial group membership (e.g., skin color) as a social construct that is associated with the allocation of resources such as education, housing, and employment, the validity of race as an indicator of genetically different population groups has been questioned widely. No racial group possesses a completely discrete set of genetic characteristics. In fact, there is significantly greater genetic variation within phenotypically defined racial groups than there is between them, with 85% variation within racial group and 15% variation between groups. All individuals are 99.0% to 99.5% identical at the DNA level. In addition, definite biologic links between racial group and disease have been found only rarely (e.g., sickle cell disease). Instead, differences in disease prevalence may be due to genetic differences; dietary, cultural, environmental, and socioeconomic factors; or a mixture of both.

As a social construct, the phenotypic expressions of race influence social interactions that predict exposure to health risks posed by environmental, social, and behavioral factors. From this perspective, health disparities are seen largely as arising from social-environmental factors (e.g., structural inequalities in access to high-quality education, employment, and housing) that influence disease susceptibility, as well as access to medical care. For example, the single most important type of structural inequality that negatively affects health may be residential segregation, which impacts access to adequate educational systems and medical care. Thus, as shown in **Figure 6-4**, structural inequalities, based on phenotypic expression of race, result in the persistence of health disparities.

What Is Ethnicity?

Although the terms "race" and "ethnicity" sometimes are used interchangeably, they actually represent two different constructs. Ethnicity, similar to race, is a social-political construct. However, ethnicity refers to sharing a common culture, language, religion, and cultural traditions.

Ethnicity embodies cultural identification. An important point to make is that such identification is fluid and may change over time. For example, a young third-generation Armenian American might culturally identify more strongly with the general American culture than with Armenian culture. However, as the person ages, he or she might adhere more strongly to the values and traditions of Armenian culture and may begin to self-identify more with Armenian culture. Ethnic self-identification becomes important during life passages such as selecting a marriage partner, becoming parents, and raising children. This means that survey results based on responses to ethnic identity may change over the life course.

The revised Directive Number 15 of the Office of Management and Budget (OMB) includes criteria to use to classify people into categories of race and ethnicity. A minimum of five separate categories is mandated for self-identified racial classification: (1) white, (2) black, African American or Negro, (3) American Indian or Alaska Native, (4) Asian, or (5) some other race. Directive Number 15 defines white as a person having origins in any of the original peoples of Europe, the Middle East, or North Africa; black, African American or Negro is defined as a person having origins in any of the phenotypically black racial groups of Africa; American Indian or Alaska Native is defined as a person having origins in any of the original peoples of North and South America, including Central America; and Asian is defined as a person having origins an any of the original peoples of the Far East, Southeast Asia, or the Indian subcontinent, including people from Cambodia, China, India, Japan, Korea, Malaysia, Pakistan, the Philippine Islands, Thailand, and Vietnam.

The application of Directive Number 15 as used in Census 2010 is shown in **Figure 6-5**. It is important to note that although most surveys of population health status and outcomes using the format mandated in Directive Number 15 include ethnic groups only for Hispanics/Latinos and Asian Americans, every racial group includes multiple ethnic subgroups. For example, among phenotypically defined European Americans, ethnic subgroups include Germans, Hungarians, Ukrainians, and so on. Among phenotypically defined African Americans, ethnic subgroups include Nigerians, Kenyans, Jamaicans, Haitians, and so on. In 2002, Ford et al. suggested that the Directive Number 15 categories be used as core modules to categorize race and ethnicity. Then, in regions of the country where larger ethnic subpopulations exist, in addition to the standardized core modules, population-specific modules could be added. This approach could allow investigators to collect data on race using a standardized format to allow cross-site comparisons of study outcomes while at the same time collecting data on population-specific ethnic subgroups whose culturally based attitudes, behaviors, and social positions related to structural inequalities could influence the outcomes under study.

HEALTH DISPARITIES IN THE UNITED STATES

The burgeoning of health disparities research was stimulated by specific mandates to address broadly adverse health outcomes, which have exposed persistent health and health care disparities. A number of policies have been instituted to support studies in examining the contributing factors and intervention targets that work toward reducing and eliminating differences in the burden of disease and medical care among population subgroups. With the high prevalence and mortality rate of specific chronic conditions across disadvantaged populations, the following disease categories exemplify health disparities that require an in-depth view and targeted efforts to make substantial impacts on health outcomes in the United States.

Cardiovascular Disease

Cardiovascular disease remains the most prevalent disease in the United States, affecting more than 83 million men and women 20 years of age and older. **Figure 6-6** shows the prevalence of CVD in adults 20 years of age and older by age and gender. Diseases such as stroke, coronary heart disease, and heart failure also contribute to the escalating numbers of individuals diagnosed with CVD. Although mortality

Reproduction of the Questions on Hispanic Origin and Race From the 2010 Census

→ NOTE: Please answer BOTH Question 5 about Hispanic origin and Question 6 about race. For this census, Hispanic origins are not races.

5. Is this person of Hispanic, Latino, or Spanish origin?

- ☐ No, not of Hispanic, Latino, or Spanish origin
- ☐ Yes, Mexican, Mexican Am., Chicano
- ☐ Yes, Puerto Rican
- ☐ Yes, Cuban
- ☐ Yes, another Hispanic, Latino, or Spanish origin — *Print origin, for example, Argentinean, Colombian, Dominican, Nicaraguan, Salvadoran, Spaniard, and so on.* ↗

[ ]

6. What is this person's race? *Mark* ☒ *one or more boxes.*

- ☐ White
- ☐ Black, African Am., or Negro
- ☐ American Indian or Alaska Native — *Print name of enrolled or principal tribe.* ↗

[ ]

- ☐ Asian Indian
- ☐ Chinese
- ☐ Filipino
- ☐ Other Asian— *Print race, for example, Hmong, Laotian, Thai, Pakistani, Cambodian, and so on.* ↗

- ☐ Japanese
- ☐ Korean
- ☐ Vietnamese

- ☐ Native Hawaiian
- ☐ Guamanian or Chamorro
- ☐ Samoan
- ☐ Other Pacific Islander — *Print race, for example, Fijian, Tongan, and so on.* ↗

[ ]

- ☐ Some other race — *Print race.* ↗

[ ]

Source: U.S. Census Bureau, 2010 Census questionnaire.

Figure 6-5. Reproduction of the questions on Hispanic origin and race from the 2010 Census (Data from Humes KR, Jones NA, Ramirez RR. *2010 Census Redistricting Data (Public Law 94-171) Summary File.* U.S. Department of Commerce Economics and Statistics Administration. U.S. Census Bureau. http://factfinder2.census.gov/main.html. Retrieved November 19, 2014.)

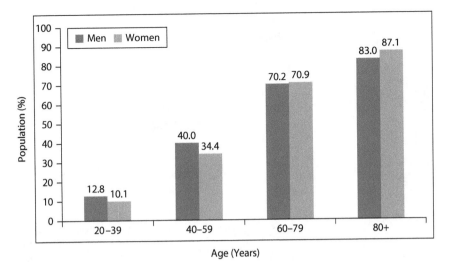

Figure 6-6. Prevalence of cardiovascular disease in adults by age and gender. (Reproduced with permission from Go AS, Mozaffarian D, Roger VL, et al. American Heart Association Statistics Committee and Stroke Statistics Subcommittee. Heart disease and stroke statistics—2013 update: a report from the American Heart Association. *Circulation.* 2013;127(1):e6-e245. © 2013 American Heart Association, Inc.)

rates have declined by one third between 2000 and 2010, CVD remains the leading cause of death in the United States, accounting for one in three deaths. **Figure 6-7** shows CVD mortality trends for men and women (United States: 1979–2010). In 2009, it was estimated that $312.6 billion was spent on CVD. A total of $192.1 billion was spent in direct patient care. By 2030, total expenditures for CVD are expected to reach more than $800 billion. See **Figure 6-8** for costs of CVD and stroke in the United States in 2010 and **Figure 6-9** for projected costs in 2015 to 2030.

Marked disparities—gender, racial/ethnic, geographic—exist in the prevalence, morbidity, and mortality associated with CVD and its related risk factors. Subgroups including African Americans, Hispanics, particularly Mexican Americans, persons with lower SES, people residing in the Southeastern United States and Appalachia, and people with lower educational levels (less than high school) tend to have a higher burden of CVD and its related risk factors. In a systematic review of racial and ethnic differences in CVD risk factors, Kurian et al. found elevated risk and higher prevalence for racial/ethnic minority groups in hypertension, diabetes, obesity, and physical inactivity. Risk and prevalence were nearly equivalent for all racial/ethnic groups in terms of assessing hypercholesterolemia and smoking status.

With a higher prevalence of CVD in the U.S. population, greater acknowledgement of differences in risk factors and medical care of those living with these chronic diseases has been the focus of much research

effort in the past 2 decades. To date, initiatives targeting reduction of adverse CVD-related outcomes lack breadth and depth among racial/ethnicity minority populations in regards to access to care, treatment intensity, risk factor management, and prevention. This subgroup layered with low SES status or rural residence places them at an even greater risk of poor CVD outcomes.

The rate of CVD mortality has likely been tempered by a range of advancements in technology, from better diagnostic and therapeutic approaches for cardiac revascularization to more effective management of CVD risk factors. Greater attention to risk factors for CVD also has resulted in substantial efforts to target smoking reduction and cessation; increase physical activity; address overweight and obesity; and control cholesterol, blood pressure, and blood glucose levels.

Diabetes

Diabetes affects 25.8 million people, or 8.3% of the United States population, and is the seventh leading cause of death in the United States. It is also the leading cause of kidney failure, nontraumatic lower limb amputations, and new cases of blindness among adults and is a major cause of heart disease and stroke. Ninety percent of all cases of diabetes are categorized as T2DM, characterized by insulin resistance rather than absolute insulin deficiency. **Figures 6-10 and 6-11** show the prevalence of diagnosed diabetes by race/ethnicity and gender and race/ethnicity and years of education, respectively.

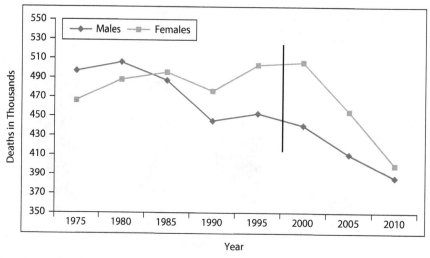

Figure 6-7. Prevalence of cardiovascular disease in men and women. (Reproduced with permission from Go AS, Mozaffarian D, Roger VL, et al. American Heart Association Statistics Committee and Stroke Statistics Subcommittee. Heart disease and stroke statistics—2013 update: a report from the American Heart Association. *Circulation.* 2013;127(1):e6-e245. © 2013 American Heart Association, Inc.)

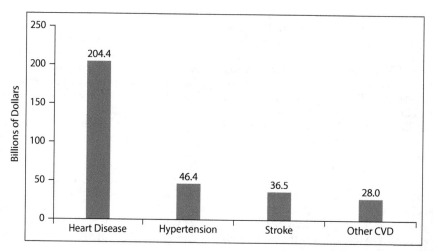

Figure 6-8. Direct and indirect costs of cardiovascular disease (CVD) and stroke (in billions of dollars), United States, 2010. (Reproduced with permission Go AS, Mozaffarian D, Roger VL, et al. American Heart Association Statistics Committee and Stroke Statistics Subcommittee. Heart disease and stroke statistics—2013 update: a report from the American Heart Association. *Circulation.* 2013;127(1):e6-e245. © 2013 American Heart Association, Inc.)

The rate of diagnosed diabetes has steadily increased and is projected to continue, creating a disease of epidemic proportions. Additionally, NHBs have poorer outcomes than NHW population across several indicators of care. **Figure 6-12** shows quality of care indicators by race/ethnicity for adults with T2DM. NHBs and Hispanics continue to receive lower quality of care than NHWs. Similarly, patients of lower SES also continue to receive poorer quality of care than those with higher SES.

Although T2DM is a concern for all racial and ethnic groups, minorities have elevated prevalence, risks from complications, and mortality rates. Compared with NHW adults, the risk of diagnosed diabetes was 77% higher among NHBs. After being diagnosed, NHBs are four times more likely to develop end-stage renal

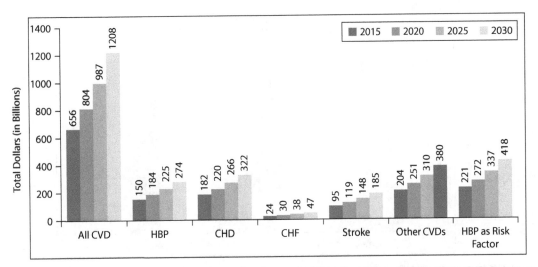

Figure 6-9. Projected expenditures for cardiovascular disease (CVD), United States, 2015 to 2030. CHD, coronary heart disease; CHF, congestive heart failure; HBP, high blood pressure. (Reproduced with permission from Go AS, Mozaffarian D, Roger VL, et al. American Heart Association Statistics Committee and Stroke Statistics Subcommittee. Heart disease and stroke statistics—2013 update: a report from the American Heart Association. *Circulation.* 2013;127(1):e6-e245. © 2013 American Heart Association, Inc.)

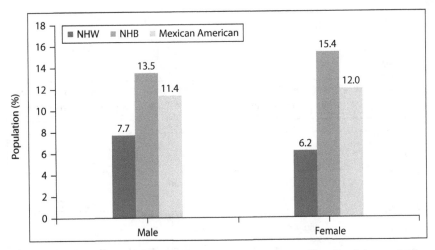

Figure 6-10. Age-adjusted prevalence of physician-diagnosed diabetes mellitus in adults age 20 years of age and older by race/ethnicity and sex. NHB, non-Hispanic black; NHW, non-Hispanic white (National Health and Nutrition Examination Survey, 2007–2010). (Reproduced with permission from Go AS, Mozaffarian D, Roger VL, et al. American Heart Association Statistics Committee and Stroke Statistics Subcommittee. Heart disease and stroke statistics—2013 update: a report from the American Heart Association. *Circulation.* 2013;127(1):e6-e245. © 2013 American Heart Association, Inc.)

disease and more likely to undergo lower limb amputations compared with NHWs. Additionally, the average life years lost by diagnosis vary by ethnicity, with NHB women losing on average 12 years compared with NHW women losing 10.3 years and NHB men losing 9.3 years compared with NHW men losing 8 years.

Ethnic differences in poor outcomes in T2DM can be attributed to patient, provider, and health systems level factors. See **Figures 6-13 and 6-14** for outcomes by race/ethnicity and race/ethnicity and income, respectively, in adult patients with diabetes. Provider and health system factors account for less

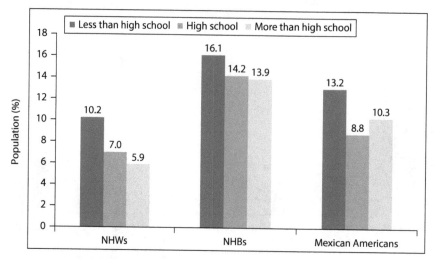

Figure 6-11. Age-adjusted prevalence of physician-diagnosed type 2 diabetes mellitus in adults 20 years of age and older by race/ethnicity and years of education. NHB, non-Hispanic black; NHW, non-Hispanic white (National Health and Nutrition Examination Survey, 2007–2010). (Reproduced with permission from Go AS, Mozaffarian D, Roger VL, et al. American Heart Association Statistics Committee and Stroke Statistics Subcommittee. Heart disease and stroke statistics—2013 update: a report from the American Heart Association. *Circulation.* 2013;127(1):e6-e245. © 2013 American Heart Association, Inc.)

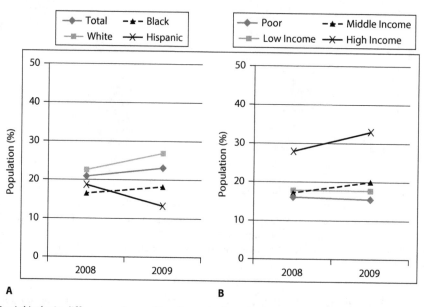

Figure 6-12. Racial/ethnic differences in quality of care indicators for adults with diabetes. Adults, age 40 and over with diagnosed diabetes who reported receiving four recommended services for diabetes in the calendar year (2+ hemoglobin A1c tests, foot exam, dilated eye exam, and flu shot) by (A) race/ethnicity and (B) income. (Reproduced from Agency for Healthcare Research and Quality. *National Healthcare Quality & Disparities Reports.* Rockville, MD; March 2012. http://www.ahrq.gov/research/findings/nhqrdr/index.html. Retrieved November 19, 2014.)

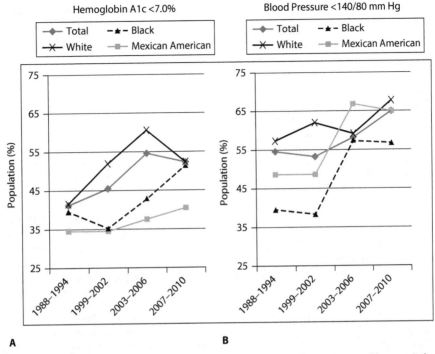

Figure 6-13. Outcomes for diabetes by race/ethnicity. (A) Glycemic (blood sugar) control by race/ethnicity based on glycosylated hemoglobin A1c <7.0%. (B) Blood pressure control by race/ethnicity based on measurement <140/80 mm Hg. (Reproduced from Agency for Healthcare Research and Quality. *National Healthcare Quality & Disparities Reports.* Rockville, MD; March 2012. http://www.ahrq.gov/research/findings/nhqrdr/index.html. Retrieved November 19, 2014.)

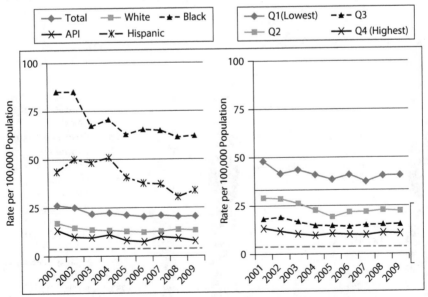

Figure 6-14. Hospitalizations for uncontrolled diabetes by race/ethnicity and area income. API, Asian Pacific Islander. (Reproduced from Agency for Healthcare Research and Quality. *National Healthcare Quality & Disparities Reports.* Rockville, MD; March 2012. http://www.ahrq.gov/research/findings/nhqrdr/index.html. Retrieved November 19, 2014.)

than 10% of variance in major diabetes outcomes, including HbA1c, lipid control, and resource use; hence, major emphasis needs to be placed on patient-level factors that have strong explanatory power. Key differences appear to be at the patient level. Of the patient-level factors, consistent differences between African Americans and European Americans with T2DM have been found in diabetes knowledge, self-management skills, empowerment, and self-efficacy or perceived control. An important area that has not been studied adequately is the contribution of social determinants of health to diabetes outcomes and how these factors explain the observed ethnic differences in key outcome variables for T2DM.

Cancer

Nearly 14 million Americans currently have a history of cancer, and another approximately 1.7 million new cases of cancer are expected to be diagnosed each year in the United States. As the second leading cause of death in the United States, about 600,000 Americans are expected to die of cancer, averaging approximately 1600 people daily. **Figure 6-15** shows the estimated cancer deaths for men and women in the United States in 2014. Additionally, the NIH estimates overall cancer costs more than $215 billion, with nearly $90 billion allocated to direct medical costs and approximately $130 billion for indirect costs.

Overall, NHB men have a 14% higher incidence of cancer compared with NHW men, and NHB women have an overall lower incidence of cancer compared with NHW women. Cancer disparities arise not only from the traditional sources of inequities, such as access, demographic characteristics, SES, and geography, among others (cultural, environmental, and so on), but also from barriers preventing high-quality care for cancer, including prevention, early detection, and treatment. People belonging to lower socioeconomic groups disproportionately have higher rates of cancer deaths than those of higher SES, and efforts to reduce the cancer death rates in persons with lower SES have been slow to occur. Evidence supports the notion that people of lower SES are more likely to engage in behaviors such as smoking, not being physically active, and eating a poor diet that increase their cancer risk (see Chapter 5). People of lower SES are also more likely to be uninsured or lack adequate health insurance coverage, which increases the likelihood of receiving a diagnosis when the cancer has already advanced, reducing viable treatment options. Ultimately, this leads to a lower 5-year survival from the cancer diagnosis.

According to the American Cancer Society (ACS), racial/ethnic cancer disparities are due largely to poverty and the barrier it poses to receiving high-quality health care services needed to successfully overcome a diagnosis of cancer. Racial and ethnic minorities, particularly NHBs and Hispanics, are more likely to live below the poverty line compared with NHWs, and as a result, they often receive lower quality care (including delayed diagnosis and less aggressive treatment),

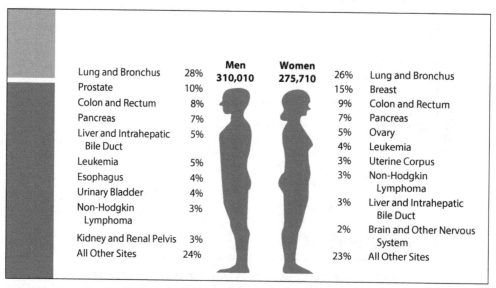

Figure 6-15. Estimated cancer deaths in the United States in 2014. (Data from Siegel R, Ma J, Zou Z, et al. Cancer statistics, 2014, *CA Cancer J Clin.* 2014 Jan-Feb;64(1):9-29.)

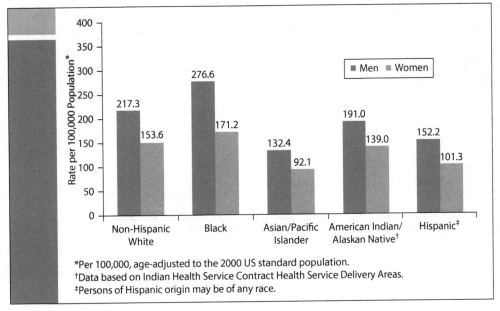

Figure 6-16. Cancer death rates by race and ethnicity. (Data from Siegel R, Ma J, Zou Z, et al. Cancer statistics, 2014, *CA Cancer J Clin.* 2014 Jan-Feb;64(1):9-29.)

resulting in higher rates of death secondary to cancer. **Figure 6-16** shows cancer death rates by race and ethnicity. Additionally, it is noteworthy to mention the Hispanic paradox that has existed historically in the United States for nearly 20 years. Despite having lower income and educational levels, Hispanics in the United States often have better health and longer life expectancies by several years compared with NHWs. Research has shown that people who have lower income and educational levels have a higher prevalence of cancer and other chronic diseases and an increased risk of death. In fact, the mortality rate for Hispanics in the United States resembles that of NHWs despite living at poverty levels and having educational levels similar to those of NHBs. The reasons for this paradox are unknown; however, the causes are thought to be multifactorial and social in origin with variations in age, gender, Hispanic subgroup, acculturation, country of birth, and cause of death postulated as associated with this consequence. In addition, cultural factors, including better health habits and stronger social support networks, within the Hispanic community are thought to confer protection against adverse outcomes such as incident disease and higher mortality rates.

In a study of more than 60,000 people to assess the impact of health care utilization and cancer susceptibility on the incidence and mortality rate of colorectal cancer, Laiyemo and colleagues found NHBs to undergo diagnostic evaluation less often and to have less follow-up for detectable abnormalities compared with NHWs. Furthermore, minority groups are more likely to develop cancer at disproportionately higher rates compared with NHWs. NHBs are more likely to develop and die from cancer than any other racial or ethnic group. NHBs have the highest incidence and mortality from colorectal cancer compared with other racial/ethnic groups. Since 1960, the mortality rate from colorectal cancer in NHB has increased by almost one third, as rates have declined by about 40% in NHWs during that same time period. As racial/ethnic cancer disparities are prominent, gender disparities are also prevalent. For example, NHB men and women have higher incidence and mortality rates from colorectal cancer compared with NHWs of the same gender. Almost a quarter million women are diagnosed with breast cancer annually, with an estimated 40,000 dying from this disease. Disparities in breast cancer exist between women, with NHW women developing it at faster rates but NHB women dying from it at faster rates. See **Table 6-1** for differences in cancer survival rates by race/ethnicity. Organizations such as the ACS must continue to advocate for and seek equitable care for populations disproportionately affected by cancer.

Table 6-1. Five-year relative cancer survival rates by race.*

Site	White	Black	Absolute Difference
All Sites	67	59	8
Breast (female)	90	79	11
Colon	65	56	9
Esophagus	18	11	7
Leukemia	56	50	6
Non-Hodgkin lymphoma	70	62	8
Oral cavity and pharynx	64	43	21
Prostate	100†	97	3
Rectum	67	61	6
Urinary bladder	78	65	13
Uterine cervix	69	59	10
Uterine corpus	84	61	23

*5-year relative survival rates based on patients diagnosed in the SEER 18 areas from 2003 to 2009, all followed through 2010.
†99.5%
Data from Howlader N, Noone AM, Krapcho M, et al. (eds). SEER Cancer Statistics Review, 1975-2011, National Cancer Institute, Bethesda, MD.

Renal Disease

According to the National Kidney Foundation Kidney Disease Outcomes Quality Initiative (KDOQI) guidelines, chronic kidney disease (CKD) is defined as the presence of markers of kidney damage, including albuminemia or a sustained reduction in estimated glomerular filtration rate (GFR), which progressively reduces over five stages. In 2005 to 2010, the prevalence of CKD was 6.3% compared with 9.3% and 8.5% for diabetes and CVD, respectively, when defined by GFR. When defined by an albumin-to-creatinine ratio, the prevalence of CKD rises to 9.2% in the general population. See prevalence estimates in **Figure 6-17**. CKD accounts for 5.7% of deaths that occur within 30 days of hospitalization for adults 66 years of age and older.

End-stage renal disease (ESRD) follows the progression of CKD and is the ultimate result of irreversible and complete damage to the kidneys, requiring hemodialysis or transplant. Being relatively stable since 2000,

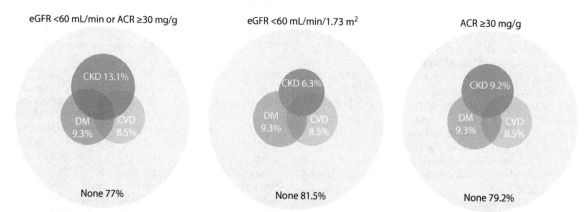

Figure 6-17. Distribution of National Health and Nutrition Examination Survey (NHANES), 2005 to 2010. ACR, albumin/creatinine ratio; CKD, chronic kidney disease; CVD, cardiovascular disease; DM, diabetes mellitus; eGFR, estimated glomerular filtration rate. (Reproduced with permission from U.S. Renal Data System. *USRDS 2013 Annual DataReport: Atlas of Chronic Kidney Disease and End-Stage Renal Disease in the United States.* Bethesda, MD: National Institutes of Health, National Institute of Diabetes and Digestive and Kidney Diseases; 2013.)

the rate of new ESRD cases per million of the general population has fallen recently, but is still prevalent in the United States, accounting for nearly $15 billion annually in Medicare and non-Medicare costs.

End-stage renal disease is mostly caused by diabetes and hypertension, disorders more prevalent in racial/ethnic minority populations and persons with lower SES. As a result, NHBs have a greater risk of CKD and over the past decade have experienced a four to six times increase in ESRD compared with NHWs. Additionally, Nicholas and colleagues found a more than 17-fold greater rate of hypertension as a cause of ESRD among NHBs. It is noteworthy to recognize also that after they have been diagnosed with CKD, NHBs and Hispanics are four times more likely to develop ESRD and more likely to undergo a lower limb amputations. Surprisingly and despite the alarming prevalence and incidence of CKD and ESRD in racial/ethnic minorities, however, NHBs and Hispanics have a greater adjusted survival rate than NHWs. Evidence shows that this paradox tends to emerge after minority populations, and particularly older members of the group (i.e., those at least 50 years of age), are on dialysis. Compared with NHWs, for example, fewer NHBs receive care from nephrologists and fewer receive referrals for peritoneal dialysis and transplantation. Despite this disparity, however, NHBs with ESRD are reported to have 13% to 45% lower mortality rates when receiving dialysis compared with NHWs. Although the cause of this disparity remains unclear, a unique relationship among multiple factors—biologic, genetic, environmental, sociocultural, and health care system levels—is considered a contributing factor. Specifically, reasons such as differential sensitivity to dialysis dosages and racial differences in nutritional status and levels of inflammation may influence this observed difference between NHBs and NHWs. Additional evidence is needed to reduce this racial/ethnic divide and improve patient outcomes in patients with CKD and ESRD.

The social determinants associated with CKD are numerous. Disparities in CKD are influenced by multiple factors, including access to care, poverty, SES, gender, dietary factors, obesity, food insecurity, and race/ethnicity. For example, Nicholas and colleagues report that women and minorities with CKD who are not on dialysis have lower rates of cardiovascular procedures than NHWs. Because women generally live longer than men, Grams and colleagues report a greater lifetime burden of CKD for women than men. Patzer and colleagues report a possible link between diet quality and SES measures, such as income and education. In a study to assess the effect of food insecurity on CKD in lower SES and poverty-stricken Americans, Crews et al. reports that food insecurity

may contribute to disparities in CKD, particularly in persons diagnosed with obesity, diabetes, and hypertension. Because it is common for many racial/ethnic minorities to live below the poverty line compared with majority NHWs, it is not surprising that racial/ethnic minorities carry a higher burden of disease and develop CKD and ESRD at higher rates.

THE CAUSES OF HEALTH DISPARITIES

Determinants of health disparities are shaped by the interaction of multiple factors such as social, environmental, biologic, and behavioral characteristics. An epidemiologic review of studies regarding deaths attributable to social factors estimated that of the nearly 3 million deaths in the United States in 2000, 9% were attributable to low education, 6% each to racial segregation and low social support, 5% to individual-level poverty, and 4% to income inequality. Collectively, these attributable factors point to several areas for intervention (e.g., access to care, quality of care, health decision making, and the legacy of distrust) where policy-, system-, and provider-level effects can impact health outcomes substantially in disadvantaged populations.

Access to Care

Access to medical care has become a consistent topic of discussion in the examination of health disparities and social determinants of health. In the United States, access to care remains suboptimal as a quarter of Americans report barriers when seeking health care. **Figure 6-18** shows the number and proportion of all access measures for which members of selected groups experienced worse, same, or better access compared with the reference group. It shows that minority groups and those classified as "poor" had worse access to care compared with the majority white population. For example, NHBs had worse access to care for 33% of the measures, and Hispanics had 70% worse access to care compared with NHWs. Asian Americans had worse access to care by 20% compared with NHWs. Additionally, those of lower SES had greater than 80% worse access to care compared with those of higher SES. Alarmingly, disparities observed in access to care are worsening, which continues to perpetuate the disparities seen in health care. **Figure 6-19** shows disparities in access to care by race and ethnicity, as well as income.

In 1993, the IOM defined access to health care as "having the timely use of personal health services to achieve the best health outcomes." The findings of many clinical studies provide evidence that racial and ethnic minorities experience significant disparities in

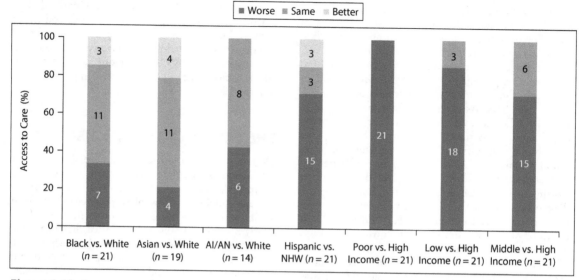

Figure 6-18. Access to care by race/ethnicity and income. AI, American Indian; AN, Alaska Native. (Reproduced with permission from Agency for Healthcare Research and Quality. *National Healthcare Quality & Disparities Reports.* Rockville, MD; 2014. http://www.ahrq.gov/research/findings/nhqrdr/index.html. Retrieved November 19, 2014.)

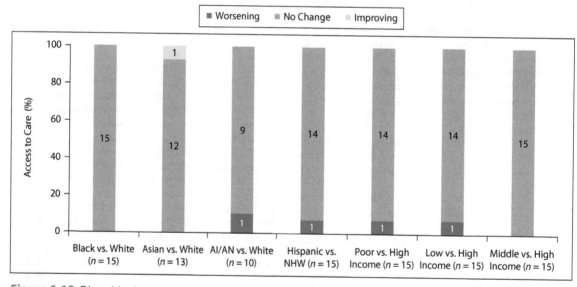

Figure 6-19. Disparities in access to care by race/ethnicity and income. AI, American Indian; AN, Alaska native; NHW, non-Hispanic white. (Reproduced with permission from Agency for Healthcare Research and Quality. *National Healthcare Quality & Disparities Reports.* Rockville, MD; 2014. http://www.ahrq.gov/research/findings/nhqrdr/index.html. Retrieved November 19, 2014.)

access to care compared with NHWs. Factors such as lower SES and lower rates of health insurance coverage among minority groups are believed to contribute to the divide seen in care. NHBs and Hispanics are more likely to enroll in managed care health plans and are less likely to have care coordinators, often referred to as "gatekeepers," and receive referrals for specialty care, when available, compared with NHWs, thus perpetuating the disproportionate access to care experienced by racial and ethnic populations.

In a study to assess racial and ethnic differences in access to medical care in managed care plans, Hargraves and colleagues examined five commonly used measures of access and utilization: having a usual source of care, having a regular provider, making visits to the physician, using emergency services, and accessing specialty care. Compared with NHWs, Hispanics had less access to care and more utilization, lacking a regular provider and frequenting the emergency department more often. Similarly, NHBs were less likely to have regular providers and more likely to seek primary care using emergency services compared with NHWs. Compared with both NHBs and NHWs, however, Hispanics did poorly in all measures of access to care, including being less likely to have terminal visits with specialists. Surprisingly, NHBs received comparable care compared with NHWs in terms of seeing a provider within the previous year and having access to specialty care.

In their study to assess racial and socioeconomic disparities in access to primary care among people with chronic conditions, Shi and colleagues found that racial disparities are associated with not having a usual source of care, provider type, or location. Minority groups were less likely to have a usual source of care and were more likely to use hospitals and facilities for care (instead of a regular physician or other health care provider). One of the goals for Healthy People 2020 is to provide comprehensive and quality health care services to all Americans. To achieve this goal, efforts must be focused on improving the health care of racial and ethnic minorities. By doing so, we may be able to achieve a second goal of Healthy People 2020, which is to reduce health disparities.

Quality of Care

Access to the health care system does not automatically assure high quality of care (see Chapter 15). Evidence exists that minorities experience a higher burden of disease and receive a lower quality of care than nonminorities. Additionally, members of minority groups have higher rates of disability and mortality than the majority population, but they are not receiving equitable and quality care.

In *Unequal Treatment: Confronting Racial and Ethnic Disparities in Healthcare*, a 2002 report by the IOM, it was documented that racial and ethnic minorities receive lower quality of health care than nonminority populations even when adjusting for factors related to access. Those belonging to minority groups often experience multiple obstacles and barriers to care despite having equivalent resources compared with NHWs. It is postulated that factors such as access, clinical appropriateness, and patient preferences are not solely responsible for the inequalities seen in health care quality. Behavioral, social, economic, cultural, biologic,

and environmental factors are all believed to contribute to disparities in quality of care.

The IOM report also suggests that disparities in health care quality are multifactorial, citing historical and contemporary inequities; financial and institutional arrangements of health care systems; and legal, regulatory, and policy environments as additional factors associated with poorer quality of care in minority populations. Furthermore, evidence suggests that provider biases (whether conscious or unconscious), behaviors, and practice patterns also contribute to disparities in quality of care. Provider preferences and practices in referral and treatment continue to perpetuate the divide in quality of care between minorities and nonminorities.

According to the National Health Disparities Report, access to care continues to worsen, while quality of care has begun to improve marginally. In 2009, about one third of all Americans reported not receiving quality care. More efforts need to be devoted to racial/ethnic minorities to improve their access to comprehensive, quality health services.

Health Decision Making

According to the medical literature, three styles of health decision making are used in clinical care. Information transferred between those making health decisions can be one way, either solely from the provider or the patient to the other, or two way, in which decision making is shared between the patient and provider. Whereas one-way information transfer from a provider to a patient is known as a paternalistic style, information from the patient to the provider is termed consumerist. When the exchange of information and deliberation of information occurs between the patient and provider, and the provider offers medical information needed for the patient to make a personal and educated decision, the transfer is known as shared decision making. In this type of health decision making, the patient is responsible for sharing information that the provider needs when suggesting an appropriate course of care. Accounting for the values and beliefs of all parties involved, shared decision making has been shown to have the most benefit in improving health outcomes; it is unclear, however, how often this type of decision making occurs and if it is even preferred by those involved in the decision-making process.

There is a paucity of research on the relationship between SES and clinical health decision making, both of which have an association with health disparities. In their study to assess whether patients received their preferred style of decision making and its association with SES and perceived quality of care, Murray and colleagues found that people of higher SES and those with a regular physician preferred shared decision making compared with those of lower SES, who preferred one of the one-way types of communication. African Americans were reported as preferring the paternalistic style of information exchange. This may result from minority patients feeling less empowered with enough information to make clinical decisions. Additionally, Dovidio and colleagues suggest that the quality of communication is lower between providers and patients with racial discordance.

Dovidio and colleagues report that providers often possess personal beliefs, perceptions, values, and biases that influence their actions in the decision-making process and ultimately contribute to the development and persistence of differences in care among groups. These biases can be explicit—personal beliefs and values known to the individual, or implicit—unintentional, or unconscious perceptions and beliefs. Providers often possess explicit and implicit biases that inherently influence their decisions when caring for patients. These biases become of particular focus and interest when providers care for those of different races and ethnicities. For example, in a landmark case assessing physician recommendations for cardiac catheterization in black versus white patients, NHBs were less likely to be referred for the procedure compared with NHWs. More recently, Dovidio and colleagues reported that minority patients are less likely to be referred by providers for various types of surgeries (i.e., oral surgery and coronary bypass surgery), procedures, and treatments (i.e., pain medications) compared with NHW patients. Furthermore, when minorities are referred to have surgery, the recommendations for surgery are frequently unnecessary and not beneficial to the patients. The researchers hypothesize that black patients are often treated differently because some physicians consider NHBs, for example, less educated and less active than NHWs.

Legacy of Distrust

The legacy of distrust that exists between minority populations and the medical community is an undeniable consequence of historical experimentation on certain groups. One of the most notorious examples was the Tuskegee Syphilis Study of 1932 that was conducted by the U.S. Public Health Service. During that 40-year study, treatment was withheld from African American men diagnosed with syphilis with the intent of gaining a better understanding of the natural history of the disease. The moral problem was that effective treatments, although not available at the outset of the study, were developed while the long-term study was ongoing. Nevertheless, curative antibiotics were never given to the subjects. Moreover, the study subjects were never even informed of the existence of effective treatments for their illnesses or of the potential harm of continuing to be untreated. The subjects were highly vulnerable because they were poorly educated, had limited access to other health care, and were living in communities and at a time when expressing concern about unfair treatment might not have been welcomed or acted upon. As a result of this type of discrimination, minorities developed a distinctive sense of medical mistrust, a legacy that continues to persist.

Evidence suggests that trust is associated with several health-related objectives, including access, routine medical care and utilization of health care services, self-management behaviors, care continuity, health care costs, and quality of care. Higher levels of trust are associated with satisfaction of care, loyalty to providers, and better self-rated health status. Additionally, patients with more distrust often experience disparities in seeking medical care and adhering to medical recommendations. To maximize trust in the patient–provider relationship, provider characteristics, patient characteristics, and factors associated with the relationship must be taken into account.

African Americans represent the minority group with the highest level of distrust in the health care system, including distrust in providers, researchers, institutions, and insurers. Variances in trust of health care providers have been associated with health disparities in race, access to care, and satisfaction with care among African Americans compared with all other racial and ethnic groups. Similarly, Hispanics report high degrees of provider and medical system discrimination when seeking medical care. Discrimination toward Hispanics and medical mistrust are often compounded when cultural issues such as language proficiency and health literacy are taken into consideration. In a study to assess the effects of race/ethnicity and SES on health information seeking, confidence, and trust, Richardson and colleagues found that NHBs, Hispanics, and those of lower SES had a lower level or trust in health care providers compared with NHWs and those of higher SES.

POTENTIAL SOLUTIONS TO HEALTH DISPARITIES

Despite the many health disparities that presently exist in the United States, potential solutions to reducing and even eliminating these disparities are on the horizon. Strategies suggested by the IOM include improved patient–provider communication, using evidence-based algorithms, diversity training for health care professionals, and greater inclusion of diverse populations in the health care workforce. Each of these potential solutions is described in greater detail below.

Reducing Health Disparities by Improving Patient–Provider Communication

In a seminal study on the impact of patient–provider communication on health disparities, Ashton et al. reviewed the literature and found that even when access to care, diagnosis, and disease severity are controlled, NHWs and Latinos use fewer services requiring a physician's order, such as hospitalization or invasive procedures, than NHWs. As these investigators argue, factors that impact patient–provider communication include a lack of shared language, using different terms to explain medical phenomena, and having different communication styles. All of these factors appear to contribute to poorer health outcomes among members of racially and ethnically diverse populations. Similarly, Levine and Ambady reviewed current literature on patient–provider communication and found that physicians tend to exhibit more disengaged nonverbal behavior with patients from different racial and ethnic groups and have a lower ability to interpret the nonverbal behaviors of these patients.

Although communication behaviors are difficult to change, it is possible for patients and physicians to be taught to communicate more effectively with each other. For example, patients could be taught to provide a health narrative, ask more questions, and express concerns during the medical visit, and physicians could be taught to engage patients by asking about what they perceive as the causes of their symptoms or the impact of the symptoms on the patient's daily life.

Reducing Health Disparities by Using Evidence-Based Algorithms

Using evidence-based algorithms could play a significant role in reducing health disparities. If algorithms that have been found to be effective in the general population were applied to members of diverse populations, then it is expected that the burden of health disparities that is borne among racial and ethnic minorities in the United States would be reduced subsequently. This assumption has been supported many times in the scientific literature across multiple disease types. For example, Graham-Steed et al. showed that in an observational cohort analysis of 1270 men diagnosed with prostate cancer and followed for 11 to 16 years at nine Veterans Health Administration (VHA) medical centers, an equal-access health care system of U.S. veterans, mortality rates among NHB and NHW men with prostate cancer were comparable.

Similarly, Lee et al. examined data from 1008 VHA patients with pancreatic adenocarcinoma, 15% of whom were NHBs. No disparities were observed in disease management or survival between the NHB

and NHW patients in the sample. Among patients with locoregional cancers, the odds of NHB patients receiving surgical resection, chemotherapy, and radiotherapy were not different from those of NHWs. The odds of receiving palliative chemotherapy were similar for NHBs with distant disease as for NHWs with distant disease. In addition, the median overall survival time did not differ between the two groups.

Likewise, Zullig et al. evaluated receipt of guideline-concordant colorectal cancer care among 2222 patients (14% of whom were NHBs) with incident colorectal cancer. No statistically significant differences were found for receipt of computed tomography scans, preoperative carcinoembryonic antigen testing, clear surgical margins, medical oncology referral for stages I and II, fluorouracil-based adjuvant chemotherapy for stage II, and surveillance colonoscopy for stages I to III.

In a study focusing on patients in the U.S. Military Health System, another equal-access health care system, Zheng et al. examined data from 10,181 patients (11% of whom were African American) with lung cancer. These investigators found that racial differences in survival were not statistically significant for adenocarcinoma, squamous cell carcinomas, or large cell carcinomas. More favorable crude survival was seen in NHB patients with small cell lung cancer than in NHWs with this disease but could not be attributed to other clinical factors. These results suggest that improving access of diverse patients to evidence-based treatment will significantly help to reduce disparities in disease outcomes.

Reducing Health Disparities through Diversity Training for Health Care Professionals

Diversity training could help to change the way health care providers interact with diverse patients. Truong et al. conducted a systematic review of cultural competency in skills development and its impact on quality of care. Typically, enhanced cultural competency results in moderate improvement in provider outcomes and health care access and use. Weaker evidence was seen for improvements in patient outcomes.

It has been suggested that medical training incorporating stories about patients that counter negative racial or ethnic stereotypes could result in more positive perceptions of members of these patient groups by medical professionals. In addition, physicians in training could be taught to recognize their own biases and then view intercultural interactions as opportunities to learn. In other words, bias can be unlearned.

A framework for redesigning medical education to meet the needs of an increasingly diverse population is presented by Alexandraki and Mooradian.

These authors advocate for patient-centered communication, which has been shown to improve health outcomes, increase patient satisfaction, and enhance patients' adherence to medical treatment regimens. Other suggestions for diversity training include interactive methods focusing on improving communication skills such as discussion groups and workshops, simulation, use of standardized patients to enhance patient–physician communication, and incorporating communication courses into medical school curricula.

Other innovative approaches for enhancing cultural sensitivity among health care providers include the use of online educational modalities; the use of community-based, longitudinal, ambulatory care training sites; and the use of interprofessional educational experiences targeted at communication, team building, and collective impact.

Reducing Health Disparities by Fostering Greater Inclusion of Diverse Populations in the Health Care Workforce

Although the percentage of medical school students and faculty who self-reported as underrepresented minorities has increased, the fact remains that the sociodemographic characteristics of the U.S. health care workforce are not reflective of the racial and ethnic diversity in the U.S. population. As noted in the Sullivan Commission's report titled "Missing Persons: Minorities in the Health Professions," diversity in the U.S. health care professions has lagged behind changing U.S. demographics, which may contribute significantly to disparities in health care access and outcomes.

In two recent observational studies with 64 primary care physicians and 489 of their patients, Thornton et al. made an interesting discovery about the impact of concordance between the physician and patient's backgrounds in terms of race, ethnicity, and SES. These investigators discovered that when social concordance between physicians and patients was low compared with when social concordance was high, patients reported less positive perceptions of care in terms of lower ratings of satisfaction with the office visit and were also less likely to refer their physician to a friend. It is possible that social concordance is a proxy for better patient–physician communication.

Enhancing diversity among medical students is a step in this direction. Greater diversity among health care providers is linked to improved access to care among racially and ethnically diverse patients and to high-quality, culturally competent health care initiatives.

In summary, developing and implementing effective strategies related to patient–provider communication, evidence-based treatment algorithms, diversity training for health care professionals, and greater inclusion of diverse populations in the health care workforce can play major roles in reducing health disparities.

SUMMARY

This chapter presents a broad overview of health disparities in the United States. The chapter begins by defining disparities in health care as racial or ethnic differences that are not a result of access-related factors, clinical needs, preferences, or appropriateness of treatment intervention. In this context, race is best characterized not as a genetic property but rather as a social construct that influences human behavior, including, at times, prejudicial treatment. Ethnicity is often confused with race but represents a separate categorization of populations based on sharing a common culture, language, religion, and traditions. Disparities in health status and health care delivery according to race and ethnicity often reflect, in part, underlying socioeconomic differences among these groups but typically are not fully explained by these factors alone.

Within the United States, there are many examples of health disparities. Risk factors for chronic diseases, such as hypertension, obesity, and physical inactivity, tend to be higher among minority populations. Diseases such as heart and vascular conditions, T2DM, renal disease, and many forms of cancer also occur with greater prevalence and mortality among minority groups.

Health disparities arise from a variety of reasons, including but not limited to differential access and quality of health care available to various population groups. Variations in behavioral, social, economic, cultural, biologic, and environmental factors also contribute to disparities in health status and quality of care. Personal beliefs, perception, biases, and values also can impact, consciously or unconsciously, how providers make treatment decisions and interact with patients.

Historical overt acts of discrimination in medical research and patient care, such as the infamous Tuskegee Syphilis Study, have produced distrust within many minority communities. Nevertheless, progress can be made in addressing health disparities by addressing provider–patient communications, increasing the diversity of the health care workforce, and incorporating cultural competency skills development in the training of health professionals.

STUDY QUESTIONS

1. Which of the following are included in the Institute of Medicine's definition of health care disparities?
   A. Clinical appropriateness
   B. Patient preferences
   C. The operation of health care systems
   D. The operation of legal and regulatory climates
   E. Discrimination: biases, stereotyping, and uncertainties
   F. B, D, and E
   G. C, D, and E
   H. B, C, D, and E
   I. All of the above

2. By the year 2050, racial and ethnic minorities will comprise which percentage of the total U.S. population?
   A. 20.0%
   B. 47.5%
   C. 67.5%
   D. 87.5%

3. All individuals are 99.0% to 99.5% identical at the DNA level.
   A. True
   B. False

4. Which of the following is an example of an ethnic group?
   A. Native Americans/American Indians
   B. African Americans
   C. Hispanics/Latinos
   D. European Americans
   E. Hmong
   F. Ukrainians
   G. A, C, D, and E
   H. C, E, and F
   I. All of the above

5. Which Directive of the Office of Management and Budget includes criteria to classify people into categories of race and ethnicity?
   A. Directive Number 15
   B. Directive Number 16
   C. Directive Number 17
   D. Directive Number 18

6. Federal policies to reduce and eliminate differences in the burden of disease and medical care among population subgroups include
   A. the Minority Health and Health Disparities Research and Education Act of 2000 Public Law 106-525.
   B. specific provisions from the Affordable Care Act.
   C. the 2010 upgrade of the NIH National Center on Minority Health and Health Disparities to full institute status as the National Institute on Minority Health and Health Disparities.
   D. A, C, and D.
   E. B and C.
   F. All of the above.

7. The causes of health disparities include racial/ethnic differences in
   A. access to care.
   B. quality of care.
   C. health decision making.
   D. legacy of distrust.
   E. A, B, and C.
   F. B, C, and D.
   G. all of the above.

8. In the United States, which percentage of Americans report barriers when seeking health care?
   A. 26.0%
   B. 36.0%
   C. 46.0%
   D. 56.0%

9. African Americans represent the minority group with the highest level of distrust in the health care system.
   A. True
   B. False

10. Potential solutions to health disparities include
    A. improving patient-provider communication.
    B. reducing use of evidence-based algorithms.
    C. diversity training for health care professionals.
    D. fostering greater inclusion of diverse populations in the health care workforce.
    E. A, B, and D.
    F. A, C, and D.
    G. all of the above.

FURTHER READING

Benz JK, Espinosa O, Welsh V, Fontes A. Awareness of racial and ethnic health disparities has improved only modestly over a decade. *Health Aff (Millwood)*. 2011;30(10):1860-1867.

Franks P, Fiscella K. Reducing disparities downstream: prospects and challenges. *J Gen Intern Med*. 2008;23(5):672-677.

Saha S, Freeman M, Toure J, Tippens KM, Weeks C, Ibrahim S. Racial and ethnic disparities in the VA health care system: a systematic review. *J Gen Intern Med*. 2008;23(5):654-761.

Washington DL, Bowles J, Saha S, Et al. Transforming clinical practice to eliminate racial-ethnic disparities in healthcare. *J Gen Intern Med*. 2007;23(5):685-691.

REFERENCES

Clinical Background

Egede LE. Race, ethnicity, culture, and disparities in health care. *J Gen Intern Med*. 2006;21(6):667-669.

Egede LE, Bosworth H. The future of health disparities research: 2008 and beyond. *J Gen Intern Med*. 2008;23(5):706-708.

Lynch CP, Strom Williams JL, Reid J, Joseph R, Keith B, Egede LE. Racial/ethnic differences in multiple diabetes outcomes in patients with type 2 diabetes in the southeastern United States. *Ethn Dis*. 2014;24(2):189-194.

Rosenstock S, Whitman S, West JF, Balkin M. Racial disparities in diabetes mortality in the 50 most populous U.S. cities. *J Urban Health*. 2014;91(5):873-885.

Strom JL, Egede LE. The impact of social support on outcomes in adult patients with type 2 diabetes: a systematic review. *Curr Diab Rep*. 2012;12:769-781.

Introduction

American Cancer Society. *Cancer Facts & Figures 2014*. Atlanta; 2014.

Ashing K, Rosales M, Lai L, Hurria A. Occurrence of comorbidities among African-American and Latina breast cancer survivors. *J Cancer Surviv*. 2014;8(2):312-318.

Barbour SJ, Schachter M, Er L, Djurdjev O, Levin A. A systematic review of ethnic differences in the rate of renal progression in CKD patients. *Nephrol Dial Transplant*. 2010;25:2422-2430.

Canetti L, Bachar E, Berry EM. Food and emotion. *Behav Processes*. 2002;60(2):157-164.

Carrillo JE, Carrillo VA, Perez HR, Salas-Lopez D, Natale-Pereira A, Byraon AT. Defining and targeting health care access barriers. *J Health Care Poor Underserved*. 2011;22:562-575.

Cheung MR. Assessing the impact of socio-economic variables on breast cancer treatment outcome disparities. *Asian Pac J Cancer Prev*. 2013;14:7133-7136.

Evans K, Coresh J, Bash LD, et al. Race differences in access to health care and disparities in incident chronic kidney disease in the US. *Nephrol Dial Transplant*. 2011;26:899-908.

Gomes C, McGuire TG. *Identifying the Sources of Racial AND Ethnic Disparities in Health Care Use*. Unpublished manuscript. Unequal Treatment, IOM Report.

Grams ME, Chow EKH, Segev DL, Coresh J. Lifetime incidence of CKD Stages 3-5 in the United States. *Am J Kidney Dis*. 2013;62(2):245-252.

Hicken MT, Lee H, Morenoff J, House JS, Williams DR. Racial/ethnic disparities in hypertension prevalence: reconsidering the role of chronic stress. *Am J Public Health*. 2014;104:117-123.

Hu R, Shi L, Rane S, Zhu J, Chen CC. Insurance, racial/ethnic, SES-related disparities in quality of care among US adults with diabetes. *J Immigr Minor Health*. 2014;16(4):565-575.

Hunt KJ, Gebregziabher M, Lynch CP, Echols C, Mauldin PD, Egede LE. Impact of diabetes control on mortality by race in a national cohort of veterans. *Ann Epidemiol*. 2013;23:74-79.

Krieger N. Defining and investigating social disparities in cancer: critical issues. *Cancer Causes Control*. 2005;16:5-14.

LaVeist T, Pollack K, Thorpe R Jr, Fesahazion R, Gaskin D. Place, not race: disparities dissipate in southwest Baltimore when blacks and whites live under similar conditions. *Health Aff (Millwood)*. 2011;30:1880-1887.

Singh GK, Azuine RE, Slahpush M. Widening socioeconomic, racial, and geographic disparities in HIV/AIDS mortality in the United States, 1987-2011. *Adv Prev Med*. 2013;2013:657961.

Smedley BD, Stith AY, Nelson AR, eds. *Unequal Treatment: Confronting Racial and Ethnic Disparities in Healthcare*. Washington, DC: Institute of Medicine; 2003.

Williams DR. Miles to go before we sleep: racial inequities in health. *J Health Soc Behav*. 2012;53:279-295.

Williams DR, Mohammed SA. Racism and health II: a needed research agenda for effective interventions. *Am Behav Sci*. 2013;57(8):1200-1226.

Wosu AC, Valdimarsdottir U, Shields AE, Williams DR, Williams MA. Correlates of cortisol in human hair: implications for epidemiological studies on health effects of chronic stress. *Ann Epidemiol*. 2013;23:797-811.

Measurement of Issues in Health Disparities Research

Beutler LE, Brown MT, Crothers L, Booker K, Seabrook MK. The dilemma of fictitious demographic distinctions in psychological research. *J Consult Clin Psychol*. 1996; 64:892-902.

Collins FS. *Cancer, Genomics, and Health Disparities: What's the Connection?* National Human Genome Research Institute, Bethesda, Maryland American Association for Cancer Research Meeting; 2007.

Egede LE, Michel Y. Medical mistrust, diabetes self-management, and glycemic control in an indigent population with type 2 diabetes. *Diabetes Care*. 2006;29:131-132.

Ford ME, Kelly PA. Conceptualizing and categorizing race and ethnicity in health services research. *Health Serv Res*. 2005;40:1658-1675.

Ford ME, Hill DD, Nerenz D, et al. Categorizing race and ethnicity in the HMO Cancer Research Network. *Ethn Dis*. 2002;12:135-140.

Freeman HP. The meaning of race in science—considerations for cancer research: concerns of special populations in the National Cancer Program. *Cancer*. 1998;82:219-225.

Fullilove MT. Deconstructing race in medical research. *Arch Pediatr Adolesc Med*. 148:1014-1015.

Humes KR, Jones NA, Ramirez RR. *2010 Census Redistricting Data (Public Law 94-171) Summary File*. U.S. Department of Commerce Economics and Statistics Administration. U.S. Census Bureau. http://factfinder2.census.gov/main.html. Retrieved November 19, 2014.

LaVeist TA. Beyond dummy variables and sample selection: what health services researchers ought to know about race as a variable. *Health Serv Res*. 1994;29:1-16.

Sawyer TC. Measuring race and ethnicity: meeting public policy goals. *American Statistician.* 1998;2:34-35.

Senior PA, Bhopal R. Ethnicity as a variable in epidemiological research. *BMJ.* 1994;309:327-330.

Baker TA, Whitfield KE. *Handbook of Minority Aging.* New York: Springer. 2013.

Williams DR. Race, socioeconomic status, and health. The added effects of racism and discrimination. *Ann N Y Acad Sci.* 1999;896:173-188.

Health Disparities in the United States

Cardiovascular Disease

Agency for Healthcare Research and Quality. *National Healthcare Quality & Disparities Reports.* Rockville, MD; 2014. http://www.ahrq.gov/research/findings/nhqrdr/index.html. Retrieved November 19, 2014.

American Heart Association. Heart disease and stroke statistics—2013 update: a report from the American Heart Association. *Circulation.* 2013;125:e6-e245.

Culter DM, McClellan M. Is technological change in medicine worth it? *Health Aff (Millwood).* 2001;20(5):11-29.

Go AS, Mozaffarian D, Roger VL, et al; American Heart Association Statistics Committee and Stroke Statistics Subcommittee. Heart disease and stroke statistics—2013 update: a report from the American Heart Association. *Circulation.* 2013;127(1):e6-e245.

Kochanek KD, Xu JQ, Murphy SL, Miniño AM, Kung HC. Deaths: final data for 2009. *Natl Vital Stat Rep.* 2011;60(3):1-116.

Kurian AK, Cardarelli KM. Racial and ethnic differences in cardiovascular disease risk factors: a systematic review. *Ethn Dis.* 2007;17:143-152.

Mensah GA, Mokdad AH, Ford ES, Greenlund KJ, Croft JB. State of disparities in cardiovascular health in the United States. *Circulation.* 2005;111:1233-1241.

Curtin LR, Mohadjer LK, Dohrmann SM, et al. National Health and Nutrition Examination Survey: Sample design, 2007–2010. National Center for Health Statistics. *Vital Health Stat.* 2013;2(160).

Sharma S, Malarcher AM, Giles WH, Myers G. Racial, ethnic and socioeconomic disparities in the clustering of cardiovascular disease risk factors. *Ethn Dis.* 2004;14:43-48.

Diabetes

Agency for Healthcare Research and Quality. *National Healthcare Quality & Disparities Reports.* Rockville, MD; 2014. http://www.ahrq.gov/research/findings/nhqrdr/index.html. Retrieved November 19, 2014.

Anderson RJ, Freedland KE, Clouse RE, Lustman PJ. The prevalence of comorbid depression in adults with diabetes: a meta-analysis. *Diabetes Care.* 2001;24(6):1069-1078.

Axon RN, Gebregziabher M, Echols C, Msph GG, Egede LE. Racial and ethnic differences in longitudinal blood pressure control in veterans with type 2 diabetes mellitus. *Medicine Gen Intern Med.* 2011;26(11):1278-1283.

Boyle JP, Honeycutt AA, Narayan KMV, et al. Projection of diabetes burden through 2050: impact of changing demography and disease prevalence in the U.S. *Diabetes Care.* 2011; 24(11):1936-1940.

Egede LE, Gebregziabher M, Lynch CP, Gilbert GE, Echols C. Longitudinal ethnic differences in multiple cardiovascular risk factor control in a cohort of US adults with diabetes. *Diabetes Res Clin Pract.* 2011;94(3):385-394.

Egede LE, Gebregziabher M, Hunt KJ, et al. Regional, geographic, and racial/ethnic variation in glycemic control in a national sample of veterans with diabetes. *Diabetes Care.* 2011;34(4): 938-943.

Egede LE, Gebregziabher M, Hunt KJ, et al. Regional, geographic, and ethnic differences in medication adherence among adults with type 2 diabetes. *Ann Pharmacother.* 2011 Feb 8. [Epub ahead of print]

Egede LE, Mueller M, Echols CL, Gebregziabher M. Longitudinal differences in glycemic control by race/ethnicity among veterans with type 2 diabetes. *Med Care.* 2010;48(6):527-533.

Egede LE, Dagogo-Jack S. Epidemiology of type 2 diabetes: focus on ethnic minorities. *Med Clin North Am.* 2005;89:949-975.

Egede LE. Diabetes, major depression, and functional disability among US adults. *Diabetes Care.* 2004;27:421-428.

Egede LE, Bonadonna RJ. Diabetes self-management in African Americans: an exploration of the role of fatalism. *Diabetes Educ.* 2003;29:105-115.

Go AS, Mozaffarian D, Roger VL, et al; American Heart Association Statistics Committee and Stroke Statistics Subcommittee. Heart disease and stroke statistics—2013 update: a report from the American Heart Association. *Circulation.* 2013;127(1):e6-e245.

Harris MI. Racial and ethnic differences in health care access and health outcomes for adults with type 2 diabetes. *Diabetes Care.* 2001;24(3):454-459.

Harris MI, Cowie CC, Howie LJ. Self-monitoring of blood glucose by adults with diabetes in the United States population. *Diabetes Care.* 1993;16(8):1116-1123.

Hofer TP, Hayward RA, Greenfield S, Wagner EH, Kaplan SH, Manning WG. The unreliability of individual physician "report cards" for assessing the costs and quality of care for a chronic disease. *JAMA.* 1999;281(22):2098-2105.

Krein SL, Hofer TP, Kerr EA, Hayward RA. Whom should we profile? Examining diabetes care practice variation among primary care providers, provider groups, and health care facilities. *Health Serv Res.* 2002;37(5):1159-1180.

National Institute for Diabetes, Digestion, and Kidney Disease. *National Diabetes Statistics, 2011.* NIH Publication 11-3892, February 2011. http://diabetes.niddk.nih.gov/DM/PUBS/statistics. Retrieved November 19, 2014.

Nwasuruba C, Khan M, Egede LE. Racial/ethnic differences in multiple self-care behaviors in adults with diabetes. *J Gen Intern Med.* 2007;22(1):115-120.

Signorello LB, Schlundt DG, Cohen SS, et al. Comparing diabetes prevalence between African Americans and European Americans of similar socioeconomic status. *Am J Public Health.* 2007;97(12):2260-2267.

Syler JS, Oddo C. Diabetes trends in the USA. *Diabetes Metab Res Rev.* 2002;18(suppl):S21-S26.

Tuerk PW, Mueller M, Egede LE. Estimating physician effects on glycemic control in the treatment of diabetes: methods, effects sizes, and implications for treatment policy. *Diabetes Care.* 2008;31(5):869-873.

Walker RJ, Smalls BL, Campbell JA, Strom Williams JL, Egede LE. Impact of social determinants of health on outcomes for type 2 diabetes: a systematic review. *Endocrine.* 2014;47(1):29-48.

Cancer

American Cancer Society. *Cancer Facts & Figures 2014.* Atlanta; 2014.

American Cancer Society. *Cancer Statistics 2014.* Atlanta 2014.

Franzini L, Ribble JC, Keddie AM. Understanding the Hispanic paradox. *Ethn Dis.* 2001;11(3):496-518.

Hunt BR, Whitman S, Hurlbert MS. Increasing black: white disparities in breast cancer mortality in the 50 largest cities in the United States. *Cancer Epidemiol.* 2014;38(2):118-123.

Laiyemo AO, Doubeni C, Pinsky PF, et al. Race and colorectal cancer disparities: health care utilization vs. different cancer susceptibilities. *J Natl Cancer Inst.* 2010;102:538-546.

Tammana VS, Laiyemo AO. Colorectal cancer disparities: issues, controversies and solutions. *World Gastroenterol.* 2014;20(4):869-876.

Zonderman AB, Ejiogu N, Norbeck J, Evans MK. The influence of health disparities on targeting cancer prevention efforts. *Am J Prev Med.* 2014;46(3 suppl 1):S87-S97.

Renal Disease

Agrawal V, Jaar BG, Frisby XY, et al. Access to health care among adults evaluated for CKD: findings from the Kidney Early Evaluation Program (KEEP). *Am J Kidney Dis.* 2012;59(3 suppl 2): S5-S15.

Barbour SJ, Schachter M, Er L, Djurdjev O, Levin A. A systematic review of ethnic differences in the rate of renal progression in CKD patients. *Nephrol Dial Transplant.* 2010;25:2422-2430.

Crews DC, Charles RF, Evans MK, Zonderman AB, Powe NR. Poverty, race, and CKD in a racially and socioeconomically diverse urban population. *Am J Kidney Dis.* 2010;55(6):992-1000.

Crews DC, Kuczmarski MF, Grubbs V, et al. Effect of food insecurity on chronic kidney disease in lower-income Americans. *Am J Nephrol.* 2014;39:27-35.

Crews DC, Pfaff T, Powe NR. Socioeconomic factors and racial disparities in kidney disease outcomes. *Semin Nephrol.* 2013;33:468-475.

Egede LE. Diabetes, major depression, and functional disability among US adults. *Diabetes Care.* 2004;27:421-428.

Evans K, Coresh J, Bash LD, et al. Race differences in access to health care and disparities in incident chronic kidney disease in the US. *Nephrol Dial Transplant.* 2011;26:899-908.

Grams ME, Chow EKH, Segev DL, Coresh J. Lifetime incidence of CKD stages 3-5 in the United States. *Am J Kidney Dis.* 2013;62(2):245-252.

KDOQI clinical practice guidelines for chronic kidney disease: evaluation, classification, and stratification. *Am J Kidney Dis.* 2002;39(suppl):S1-S266.

Kucirka LM, Grams ME, Lessler J, et al. Association of race and age with survival among patients undergoing dialysis. *JAMA.* 2011;306(6):620-626.

Nicholas SB, Kalantar-Zadeh K, Norris KC. Racial disparities in kidney disease outcomes. *Semin Nephrol.* 2013;33:409-415.

Norris KC, Agodoa LY. Unraveling the racial disparities associated with kidney disease. *Kidney Int.* 2005;68:914-924.

Palmer Alves T, Lewis J. Racial differences in chronic kidney disease (CKD) and end-stage renal disease (ESRD) in the United States: a social and economic dilemma. *Clin Nephrol.* 2010;74(suppl 1):S72-S77.

Patzer RE, McClellan WM. Influence of race, ethnicity and socioeconomic status on kidney disease. *Nat Rev Nephrol.* 2012; 8:533-541.

Plantinga LC. Socio-economic impact in CKD. *Nephrol Ther.* 2013;9:1-7.

U.S. Renal Data System. USRDS 2013 Annual Data Report: Atlas of Chronic Kidney Disease and End-Stage Renal Disease in the United States. Bethesda, MD: National Institutes of Health, National Institute of Diabetes and Digestive and Kidney Diseases; 2013.

The Causes of Health Disparities

Access to Care

Agency for Healthcare Research and Quality. *National Healthcare Quality & Disparities Reports.* Rockville, MD; 2014. http://www.ahrq.gov/research/findings/nhqrdr/index.html. Retrieved November 19, 2014.

Hargraves JL, Cunningham PJ, Hughes RG. Racial and ethnic differences in access to medical care in managed care plans. *HSR: Health Serv Res.* 2001;36(5):853-868.

Institute of Medicine, Committee on Monitoring Access to Personal Health Care Services. *Access to Health Care in America.* Washington, DC: National Academies Press; 1993.

Mayberry RM, Mili F, Ofili E. Racial and ethnic differences in access to medical care. *Med Care Res Rev.* 2000;57:108-145.

Shi L, Chen C, Nie X, Zhu J, Hu R. Racial and socioeconomic disparities in access to primary care among people with chronic conditions. *J Am Board Fam Med.* 2014;27:189-198.

U.S. Department of Health and Human Services, Office of Disease Prevention and Health Promotion. *Healthy People 2020. Healthy People in Healthy Communities.* Washington, DC: Government Printing Office. http://www.healthypeople.gov. Retrieved November 19, 2014.

Quality of Care

Agency for Healthcare Research and Quality. *National Healthcare Quality & Disparities Reports.* Rockville, MD; 2014. http://www.ahrq.gov/research/findings/nhqrdr/index.html. Retrieved November 19, 2014.

Anderson RJ, Freedland KE, Clouse RE, Lustman PJ. The prevalence of comorbid depression in adults with diabetes: a meta-analysis. *Diabetes Care.* 2001;24(6):1069-1078.

Beach MC, Cooper LA, Robinson KA, et al. *Strategies for Improving Minority Healthcare Quality 2004.* Evidence Report/Technology Assessment No. 90. Rockville, MD: Agency for Healthcare Research and Quality. http://www.ahrq.gov/clinic/epcsums/minqusum.htm. Retrieved November 19, 2014.

Beach MC, Gary TL, Price EG, et al. Improving health care quality for racial/ethnic minorities: a systematic review of the best evidence regarding provider and organization interventions. *BMC Public Health.* 2006;6:104-115.

Dovidio JF, Fiske ST. Under the radar: how unexamined biases in decision-making process in clinical interactions can contribute to health car disparities. *Am J Public Health.* 2012; 102(5):945-952.

Mayberry RM, Mili F, Ofili E. Racial and ethnic differences in access to medical care. *Med Care Res Rev.* 2000;57:108-145.

Paez KA, Allen JK, Carson KA, Cooper LA. Provider and clinical cultural competence in a primary care setting. *Social Sci Med.* 2008;66:1204-1216.

Smedley BD, Stith AY, Nelson AR. *Unequal Treatment: Confronting Racial and Ethnic Disparities in Healthcare.* Washington, DC: Institute of Medicine, National Academies Press; 2003.

Wennberg DE. Variation in the delivery of health care: the stakes are high. *Ann Intern Med.* 1998;128:866-868.

Health Decision Making

Alden DL, Friend J, Schapira M, Stiggelbout A. Cultural targeting and tailoring of shared decision making technology: a theoretical framework for improving the effectiveness of patient decision aids in culturally diverse groups. *Social Sci Med*. 2014;105:1-8.

Bouma AB, Tiedje K, Poplau S, et al. Shared decision making in the safety net: where do we go from here? *J Am Board Fam Med*. 2014;27:292-294.

Dovidio JF, Fiske ST. Under the radar: how unexamined biases in decision-making process in clinical interactions can contribute to health car disparities. *Am J Public Health*. 2012; 102(5):945-952.

Legare F, Turcotte S, Stacey D, Ratte S, Kryworuchko J, Graham ID. Patients' perceptions of sharing in decisions. A systematic review of interventions to enhance shared decision making in routine clinical practice. *Patient*. 2012;5(1):1-19.

Murray E, Pollack L, White M, Lo B. Clinical decision-making: patients' preferences and experiences. *Patient Educ Couns*. 2007;65:189-196.

Schulman KA, Berlin JA, Harless W, Kerner JR, Sistrunk S, Gersh BJ. The effect of race and sex on physicians' recommendations for cardiac catheterization. *N Engl J Med*. 1999;340:618-626.

Legacy of Distrust

Armstrong K, McMurphy S, Dean LT, et al. Differences in the patterns of health care system distrust between African Americans and European Americans. *J Gen Intern Med*. 2008;23(6):827-833.

Boulware LE, Cooper LA, Ratner LE, LaVeist TA, Powe NR. Race and trust in the health care system. *Public Health Rep*. 2003;118:358-365.

Brandon DT, Isaac LA, LaVeist TA. The legacy of Tuskegee and trust in medical care: is Tuskegee responsible for race differences in mistrust of medical care? *JAMA*. 2005;97(7):951-956.

Clayman ML, Manganello JA, Viswanath K, Hesse BW, Arora NK. Providing health messages to Hispanics/Latinos: understanding the importance of language, trust in health information sources, and media use. *J Health Commun*. 2010;15(suppl 3): 252-263.

Dovidio JF, Penner LA, Albrecht TL, Norton WE, Gaertner SL, Shelton JN. Disparities and distrust: the implications of psychological processes for understanding racial disparities in health and health care. *Social Sci Med*. 2008;67:478-486.

Jacobs EA, Mendenhall E, Mcalearney AS, et al. An exploratory study of how trust in health care institutions varies across African American, Hispanic and white populations. *Commun Med*. 2011; 8(1):89-98.

Ozawa S, Sripad P. How do you measure trust in the health system? A systematic review of the literature. *Social Sci Med*. 2013; 91:10-14.

Richardson A, Allen JA, Xiao H, Vallone D. Effects of race/ethnicity and socioeconomic status on health information-seeking, confidence, and trust. *J Health Care Poor Underserved*. 2012;23(4):1477-1493.

Shenolikar RA, Balkrishnan R, Hall MA. How patient-physician encounters in critical medical situations affect trust: results of a national survey. *BMC Health Serv Res*. 2004;4:24.

Trachtenberg F, Dugan E, Hall MA. How patients' trust related to their involvement in medical care. *J Fam Pract*. 2005;54(4): 344-352.

Potential Solutions to Health Disparities

Smedley BD, Stith AY, Nelson AR, eds. *Unequal Treatment: Confronting Racial and Ethnic Disparities in Healthcare*. Washington, DC: Institute of Medicine; 2003.

Reducing Health Disparities by Improving Patient–Provider Communication

Ashton CM, Haidet P, Paterniti DA, et al. Racial and ethnic disparities in the use of health services: bias, preferences, or poor communication? *J Gen Intern Med*. 2003;18:146-152.

Kagawa-Singer M, Kassim-Lakha S. A strategy to reduce cross-cultural miscommunication and increase the likelihood of improving health outcomes. *Acad Med*. 2003;78:577-587.

Levine CS, Ambady N. The role of non-verbal behavior in racial disparities in health care: implications and solutions. *Med Educ*. 2013;47:867-876.

Reducing Health Disparities by Using Evidence-Based Algorithms

Alexandraki I, Mooradian AD. Redesigning medical education to improve health care delivery and outcomes. *Health Care Manager*. 2013;32:37-42.

Graham-Steed T, Ulchio E, Wells CK, Aslan M, Ko J, Concato J. "Race" and prostate cancer mortality in equal-access healthcare systems. *Am J Med*. 2013;126:1084-1088.

Greenfield S, Kaplan S, Ware JE. Expanding patient involvement in care. Effects on patient outcomes. *Ann Intern Med*. 1985;102:520-528.

Klocko DJ, Hoggatt Krumwiede K, Olivares-Urueta M, Williamson JW. Development, implementation, and short-term effectiveness of an interprofessional education course in a school of health professions. *J Allied Health*. 2010;41:14-20.

Lee S, Reha JL, Tzeng CW, et al. Race does not impact pancreatic cancer treatment and survival in an equal access federal health care system. *Ann Surg Oncol*. 2013;13:4073-4079.

Levine CS, Ambady N. The role of non-verbal behavior in racial disparities in health care: implications and solutions. *Med Educ*. 2013;47:867-876.

Lieberman SA, McCallum RM, Anderson GD. A golden opportunity: the coevolution of medical and education homes. *Acad Med*. 2011;86:1342.

Ross PT, Wiley CC, Bussey-Jones J, et al. A strategy for improving health disparities education in medicine. *J Gen Intern Med*. 2010;2(suppl):S160-S163.

Truong M, Paradies Y, Priest N. Interventions to improve cultural competency in healthcare: a systematic review of reviews. *BMC Health Serv Res*. 2014;14:99.

Welch VA, Petticrrew M, O'Neill J, et al. Health equity: evidence synthesis and knowledge translation methods. *Syst Rev*. 2013; 2:43.

Zheng L, Enewold L, Zahm SH, et al. Lung cancer survival among black and white patients in an equal access health system. *Cancer Epidemiol Biomarkers Prev*. 2012;10:1841-1847.

Zullig LL, Carpenter WR, Provenzale D, Weinberger M, Reeve BB, Jackson GL. Examining potential colorectal cancer care disparities in the Veterans Affairs health care system. *J Clin Oncol*. 2013;28:3579-3584.

Reducing Health Disparities by Fostering Greater Inclusion of Diverse Populations in the Health Care Workforce

Association of American Medical Colleges. *Striving Toward Excellence: Faculty Diversity in Medical Education*. Washington, DC. 2009.

Guevara JP, Adanga E, Avakame E, Carthon MB. Minority faculty development programs and underrepresented minority faculty representation at US medical schools. *JAMA*. 2013;310:2297-2304.

Perez T, Hattis P, Barnett K. *Health Professions Accreditation and Diversity: A Review of Current Standards and Processes*. Battle Creek, MI: W.K. Kellogg Foundation; 2007.

Price SS, Crout RJ, Mitchell DA, Brunson WD, Wearden S. Increasing minority enrollment utilizing dental admissions workshop strategies. *J Dent Educ*. 2008;72:1268-1276.

Smedley BD, Butler AS, Bristow LR, eds. *In the Nation's Compelling Interest: Ensuring Diversity in the Healthcare Workforce*. Washington, DC: Institute of Medicine; 2004.

Thornton RL, Powe NR, Roter D, Cooper LA. Patient-physician social concordance, medical visit communication and patients' perceptions of health care quality. *Patient Educ Couns*. 2011; 85:301-208.

SECTION II
Collecting Evidence for Medical Practice

Clinical Trials

Valerie L. Durkalski-Mauldin and Kathleen T. Brady

HEALTH SCENARIO

Stroke is a potentially debilitating medical event that affects approximately 800,000 people in the United States each year, leaving as many as 30% of survivors permanently disabled. Given this impact, there is great demand for treatments that significantly improve functional outcome after a stroke. To date, few clinical trials for the treatment of acute stroke have succeeded. Suppose you and a team of collaborators have a new treatment that you would like to test for use in patients who have had strokes. Where do you begin? How many patients do you need to sample to know if your treatment is safe and effective? How do you choose a comparison group and allocate treatment? How do you choose the outcome of interest and conduct the analysis of your data? These questions will be addressed in the following sections.

INTRODUCTION

A clinical trial is a prospective research study conducted in humans to assess the impact of an experimental intervention. The intervention can be a drug product, a device such as a surgical stent or diagnostic tool, a procedure such as a surgical treatment, or a behavioral intervention. Clinical trials are a critical step to therapeutic development because they provide the necessary methodology to make inferences with minimal bias and the best possible precision. Clinical trials have been in existence since the 1700s, although the primary

concepts and terminology of trials were not identified until much later (**Figure 7-1**, Timeline), and clinical trial methods and regulations continue to be developed.

The history of clinical trials is important for understanding the impetus for good clinical practice guidelines, as well as the evolution of the drug and device development process. On average, the typical time from initial development to introduction into clinical practice for a drug in the United States is 15 years (Woosley and Cossman, 2007). Because therapeutic development is a time-consuming and costly process, it is important to take the time to develop the most appropriate study design and ensure proper conduct and analysis of the trial. There are plenty of examples of failed clinical trials, and the cause is not necessarily the absence of a treatment effect. For example, several trials were conducted in acute stroke only to conclude that patients may not have been treated early enough after the injury. Similarly, hundreds of AIDS trials were conducted before it was determined that CD4 cell levels might not be a reliable surrogate for AIDS. There are examples in areas where technology is evolving quickly in which the intervention under study becomes outdated by the end of the trial. Some of these failures can be avoided with the appropriate trial design.

A successful trial depends not only on the right design but also on the right team. Clinical trials demand a team approach, which includes, at a minimum, the clinical researcher, biostatistician, study coordinator, and patients. This chapter provides an introductory view of clinical trials, including study design, study

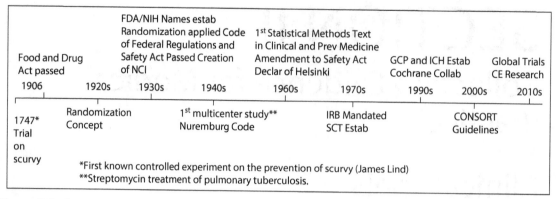

Figure 7-1. Clinical trial history. CE, Comparative Effectiveness; CFR, Code of Federal Regulations; CONSORT, Consolidated Standards of Reporting Trials; FDA, Food and Drug Administration; GCP, Good Clinical Practice; ICH, International Conference on Harmonization; IRB, Institutional Review Board; NCI, National Cancer Institute; NIH, National Institutes of Health; SCT, Society for Clinical Trials.

population, randomization and blinding methods, sample size estimation, and outcomes and analyses.

CLINICAL TRIAL DESIGNS

There are a variety of clinical trial designs. The best design for any specific study depends on a number of issues, including the research question to be addressed, the type of treatment under investigation, and characteristics of the patient population being studied. Although we often think of clinical trials as a method for investigating new therapeutic interventions, clinical trials can also investigate prevention strategies, screening and diagnostic efforts, or supportive care designed to lessen symptom severity and improve quality of life rather than to cure disease.

Sound scientific clinical investigation almost always requires that a control group be used against which the experimental intervention can be compared. To control for expectations and some of the "nonspecific" therapeutic benefit of contact with professionals, many medication trials use a **placebo**, *a biologically inactive substance that is identical in appearance to the medication under investigation.* In trials of therapeutic devices, there is usually some attempt made to mimic the device application while not delivering the therapeutic elements of treatment (e.g., sham transcranial magnetic stimulation in which the device is applied but no current is delivered). In some disease states, the use of a placebo is considered unethical because there are known efficacious therapies and to deny a participant access to these treatments places them at unnecessary risk for harm. In these cases, an active control group receiving an existing standard treatment typically is used.

As recently as 50 years ago, the primary means of evaluating a new treatment was to compare a group of individuals treated with the new method to outcomes observed in the past from a group of individuals who received standard therapy, referred to as "historical controls." There are several problems inherent in this approach. The primary problem is that it does not allow the investigator to control for the effects of important potential prognostic characteristics of the groups over time (e.g., age, sex, socioeconomic factors). In addition, there could be important variations in the disease state depending on seasonal variation, changes in environmental determinants, and so on over time. In addition, diagnostic criteria and sensitivity of methods for diagnosis of various disease states may change over time, making historical controls a less valid comparison group. For example, improved detection methods may result in earlier stage, more treatable extent of disease than existed historically.

As such, a randomized, controlled clinical trial is often considered to be the "gold standard" for testing a new medication or therapeutic device. Other common designs include pre-/post-, crossover and factorial (**Figure 7-2**). These are generally conducted using a parallel group design in which two or more treatment groups are treated at approximately the same time and directly compared (**Figure 7-2**). In a pre-post comparison study design, individuals serve as their own controls with a basic comparison made before and after treatment. In a **cross-over study** design, *each participant also serves as his or her own control, but subjects are randomized to sequences of treatments.* For example, at random, half of subjects receive treatment A followed by treatment B, and the other half at random receive treatment B followed by treatment A. Varying the order in which the subjects receive the treatment

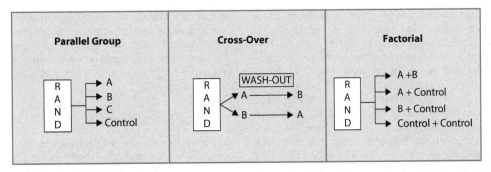

Figure 7-2. Study design examples.

allows for investigation of whether there is any impact of the order in which the treatments are delivered on the treatment outcome. A "wash-out" period or time between treatment periods is also often used to minimize the likelihood that the treatment in the first period will impact the outcomes of the treatment in the second period ("carry-over effect"). A cross-over design study can have more than two treatment periods. There are several advantages to the cross-over design. Because each subject is used as his or her own control, the treatment comparison has only within-subject variability compared with between-subject variability, allowing a smaller sample size to be studied. There are, however, a number of disadvantages. It is most suitable for studying chronic conditions (e.g., diabetes mellitus) that can be expected to return to a baseline level of severity at the beginning of the second treatment period and is not a suitable design for the study of any disease states that may be cured during the first treatment period (e.g., many acute infections). In addition, the assumption that the effects of intervention during the first period will not carry over into subsequent periods must be valid. In addition, subject drop-out (i.e., voluntarily or involuntarily discontinuing participation) before the second treatment period can severely limit the validity of the results.

The **factorial** design (**Figure 7-2**) attempts to *evaluate two interventions compared with a control within a single trial.* Given the cost and effort involved in recruitment for clinical trials, this is an efficient and attractive proposition. If it can be validly assumed that there is no interaction between the two interventions being compared, with only a modest increase in sample size, two experiments can be conducted simultaneously. However, one concern with factorial design is the possibility of an interaction between the two interventions being compared. An **interaction** exists *when the two treatments administered together have a greater effect than would be expected from the combination of the separate effects of the treatments when administered individually.* An interaction may arise

when the two treatments impact on different biological processes, thereby amplifying each other's effect. When interaction is present, the sample size must be increased to account for the interaction. As such, the factorial design can be particularly appropriate and efficient either when there is no interaction expected or when the interaction between two treatments is an important focus of the study.

Other types of designs include cluster randomized trials, equivalence trials and adaptive trials. These designs address a specific study setting as described herein. In group allocation or **cluster randomization** designs, *a group of individuals (e.g., those attending a clinic, school, or community) is randomized to a particular intervention or control.* In this type of design, the basic sampling unit is the group, not individual participants, and the overall sample size needs be inflated accordingly. Cluster randomized designs are a good option when one is concerned with contamination across treatment groups. For example, a trial on a new educational program should be concerned with **contamination** (*those not intended to have the experimental treatment receiving it inadvertently because of proximity and sharing with the experimental subjects*) within the same school or same grades. Therefore, one would consider randomizing by grades or schools rather than by individual students.

In studies of **equivalency**, or noninferiority trials, *the objective is to test whether a new intervention is as good as or no worse than an established one.* The control or standard therapy in such a trial must have established efficacy. The investigator must specify what is meant by equivalence because it cannot be proven that two therapies have absolutely identical effects, as an infinite sample size would be required to prove equivalence. In this situation, outcomes other than the primary become important as frequency, and severity of adverse events (AEs), quality of life measures, ease of use, and costs may be important secondary bases of comparison in preferring one treatment over another.

An **adaptive** design *allows predefined design adaptations to be made to trial procedures of ongoing clinical trials.* In adaptive trials, as the trial progresses, the collected data are used to guide the predefined adaptation of the trial during its progress. The adaptations can be to drop a treatment arm that is not effective, alter dose levels, or increase the trial size if pretrial assumptions are not as predicted. This means that the dosing, eligibility criteria, sample size, or treatment settings can be adjusted during the course of the trial as evidence accumulates. The most important aspect of these designs is that the adaptations must be defined before the onset of the trial so that the statistical team can assess the impact of the changes on trial operating characteristics such as sample size and the possibility of a false conclusion. Adaptive designs have the potential to accelerate therapeutic development, but there are methodologic and implementation challenges in terms of randomization and statistical analysis that are specific to adaptive design clinical trials.

One of the motivations for conducting clinical trials is the persistent and unexplained variability in clinical practice (see Chapter 16) and high rates of care for which evidence of effectiveness is lacking (see Chapter 11). The increasing cost of health care has fueled an increasing demand for evidence of clinical effectiveness (see Chapter 11). *Clinical trials that are developed specifically to answer the questions faced by clinical decision makers are called* **pragmatic** or **practical clinical trials** (PCTs). PCTs often address practical questions about the risks, benefits, and costs of interventions as would occur in routine clinical practice. In general, PCTs focus on a relatively easily administered intervention and an easily ascertained outcome. Characteristic features of PCTs are that they compare clinically relevant alternative interventions, include a diverse population of study participants, recruit from heterogeneous practice settings, and collect data on a broad range of health outcomes (Tunis et al., 2003).

CLINICAL TRIAL PHASES

Clinical studies conducted to evaluate the therapeutic potential of a compound for a given illness have been divided into four phases. Before clinical studies, one often begins with translational research that brings the laboratory bench science and preclinical studies to the bedside so that new interventions (e.g., drugs, devices, behavioral interventions) can be further studied to develop promising new treatments. Clinical studies generally begin cautiously. As experience with the agent grows, the questions expand from tolerable dose to safety and then to efficacy. The number of subjects studied at each phase and the duration of studies can vary significantly depending on statistical considerations, the prevalence of the disease under consideration, and the agent under investigation. There are, however, some general principles and procedures regarding the four phases of clinical testing described below.

Phase I Clinical Trials

In **phase I trials,** *the compound under investigation is administered to humans for the first time.* Phase I studies generally are conducted in a hospital setting with close medical monitoring. When possible, phase I studies are conducted in normal, healthy volunteers to allow for the evaluation of the effects of the drug in a subject with no preexisting disease conditions. In some situations when it is not ethical to use normal human volunteers (e.g., testing oncology drugs, which are highly toxic), testing may be done in volunteers who have the disorder under investigation and have exhausted all other available treatment options.

The purpose of a phase I trial is to determine basic safety, pharmacokinetic, and pharmacologic information. These studies generally share certain characteristics. A series of ascending dose levels is used, with initial doses determined by extrapolation from animal data, beginning with a low dose and proceeding until a dose range suitable for use in later trials is identified. A small group of subjects is treated concurrently and may receive one dose of medication or several doses in a series of consecutive treatment periods. Data from each set of studies are generally collected and assessed before choosing the next set of doses for administration. Adverse Events (AEs) are investigated intensively in phase I trials. In some cases, such as the investigation of oncology drugs, dose escalation is continued until limited by toxicity for the determination of a maximally tolerated dose (MTD). Although clinical monitoring for AEs is one of the critical elements of all first-in-human studies, the MTD is not the universal endpoint of phase I investigation, and when appropriate, the endpoint for dose escalation may be a given plasma concentration or a biomarker for some indication of the action for the agent (Collins, 2000).

A diversity of procedures can be used in phase I trials. For many compounds, it is anticipated that AEs will not be a major limiting concern. In this case, AEs are monitored, but the principal observations of interest are pharmacokinetic and pharmacodynamic endpoints. Parameters repeatedly assessed during most phase I trials include vital signs, physical and neurologic status, laboratory testing (in particular hepatic, renal, hematopoietic function), cardiac conduction (serial electrocardiography [ECG] or telemetry), and AEs. Pharmacokinetic parameters after single, repeated, and a range of doses are assessed.

Assessments include maximal plasma concentrations, time to maximal plasma concentration, time to steady state, elimination half-life, plasma accumulation, and total drug exposure to test for dose-plasma level proportionality. Studies investigating bioavailability, particularly by the oral route of administration, food effects on absorption, and relative bioavailability studies of different formulations (e.g., capsule and solution), are also conducted. The metabolic profile and elimination pathways also are determined.

Phase II Clinical Trials

Phase II clinical trials range from small, single-arm studies to randomized trials comparing a control treatment with the experimental drug in either a single dose or at several doses. Because these studies vary considerably in size and study objectives, the study designs are quite heterogeneous. In phase II studies, the study subjects are the patient population that has the disorder of interest. *There is an assessment of treatment efficacy as well as safety.* Phase II trials are designed to extend the safety database and provide initial evidence for efficacy of the compound. Phase II trials are not designed to give definitive evidence of efficacy, and the goal of the trial is to lead to a decision concerning further (phase III) testing rather than regulatory submission. Although the focus of a phase II study is efficacy, further information about drug delivery, protocol feasibility, dosing, and AEs are gathered. As in phase I, data collected may include pharmacokinetics, repeated physical and neurologic examinations, comprehensive laboratory testing, cardiac conduction (ECG), and vital signs. The primary outcome variables typically are focused on the target condition. These usually include relevant illness appropriate rating scales such as the Clinical Global Impression (CGI) rating for mental health studies, the modified Rankin scale (mRS) for stroke, and so forth. There is an emphasis on adverse effects and compliance, usually determined by both pill count and pharmacokinetic parameters. Frequency of visits depends on the target condition and the agent under investigation. There may be a required period of "in-clinic," close medical assessment after administration of the initial dose(s) of the compound in situations when there are some acute effects of concern.

Phase III Clinical Trials

Phase III trials *are large clinical studies that can involve the treatment of several hundred subjects from multiple centers with a goal of assessing therapeutic benefit.* The large number of patients involved allows for the development of a broad database of information about the safety and efficacy of the drug candidate.

Despite the large numbers of patients studied, the exclusion criteria for phase III trials are stringent. As in phase II trials, subjects with comorbid conditions other than the target condition under investigation generally are excluded.

Study designs used in phase III trials are less heterogeneous than those used in phase II because of the need to meet defined regulatory standards for the New Drug Application (NDA) to the Food and Drug Administration (FDA). The study duration is variable depending on the therapeutic area. The assessments of laboratory data and physical and neurologic examination are less frequent than in the phase I and II trials and outcome measures generally include assessment of the primary outcome (target condition) using disease-specific measures (e.g., reducing symptoms, arresting or reversing an underlying pathologic process, decreasing complications of the illness) and secondary outcome measures such as quality of life and disability measures.

Phase III trials often include fixed-dose studies, flexible dose studies, and studies that include the comparison of a "gold standard" treatment along with the experimental agent and placebo. The large group of geographically and demographically diverse participants may allow for the identification of rare AEs that only affect a few patients. Despite the earlier testing, approximately one in five potential drugs are eliminated during phase III of testing. However, if a drug candidate is successful in phase I and II, some of the phase III studies will be "pivotal" studies that will serve as the basis for FDA approval.

Phase IV Clinical Trials

Phase IV trials are initiated after a drug has been approved by the FDA. These trials are also referred to as postmarketing studies. *They are generally conducted for the approved indication, but they may evaluate different doses, the effects of extended therapy, or the safety of the agent in patient populations that were not studied in the premarketing clinical trials.* Phase IV trials may be initiated by the sponsor in an attempt to gather more information on the safety and efficacy of the drug, or they may be requested by the FDA. To evaluate the risk of rare side effects, phase IV trials often involve very large and diverse study populations.

STUDY PARTICIPANT SELECTION

The study population is a subset of individuals with the condition or characteristics of interest as defined by study eligibility criteria. The types of characteristics typically used for eligibility criteria include stage or severity of illness, age and gender of patients, absence of other comorbid conditions, and ease of follow-up. Careful consideration of study eligibility criteria is essential because it will impact the generalizability (extent to which results can be extrapolated to other patients) and utility of the study. In general, eligibility criteria are related to participant safety and the anticipated effect of the intervention. If the study population is very homogeneous with highly selective inclusion and exclusion criteria, the decreased variability in response means that a treatment effect is more likely to be detected if one truly exists. However, with a narrowly defined study population, the study results will not be as easily generalized to the entire universe of individuals with the disease state in question. However, if the study population is heterogeneous with few exclusion criteria, the variability in response may make it more difficult to discern a treatment effect, but the results of the study will have broad generalizability. It is of critical importance that the investigators give a careful and detailed description of the study population so that readers can fully assess the applicability of the findings to their patient populations. When defining the eligibility criteria, it is important to consider who will potentially benefit from the proposed experimental intervention, who will have minimal risk, and who will adhere to the intervention.

Choosing the right study population is important; however, it is just as important to ensure that certain populations are not neglected or coerced to participate and that there is an equitable selection of participants. For example, in the history of clinical research, it has been argued that women, children, and disadvantaged ethnic groups have either been harmfully neglected or exploited in clinical studies. These populations are referred to as *vulnerable populations*, a category of participants subject to an inequity in research. This category includes children, prisoners, pregnant women, disadvantaged ethnic groups, and persons with physical or mental disabilities. Great care should be taken when designing a clinical trial to ensure minimal risk to the participating population and equity in participant selection. This is why clinical research has a participant consent process referred to as the *informed consent* process. One main requirement when conducting a clinical trial is that all participants are fully informed about the trial. This includes understanding the intervention they may be given, what they will have to do if they take part in the trial, what benefit they might gain or what harm may come to them, what will happen to them after the trial is over, and what their rights may be to other treatments. When obtaining consent from minors or mentally impaired populations, there must be a person who is permitted to give consent on the participant's behalf such as a parent or a legally authorized representative.

RANDOMIZATION AND BLINDING

Randomization of study participants is a key component of clinical trials with multiple treatment arms. *The goal of randomization is to establish comparable groups with respect to both known and unknown prognostic factors, to minimize selection and accidental biases, and to ensure that appropriate statistical tests have valid significance levels.* An important question regards how to randomize. Several randomization methods are available. Fixed allocation schemes, including simple randomization, blocked randomization, and stratified randomization, assign the intervention with a prespecified probability (equal or unequal) that remains constant during the study period. Simple randomization is analogous to flipping a coin when the rules are prespecified (e.g., heads = experimental; tails = control). Although easy to implement and provides random treatment assignment, simple randomization does not take into account important prognostic variables, so the balance of these variables across treatment arms is not guaranteed.

Constrained randomization, which includes blocked and stratified schemes, addresses this potential limitation of simple randomization. Using a blocked scheme, randomization is done within small subsets (small blocks). Block size is determined by the number of treatment arms and must be an exact integer multiple of the number of arms. For example, if a trial with two treatment arms has a chosen block size of four, then there are six possible permutations of treatments (ABAB, AABB, and so on). A list of blocks can be pregenerated, and when enrollment begins, blocks are randomly selected. It is important to completely fill a block before using another block because complete blocks ensure balance in treatment assignments. Although blocking does not ensure balance of important prognostic factors, this can be achieved by adding stratification. For example, if gender impacts the outcome of interest, the researcher should ensure that males and females receive equal treatment assignments. In a blocked stratified scheme, blocks would be set up within each stratum (i.e., male, female) to provide treatment assignment balance within each stratum. Although blocked, stratified schemes have been used commonly in trials (mainly because of their ease of implementation); there are cons to this approach. Specifically, one loses randomness in the assignment as a block fills, and the assignment becomes deterministic by the end of a block. As randomization methodologies expand, there are alternatives to fixed and constrained allocation schemes such as adaptive randomization schemes. Adaptive schemes allocate patients with a changing probability and include number adaptive, baseline adaptive, and response (outcome) adaptive. Although the various adaptive schemes can be more complex to implement, the advantages include minimized deterministic assignments and maintenance of the randomness of assignments. Schemes include minimization, minimal sufficient balance, and play the winner.

In addition to randomization, **blinding**, *which means keeping the identity of treatment assignment hidden*, is another important aspect of a clinical trial design. When the identity of treatment assignment is kept from the investigator and the evaluation team as well as the participant, this is referred to as a *double-blind* trial. Although not always feasible, blinding has several important features. It minimizes the potential biases resulting from differences in patient management, treatment, or interpretation of results and the influence of patient expectation, and it avoids subjective assessment and decisions that could occur if investigators or participants are aware of the treatment assignment.

Ideally, the participant, investigator, and evaluation team should be blinded to the treatment allocation, and it is important to ensure that the treatment assignment information remains confidential until the end of the trial. For example, if a participant is made aware that the next treatment assignment is to a placebo control arm, then he or she may decline participation, which may lead to a selection bias in the study population. If the investigator is made aware of the next treatment assignment, then he or she may decide to not enroll the next patient because of a specific patient characteristic such as disease severity, which also could produce selection bias. Similarly, if the various parties are blind to treatment allocation but are made aware after the assignment, then they may withdraw consent, or the care of that participant may be impacted if the evaluating team knows what intervention the patient received.

As previously mentioned, blinding is not always feasible. When considering the feasibility of blinding, ethics and practicality must be examined. The investigator needs to ensure that implementation of a blinding scheme will not result in harm to the participants. In terms of practicality, surgical trials, diagnostic studies, and behavioral studies often struggle with implementing blinding because the person delivering the intervention knows the assignment. Blinding of the allocation can still be maintained; however, at a minimum, the post-intervention evaluation should be done by a person(s) who is (are) blind to individual treatment assignment. This situation is often called a *single-blind* trial.

SAMPLE SIZE ESTIMATION

For every clinical trial, sample size must be determined to ensure adequate statistical power (ability to discern an effect, if present) for the proposed analysis plan. The question that is answered by sample size estimation is, "How many participants are needed in order to ensure a certain probability of detecting a clinically relevant difference at a defined significance level?" The overall goal of sample size estimation is to achieve reasonable precision in estimating the outcome of interest. That is to say, one should characterize the treatment effect within an acceptably narrow range of values consistent with the data. The study sample size should reflect what is needed to address the primary objective of the trial and the analysis of the outcome and should be enough to examine the secondary outcomes. Just as important, sample size needs to be determined so that a budget can be derived. The estimation of study sample size starts with the primary outcome. One needs to define the quantitative measure (outcome) and determine how to analyze it in order to estimate sample size. When there is a dichotomous (yes/no) outcome from a paired sample (McNemar test) but the sample size is estimated for an independent outcome (chi-square test), an incorrect sample size will be estimated and the trial is threatened to be underpowered to detect the relevant differences.

When calculating sample size, four parameters need to be predefined: the probability of a type I error, the probability of a type II error, the standard deviation of the outcome measure, and what you determine to be the clinically relevant difference between the experimental intervention and the control intervention. The type I error occurs when a null hypothesis is falsely rejected; for example, when testing to see if the experimental intervention is superior to the control intervention, a type I error occurs when there is a false claim of superiority. The probability of a type I error is referred to as the significance level of a test. Common values for a significant level are 0.05 or 0.10. A type II error occurs when one fails to reject the null hypothesis (e.g., in the superiority setting, this is falsely claiming no difference when in fact a true difference exists). Common values for type II error probabilities are 0.10 and 0.20. One minus type II error is the statistical power of the trial.

Clinical trials are concerned about power because the statistical power of the test tells us how likely we are to reject the null hypothesis given that the alternative hypothesis is true. If the power is too low (<80%), then we have insufficient chance of detecting the predefined clinically relevant difference. Invariably, the cause of low power is inadequate sample size. Just as important, though, is that we must acknowledge that statistical significance does not imply clinical significance. With unlimited funds, one could have a large enough study to have adequate power to detect a difference that is so small that it does not have any clinical meaning. For example, if one could afford to conduct a 10,000-patient trial and detected less than 1-point change in a continuous outcome scale, there is reason to doubt whether that 1-point change is clinically meaningful. Will the difference detected change practice? That is the most important question for the clinical researcher to bring to the table for sample size estimation.

The clinically relevant difference for trials is either defined as the absolute difference or the relative difference between the experimental treatment and control (i.e., how much difference should there be in order to change practice). In trials for acute spinal cord injury, the primary outcome is often the mean American Spinal Injury Association (ASIA) motor score at 12 months after randomization. When estimating sample size for a two-arm trial, we turn to the literature on the ASIA motor score for this population to guide us in determining the expected 12-month mean ASIA motor score for standard of care. If we assume that the control arm (standard of care) is going to have a mean score of 25 with a standard deviation of 15, then we need to determine what absolute difference should be detected in order to state the experimental treatment is beneficial compared with control. This is not an easy task and requires a combination of literature review, clinical expertise, and consensus. This is similar when the outcome is a proportion. Consider a trial with a primary outcome of proportion of successes in which success is defined by a certain predefined threshold of improvement. If we assume the proportion of successes in the population that is receiving the control is 30%, then how much better (e.g., 40%, 50%) does the proportion need to be in the experimental arm in order to claim it is better? This can be defined in absolute or relative terms. On an absolute scale, we can state that the experimental arm must have at least an absolute increase of 30%. We can take that same difference and turn it into a relative scale; the experimental arm must have a 50% relative increase in the success rate compared with the control. Both are acceptable approaches to defining the clinically relevant difference, but it is important to be clear which scale you are basing your sample size calculations on because you can get very different results if you mistakenly used the 50% absolute difference rather than the intended 30%.

OUTCOMES AND ANALYSIS

Research studies start with a question, which leads to study objectives, which lead to the definition of outcomes. Researchers often have multiple questions, and it is the responsibility of the study team to determine the primary versus the secondary and tertiary questions. The reason to delineate the major hypothesis is because in clinical trials, the primary question drives the various aspects of the study design, including sample size, study population, study procedures, and data analyses. Consider common questions in a clinical trial setting: What dose of a new experimental anticlotting drug is safe and well tolerated in patients with thrombotic strokes? Is an innovative surgical stenting procedure safe and effective in patients with carotid artery blockages? Is another new drug showing a signal of efficacy in preventing strokes in patients with transient ischemic attacks? These questions lead to objectives: to determine safety, to determine dose, and to determine efficacy. After one has the question and objectives, then one can determine the outcomes that need to be measured.

Outcomes, also referred to as endpoints, *are the quantitative measures that correspond to the study objectives*. The outcome can be continuous, categorical, ordinal, nominal, or a time to an event, or the outcome can be a composite measure. When choosing the study outcome, it is desirable for the outcome to have the following properties: valid and reliable, capable of being observed for every trial participant, free of measurement error, and clinically relevant. All of these properties are important, and the combination of the literature and the features of the disease that the intervention is targeting to improve should be used to help decide the best outcomes for the clinical trial. For example, in acute spinal cord injury trials, researchers examine mean ASIA motor scores to interpret treatment effects. For oncology trials, a common study outcome is a time to event such as overall survival or time to tumor progression. In acute stroke and cardiovascular disease trials, the outcome often is a proportion of good or bad outcomes as defined by dichotomizing the modified Rankin scale for stroke and reporting the proportion of nonfatal myocardial infarctions or the total mortality rate for cardiovascular disease. After the outcomes are defined, then one can consider the analysis plan.

If the primary outcome is a categorical variable, then an appropriate analysis for categorical outcomes must be used. For example, a simple dichotomous outcome (e.g., success or failure; yes or no) could be analyzed using a chi-square test. If a cell size is small, however, then the analysis may use Fisher's exact test, or if data are not independent (e.g., each participant receives both treatment A and treatment B), then McNemar's test for paired data should be used. **Table 7-1** provides an example of how to display the data for a dichotomous outcome. When reporting results from a trial, it is very important to report both the point estimate of the treatment effect with the appropriate confidence interval (CI) and the *P* value produced from the statistical test. The CI includes the range of values that are consistent with the data observed at a defined level of statistical

Table 7-1. Results of a hypothetical trial concerning the 12-month outcome of success or failure in patients with the targeted disease.

| | Treatment | | |
	Experimental	Control	Total
Success	34	25	59
Failure	107	116	223
Total	141	141	282

precision (e.g., 95%). This information will give the audience a more complete picture of the benefit of the experimental treatment. For example, based on the data in **Table 7-1**, we see that the experimental arm had 34 successes out of 141 randomized into that arm (proportion of success, p_e, of 0.24), and the control arm had 25 successes out of 141 randomizations ($p_c = 0.18$). The treatment effect of this trial can be reported as a 6% absolute risk difference ($0.24 - 0.18$) with a 95% CI of -3.1%, 15.8% between the proportion of success in the experimental arm compared with the control arm. This point estimate can be supported by conducting a chi-square test and reporting a test statistic of 1.74 and a P value of 0.19. Note that the 95% CI included the value of no effect (0% difference). This tells us that the point estimate of 6% difference is not statistically significant at the 5% level ($P > 0.05$). In other words, we cannot exclude chance as an explanation for treatment differences of this magnitude with a sample of this size.

Alternative approaches of reporting the treatment effect include percentage absolute risk reduction (or benefit), relative risk or number needed to treat (NNT), which is the number of patients needed to be treated with the experimental treatment rather than the control treatment for one additional patient to benefit. Using the data in **Table 7-1**, we can calculate these measures as follows:

Percent absolute risk reduction or Benefit

$$= \frac{P_e - P_c}{P_c} \times 100\% = \frac{(34/141 - 25/141)}{25/141} \times 100\% = 36\%$$

This means that the experimental group had about a one third improvement in response likelihood compared with the baseline response among controls.

$$\text{Risk ratio} = \frac{P_e}{P_c} = \frac{0.241}{0.177} = 1.36$$

This means that the likelihood of a successful response was 36% higher within the experimental group when compared with the control group.

$$\text{NNT} = 1/\text{ARR} = \frac{1}{0.241 - 0.177} = 15.7$$

Where ARR is the Absolute Risk Reduction. This means that almost 16 patients need to be treated with the experimental method in order to have one more patient respond than would otherwise.

All of these summary measures are acceptable for reporting clinical trial data. For this particular example, the measures should be interpreted as follows: being treated with the experimental therapy provides about one third more successful outcomes than the control therapy, the risk of having a beneficial (successful) outcome in the experimental treatment group is about one third greater than in the control group, and the experimental treatment will lead to one more success for every 16 patients treated. Choosing which metric to report is a decision that should be based on what the study team believes is most important for their audience to know in order to understand the magnitude of the treatment effect. Sometimes a combination of the measures is provided. In addition to these various point estimates, the reported value should be accompanied by a two-sided CI to show the uncertainty in the estimate. Although the point estimate tells us something about the treatment effect, the point estimate alone does not provide information on whether this value is statistically different from no effect. By including the CI, we are providing valuable information on the statistical precision of our estimate. For example, the risk ratio is 1.36 in the above example and has a 95% CI of 0.86, 2.16. A risk ratio of 1 indicates that there is no difference between the two treatments ($P_e = P_c$) and as it moves away from 1 we begin to see greater differences in outcomes between the groups. The CI provides a range of plausible values for the risk ratio, and because the interval includes 1, we can conclude that there is no statistical difference (at $P < 0.05$) between the two treatment arms. A similar approach can be seen with the reported interval for the absolute risk reduction (ARR) or benefit. In that scenario, an interval that contains zero indicates no risk difference between the two treatment arms ($p_e = p_c$).

It should be noted that odds ratios (ORs) were not part of the above approaches. Although ORs are valid measures and sometimes reported in clinical trials, the data from trials are often interpreted as the proportion that "do better" on treatment compared with control. This is the interpretation of a risk ratio, not an OR. The OR, often used for case control studies (see Chapter 9), provides the relative odds that a patient would "do better" if he or she received the treatment compared with the control and is calculated as follows:

$$OR = \frac{p_e/(1-p_e)}{p_c/(1-p_c)} = \frac{0.317}{0.215} = 1.47$$

Odds ratios and risk ratios give similar values only when the proportion of events is small, but as that proportion increases, the two values can give very different results. The OR for the data in **Table 7-1** is 1.47, which is slightly larger than the reported risk ratio of 1.36. Although both measures are valid, the interpretation of the results guides which relative measure to report. In trials, we commonly report the risk ratio or absolute risk reduction or benefit.

Often clinical trial analyses include a known *prognostic variable*, a variable that impacts outcome regardless of treatment. For example, in certain acute neurologic diseases such as stroke, traumatic brain injury, and spinal cord injury, the baseline severity of the injury impacts outcome such that more severe cases tend to have worse functional outcomes. The analysis for these outcomes often includes an adjustment for baseline severity to account for the impact of severity on outcome because our true focus is the impact of treatment on outcome regardless of severity. The treatment effect within each subgroup of severity may be of secondary interest; however, the study often lacks sufficient statistical power for subgroup analysis. Overall, if the incorrect analysis method is used, then correct inferences about treatment effect cannot be made, and the trial will lack validity. **Table 7-2** provides a basic guide for analysis choices.

In addition to choosing the correct analysis, it is important to analyze the correct population.

In randomized clinical trials, the primary analysis should be conducted on the intent-to-treat population, which is defined by the randomization assignment. If a participant was randomized to receive the experimental treatment and it is known that he or she ended up never receiving it, that participant should still be analyzed as part of the experimental arm. Although this may seem illogical at first, the intent-to-treat population is a more unbiased representation of the population with the disease being studied. The reason it is less biased is that there are several scenarios in which a participant may not receive the assigned treatment, including clinical errors and participant choice if the experimental treatment has negative side effects or if the participant forgets to take the treatment or drops out of the study. Not receiving the experimental therapy can be similar, in some situations, to being in the control arm. We do not want to analyze the data by moving those individuals to the control arm, however, because then we lose the benefits of randomization as described earlier. In addition, these scenarios can occur outside of the trial in the general population with the disease. When we interpret results from a trial, particularly a phase III definitive trial, we want the results to be generalizable to patients outside of the trial. Accordingly, it is recommended to be conservative in the estimate of a treatment effect and report the results using the intent-to-treat population.

Another important aspect of outcomes and analysis is the handling of missing data. In clinical trials, missing outcome data is to be expected. Study participants may miss a follow-up visit, may withdraw consent, or may move and be unable to be followed for the remainder of the study. All of these scenarios can

Table 7-2. Outcomes and common analyses.

Data Type	Examples	Common Tests for Differences
Categorical	Nominal, dichotomous, and nondichotomous—success or failure, present or absent, nationalities	Test for binomial proportions (one sample or two independent samples) Chi-square test (independent data) McNemar's test (matched paired data) Sign test (nonparametric)
Ordinal	Values that have a natural ordering (e.g., dislike, neutral, like); rating of 1 to 5	Trend test Sign-rank test (nonparametric paired samples) Rank sum test (nonparametric independent samples)
Continuous	Comparison of means or medians	Student's t-test (one sample or two independent samples) Paired t-test (two dependent samples) Rank sum test (non-normal data) ANOVA (more than two independent samples) Sign-rank test (nonparametric paired samples) Rank sum test (nonparametric independent samples)
Time to event	Comparison of survival curves	Log-rank test

contribute to missing data, which impacts the data analysis. As mentioned earlier, in an intent-to-treat analysis, we would not remove participants with missing outcome data from the analysis. Instead, we have to keep them in the analysis population in order to reduce the potential bias of our treatment estimate. There are several methods for imputing data for missing observations, but this is beyond the scope of this chapter. The overall goal in the design and conduct of a trial is to minimize the amount of missing data by ensuring that outcomes of interest can be measured in all participants, the length of participant follow-up is reasonable, and there is frequent contact with the participants throughout the follow-up period.

One other point to consider is categorizing a continuous endpoint. Although dichotomous outcomes may in some situations provide simplified clinical interpretation, categorization comes with a price. Knowledge of the correct categories is not always available and thus could lead to incorrect results. Caution should be taken when attempting to categorize a continuous outcome. If possible, the existing literature should be reviewed, and the properties of an ideal outcome should be considered.

CONCLUSIONS AND LIMITATIONS

Although clinical trials are an invaluable source of information to drive innovation and improvements in clinical practice, there are a number of challenges facing the clinical research enterprise (Sung et al., 2003). In recent years, there have been concerns expressed over the disconnect between the promise of basic science discovery and the delivery of better health care. This is, in part, due to the failure to translate the findings from clinical trials, often conducted in highly controlled environments, into everyday clinical practice. The reasons for this failure are multifaceted and have led to a new area of research known as implementation and dissemination science (see Chapter 17). In addition, there are problems with the clinical research environment. It is burdened by rising costs, increasing regulatory controls, and a shortage of qualified investigators and research participants. It is important to engage the public more effectively in clinical research, both as research participants and advocates for research funding. In addition, wider participation of diverse populations in clinical trials will improve the generalizability and applicability of the information gained from the trials. Adaptive trials and PCTs address some of these issues, but there still is a need to develop new clinical trial methodologies and creative approaches to the use of data to examine and improve clinical practice

in a timely manner. In addition, efforts to standardize and streamline regulatory processes are critical to improving the efficiency and cost-effectiveness of clinical trials. In conclusion, clinical trials have contributed tremendously to evidence-based clinical practice. Improvements in the approach to clinical trial design and analysis will help to make the information gained through clinical trials even more relevant to efforts to improve clinical practice and health outcomes.

SUMMARY

In summary, a well-designed and conducted clinical trial is essential for therapeutic development. The various clinical trial phases are a gradual progression to addressing the overall question of safety and efficacy. Phase I designs focus on finding the correct dose or treatment regimen to move forward in future studies. Phase II designs focus on further assessment of safety and identifying a signal of efficacy. Phase III designs continue to assess safety and focus on determining efficacy. Phase IV or postmarketing trials further refine safety and efficacy in large clinical populations. There are several study designs to choose from for each trial phase, and the choice should be driven by the primary study question and the goal of reducing biases in order to make correct inferences from the collected data. Features of good trial design include use of a concurrent control group, implementation of randomization and blinding when the design includes two or more treatment arms, a primary outcome that is valid and reliable, sample size estimation that is based on the primary outcome and the clinically relevant difference of interest, and a study population that represents the patient population of interest. In addition to good design, the analysis should complement the design in terms of accounting for the correct variability (e.g., independent vs. paired outcomes) and inclusion of important prognostic variables. The combination of appropriate trial design and analysis promotes unbiased inference of the treatment effect with the best possible precision.

The design and conduct of trials is a team effort composed not only of the clinician but also the statistician, study coordinator, and patients. This chapter introduces readers to key concepts of clinical trials and hopefully provokes further interest in the topic. Clinical trials are quite complex, and design methodology continues to be developed to improve the efficiency of these research studies. The best clinical trial lesson is to become involved in the design and conduct of a trial after becoming familiar with the basic terminology and concepts. Each trial introduces a new lesson on the methodology as well as the practical aspects of conducting a clinical trial.

STUDY QUESTIONS

1. What are the properties that classify research as a clinical trial?

    A. A prospective experiment of an intervention with a control group that is conducted in humans

    B. The retrospective analysis of data that was collected on humans exposed to a certain intervention

    C. The testing of a new intervention on humans or animals

    D. None of the above

2. What type of design would allow one to study an interaction effect?

    A. Crossover design

    B. Parallel design

    C. Adaptive design

    D. Factorial design

3. Why do we randomize trials?

    A. To avoid selection bias

    B. To ensure treatment assignment balance within a certain prognostic variable

    C. To ensure valid statistical tests

    D. All of the above

4. What makes an ideal primary outcome?

    A. One that can be easily dichotomized

    B. One that is a short-term endpoint

    C. One that is valid and reliable

    D. Both A and C

5. What phase of clinical trial development assesses what dose to use?

    A. Phase III

    B. Translational

    C. Phase II

    D. Phase I

6. Women are considered a vulnerable population.

    A. True

    B. False

7. A prognostic variable is

    A. a variable that impacts the outcome regardless of treatment.

    B. something to be avoided in trials.

    C. a variable that impacts the outcome because of treatment.

    D. none of the above.

8. Sample size estimation is based on

    A. the primary outcome.

    B. the subgroup of interest.

    C. all of the outcomes one wants to examine.

    D. both A and B.

9. The statistical power of a trial is the likelihood of detecting a difference if one truly exists.

    A. True

    B. False

10. The most important data point an investigator can contribute for sample size estimation is

    A. type I error rate.

    B. variance of the outcome measure based on the literature.

    C. the clinically relevant difference.

    D. the dollar amount that he or she has to spend on the trial.

FURTHER READING

Chan AW, Tetzlaff JM, Gøtzsche PC, et al. SPIRIT 2013 explanation and elaboration: guidance for protocols of clinical trials. *BMJ.* 2013;346.

Lambert J. Statistics in brief: how to assess bias in clinical studies? *Clin Orthop Relat Res.* 2011;469(6):1794-1796.

Little RJ, D'Agostino R, Cohen ML, et al. The prevention and treatment of missing data in clinical trials. *N Engl J Med.* 2012;367:1355-1360.

Schulz KF, Altman DG, Moher D; CONSORT Group. CONSORT 2010 statement: updated guidelines for reporting parallel group randomized trials. *Ann Intern Med.* 2010;152(11):726-732.

Senn S. Seven myths of randomisation in clinical trials. *Stat Med.* 2013;32(9):1439-1450.

Pocock SJ, Assmann SE, Enos LE, Kasten LE. Subgroup analysis, covariate adjustment and baseline comparisons in clinical trial reporting: current practice and problems. *Stat Med.* 2002;21(19):2917-2930.

Zarin DA, Tse T, Williams RJ, Califf RM, Ide NC. The ClinicalTrials.gov results database—update and key issues. *N Engl J Med.* 2011;364:852-860.

Web Resources

Clinicaltrials.gov

Cochrane Library. http://www.cochrane.org.

Consort Guidelines. http://www.consort-statement.org.

International Conference on Harmonization. http://www.ich.org.

REFERENCES

Introduction

Woosley RL, Cossman J. Drug development and the FDA's Critical Path Initiative. *Clin Pharmacol Ther.* 2007;81(1):129-133.

Clinical Trials Design

Tunis SR, Stryer DB, Clancy CM. Practical clinical trials increasing value of clinical research for decision making in clinical and health policy. *JAMA*. 2003;290(12):1624-1632.

Phase I Clinical Trials

Collins JM. Innovations in phase 1 trial design: where do we go next? *Clin Cancer Res*. 2000;6(10):3801-3802.

Conclusions and Limitations

Sung NS, Crowley WF Jr, Genel M, et al. Central challenges facing the national clinical research enterprise. *JAMA*. 2003;289(10), 1278-1287.

Cohort Studies

8

Raymond S. Greenberg and Daniel T. Lackland

HEALTH SCENARIO

Staff Sergeant P. was a 34-year-old veteran of the United States Army, having served two tours of duty in Operation Enduring Freedom in Afghanistan. During his second tour of duty, his squadron of nine soldiers was attacked with an improvised explosive device, resulting in the deaths of two soldiers and injuries to three others, including Staff Sergeant P. The explosion resulted in a traumatic brain injury (TBI) to Staff Sergeant P., which produced persistent headaches, trouble concentrating, fatigue, sleep disturbance, irritability, depression, and anxiety. He was evaluated by an Army physician and found to be unfit for military service, ultimately resulting in a medical discharge.

Upon returning from military service, Staff Sergeant P. married his high school girlfriend and was employed as a security guard. He had difficulty adjusting to civilian life and began experiencing recurrent nightmares, emotional detachment, and conflict with his wife and coworkers. He began abusing alcohol and a variety of other substances. Staff Sergeant P. was seen at a Department of Veterans Affairs clinic and diagnosed with posttraumatic stress disorder (PTSD) for which he was prescribed cognitive behavioral therapy.

Persistent violent outbursts led first to Staff Sergeant P.'s termination from work and then to his separation and eventual divorce from his wife. He became increasingly isolated, with few friends, diminishing financial resources, and few prospects for employment. On the first anniversary of his divorce, he ended his life with a self-inflicted gunshot wound.

CLINICAL BACKGROUND

Suicide is the 10th leading cause of death in the United States, accounting for nearly 40,000 fatalities or about 1.5% of all deaths. Globally, suicide is the 16th most common cause of death, with an estimated million lives lost to it each year. The risk of suicide is highly age dependent, rising rapidly in the teen years and continuing to rise through young adulthood, peaking in the 45- to 54-year age group. For persons age 15 to 24 years, suicide trails only unintentional injuries and homicide as a cause of death, and among those age 25 to 34 years, suicide is second only to unintentional injuries as a cause of death.

Although females are more likely than males to have had suicidal thoughts, completed suicides are four times more likely among males than among females. Non-Hispanic whites have the highest death rate from suicide followed by American Indians/Alaska Natives, with comparatively low rates among blacks, Hispanics, and Asian Americans. Suicide rates declined over the latter years of the 20th century but have increased steadily since the year 2000. The largest increases over time have been seen among adults age 45 to 64 years, with decreases observed among elderly adults.

Among males, firearms are the most common method of suicide (56%) followed by suffocation or hanging and then poisoning. In contrast, among females, poisoning is the most common method (37%) followed in turn by firearms and suffocation or hanging. Approximately one third of all suicides involve alcohol consumption, one quarter involve antidepressants, and one fifth involve opiates.

A number of risk factors for suicide have been identified, the strongest of which is a prior history of an attempted suicide. Those who have previously attempted unsuccessfully to end their lives are at about a 40-fold increased risk of suicide compared with persons who have never made such an attempt. Another compelling risk factor for suicide is a history of mental illness, including substance abuse. Approximately, 90% of suicides occur in persons with a psychiatric illness, of which almost two thirds are mood disorders. It is important to recognize, however, that mood disorders are common, and only a small percentage of affected persons will ever attempt or commit suicide.

Another widely accepted risk factor for suicide is stress, which can be either acute (e.g., family or romantic conflicts, bereavement, or legal or disciplinary problems) or chronic (e.g., persistent physical pain illness). Other predisposing factors include childhood abuse, impulsive or aggressive behavior, and a family history of mental illness or suicidal behavior. A variety of psychological characteristics (e.g., decision-making abilities, problem-solving skills, and cognitive control) also have been linked to risk of suicide. Finally, a variety of social factors have been linked to risk of suicide. These factors include, among others, not being married, not having children, living alone, being unemployed or working in a low-status job, experiencing economic hardship, and being a victim of interpersonal violence.

A number of psychological attributes have been shown to be associated with a reduced risk of suicide. Among these characteristics are resilience to adverse circumstances, stoicism, high satisfaction with life, and high self-esteem, as well as the capacities for hope, gratitude, and reciprocated relationships. Several strategies have been linked with a lowering of suicide risk. The preventive measures include limiting access to lethal means, preserving contact with persons who have made prior unsuccessful attempts, and implementing crisis intervention call centers. In contrast, other strategies to reduce risk have shown little or no benefit. These include training of primary care providers to screen for at-risk patients, school-based interventions, and public information campaigns.

A recent area of public attention and research focus has been suicide rates among active duty military personnel and veterans. Historically, these groups have experienced a lower risk of suicide, probably in part because of the screening processes to limit the entrance into the military of candidates who would be at high risk of mental health concerns. Persons with predisposing factors, such as prior mental illness or criminal history, are precluded from service, leading to the preferential enrollment of lower risk individuals. This barrier to entry has given rise to what is sometimes referred to as the "healthy warrior effect."

The suicide rates among active duty and former U.S. military personnel experienced about a 50% increase between 2005 and 2008, overtaking the corresponding rates in nonmilitary populations when adjusting for age, race/ethnicity, and gender. This alarming increase, to the point at which the risk of taking one's own life exceeded the risk of death in combat, has been the subject of intense investigation. The research published to date affirms that risk factors seen in nonmilitary populations, such as male gender, depression, and heavy alcohol consumption, also predict risk within the military. Certain aspects of military service, such as combat experience, number of deployments, and days of deployment, are not associated with suicide risk. However, other types of military service, such as serving in the infantry or on gun crews, are associated with suicide risk. Suicides tend to occur with higher frequency during the first year of service and among those who have been demoted or not progressed in rank as expected.

Traumatic brain injury has become an increasingly frequent type of casualty of military service, affecting an estimated 8% to 20% of U.S. personnel deployed in Iraq or Afghanistan. TBI is associated with PTSD, depression, diminished problem-solving ability, and impaired social functioning, all of which increase the risk of suicide. Even after adjusting for these effects, however, the number of TBI events is associated with suicide risk.

The individual in the Health Scenario had many of the personal attributes associated with suicide. He was a young man with a history of substance abuse, interpersonal conflict, aggressive and violent behavior, social isolation, unemployment, and military service resulting in a TBI and PTSD. Although he had access to care, including mental health professionals, ultimately this was not sufficient to prevent his eventual suicide. The early death of a person who has served his country at great personal sacrifice provides ample cause to better understand how such tragedies might be prevented in the future.

OBSERVATIONAL STUDIES

Chapter 7 introduced randomized controlled clinical trials. These studies typically are considered to provide the strongest or most compelling evidence of cause-and-effect relationships. Unfortunately, it is not always possible to conduct a randomized controlled clinical trial. For example, if one is studying potential risk factors for suicide, it would be impossible to randomly assign to subjects attributes related to age, gender, race/ethnicity, family history, genetic profiles, or psychological and behavioral attributes. Moreover, it would be unethical to enroll subjects in a trial in which the outcome of interest is intentional self-inflicted fatal injury.

When a clinical trial cannot be performed, an alternative is to study risk factors as they occur naturally and then follow the subjects to learn their subsequent outcomes. We refer to such a study as **observational** because the role of the investigator is not to determine who is exposed and who is not but rather to observe the exposures and outcomes as they occur within the population of interest. One such type of observational study is the cohort study, so named because it starts with a group (cohort) of subjects defined by exposure status. The subjects are then traced over time to determine their ultimate outcomes with respect to the disease of interest. For example, if one was interested in studying low levels of social interaction among

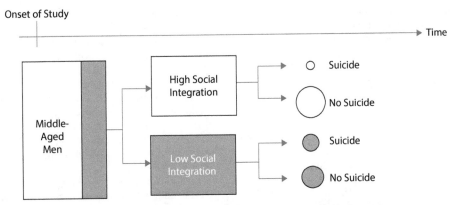

Onset of Study

Time

Figure 8-1. Schematic diagram of a cohort study of the relationship between low social integration (unexposed) and risk of suicide. The shaded areas represent the unexposed persons (those with low levels of social integration).

middle-aged men in relation to suicide risk, one might design a cohort study along the lines of the schematic illustration in **Figure 8-1**. One begins at the left of the diagram by identifying the source population of middle-aged men. Next, the men are classified as having low social integration (unexposed and shaded in the diagram) or high social integration (exposed and unshaded in the diagram). The subjects are followed for the subsequent development of the outcome, in this instance, suicide.

Example: The design of a cohort study is well illustrated by an investigation of social integration and risk of suicide conducted by Tsai and colleagues (2014). This research began in 1986 as the Health Professionals Follow-up Study (HPFS). In brief, men age 40 to 75 years who were dentists, optometrists, osteopathic physicians, pharmacists, podiatrists, or veterinarians were eligible for participation and enrolled if they completed a baseline questionnaire. The subjects were followed every 2 years with updated questionnaires. The first follow-up questionnaire in 1988 included questions on social interactions, so that became the baseline for exposure classification and follow-up. Answers to seven questions allowed the researchers to classify subjects into four levels of social integration. These questions related to marital status, size of the subject's social network, frequency of interaction with social contacts, and participation in religious or other social groups. The responses to these questions created a summary score ranging from 1 to 12, which was then used to divide subjects into four ordinal categories of social integration. Of the 34,901 subjects who completed the social integration questions in 1988, 2937 (8%) were classified into the lowest level and 14,476 (41%) were classified into the highest level, with the remainder falling into the two intermediate categories. Subjects were followed

through February 1, 2012, to determine their outcome, with particular focus on suicides.

The HPFS large cohort study was designed as an all-male complement to the all-female Nurses' Health Study (NHS). The widely cited NHS, now in its third iteration, has greatly advanced knowledge about a number of risk factors for leading chronic diseases. Originally designed in 1976, the primary goal was to assess the health impact of oral contraceptive use. Nurses were targeted for enrollment because it was anticipated that they would be motivated to participate in health research and had the technical knowledge to accurately report medication and other exposures.

The first NHS enrolled more than 120,000 nurses from 11 states who were between the ages of 30 and 55 years old. After completing a baseline questionnaire, subjects were followed with repeat questionnaires every 2 years. A second NHS was launched in 1989, this time enrolling slightly younger women, age 25 through 42 years, and again resulting in a baseline study population of nearly 120,000 women. The questionnaires focused again on oral contraceptive use but also on a variety of other lifestyle factors, including diet.

The many analyses from the NHS have produced a host of important findings. Current oral contraceptive use, for example, was linked to risk of breast cancer and cardiovascular disease but was associated with a reduced risk of colon cancer. Postmenopausal hormone use was associated with lower risk of colon cancer and hip fracture but was also associated with an increased risk of stroke and with prolonged exposure, breast cancer. Dietary analyses revealed that a Mediterranean-type diet reduced the risk of heart disease and stroke. High levels of red meat consumption were linked to both premenopausal breast and colon cancer risk. Intakes of folate, vitamin B_6, calcium, and vitamin D were all seen to lower the risk of colon cancer. These are just a sample of the findings related to this long-standing research effort.

TIMING OF MEASUREMENTS

Typically, a cohort study is **prospective**, meaning that the study is launched, and then exposure status is assessed in subjects followed by subsequent development of disease. All of the events of interest occur after the study begins. In the previously cited HPFS, for instance, the study was launched in 1986, exposure was defined by questionnaire responses in 1988, and subjects were followed to determine their suicide risk until 2012. Other names for this type of research design are **longitudinal** or **follow-up** studies because the events of interest are measured across time.

An alternative approach is the so-called **retrospective** (or **historical**) cohort study in which all of the events under investigation have occurred before the onset of the study. In this version of the cohort study, one typically accesses historical records to determine exposure status and disease outcome. Here, for example, the investigator might launch the study in 2012, going back to archived records in 1988 to define exposure (e.g., social integration), and then follow death records up to 2012 to determine health outcomes.

The rationale for conducting a retrospective cohort study may not be immediately obvious. If one considers the challenges in studying a disease that requires many years from exposure to development, however, the advantages become more apparent. For a slowly developing disease, such as cancer or heart disease, a prospective study might require decades to complete, with the answer to the research question remaining uncertain until the study could be concluded. It would be much quicker to simply avail oneself of historical information and avoid having to wait years for outcomes to occur or not. Moreover, for exposures that no longer occur, it would not be possible to conduct a prospective cohort study, and one is limited to the retrospective approach.

The principal advantages of the retrospective cohort study design are that it provides more rapid results and that it is generally less expensive because it relies on information that is already available. The downsides of a retrospective cohort study are that historical information, whether from archived records or personal recall, may be incomplete, inaccurate, or both. Moreover, a retrospective cohort study would not be useful for evaluating a new or emerging exposure.

Regardless of whether it is conducted in a prospective or a retrospective fashion, a cohort study often requires a large sample size, especially if the outcome of interest is uncommon. This point is well illustrated by the HPFS cited earlier in which the evaluation of social integration and suicide risk involved nearly 35,000 persons. Even with a sample size that large and nearly a quarter of a century of follow-up, only 147 suicides were observed in this study.

The size of such a study creates many logistical challenges and can be quite expensive to conduct even if efficient methods are used to collect data, such as self-administered questionnaires and linkage to existing record sources. Attempting to follow subjects over several decades has its own logistical challenges. Individuals may move, change their names (a particular issue when following adult women, who may change their names upon marriage or divorce), elect to discontinue participation, or die from some other cause. To the extent that people who have incomplete follow-up differ from those who are successfully followed, the results of the study could be distorted. Another challenge can arise if exposure status changes during the course of the follow-up. This phenomenon was observed in the HPFS, in which 27% of the subjects traced through 8 years had decreased their level of social integration, while another 18% had increased their level of social integration. With nearly half of the subjects changing their exposure status after entry, it was important for the investigators to account for both the initial and changed exposure status in their analysis.

SELECTION OF SUBJECTS

In some situations, such as the HPFS, the subjects for a cohort study are sampled without regard to exposure status. In the HPFS, subjects had to be (1) male, (2) between the ages of 40 and 75 years old at study onset, (3) resident in the United States, and (4) a member of one of six specified health professions. In addition, subjects had to agree to participate and complete the requisite data collection instruments. A typical exclusion from a cohort study would be anyone with the outcome of interest, which in this example would not be an issue because the outcome was suicide. In other situations when the outcome of interest is not a fatal event, it would be important to exclude affected individuals. Failure to do so might distort the results or lead to mistaken inferences about the temporal sequence between exposure and disease development.

EXPOSURE STATUS

When the exposure of interest is relatively common, a general population group, such as health professionals, may be selected. In other situations, the exposure of interest may be less frequent, necessitating a strategy to enrich the study sample with exposed persons. For example, if one is interested in a study of prior suicide attempts as a risk factor for subsequent completed suicide, a general population sample likely has too few exposed individuals (prior suicide attempters). Under such circumstances, one might want to access emergency departments and mental health facilities to identify the suicide attempters to enroll in the study.

Because the subjects in a cohort study likely will have to be followed for some time, the investigator would be well served in identifying persons who are motivated to participate and are unlikely to withdraw subsequently. The example of studying prior suicide attempters illustrates the challenges that an investigator might face in following subjects because these individuals may not be motivated to participate and may have predisposing mental health issues, social instability, and other characteristics that make them difficult to enroll and follow.

For some exposures, it may be sufficient or necessary to classify subjects into just two levels of exposure (exposed vs. not exposed). For instance, either someone has previously attempted suicide or has not. For other situations, such as the social integration HPFS study, the exposure has multiple levels. Social integration was measured on an ordinal scale with four levels from lowest to highest. An advantage of the multiple level exposure classification is that it allows a determination of whether any association with the outcome varies in a graded fashion. Such a dose-response relationship can be useful in making inferences about whether an association is likely to be one of cause and effect. The presence of a dose-response gradient is a feature that supports a causal inference.

The accuracy and reliability of information on exposure also is critical to reaching a valid conclusion from a cohort study. In some instances, the exposure may be assessed by a biologic marker, such as blood levels of serotonin or its metabolites in relation to suicide risk. Such measures have the advantage of being objective, and their reproducibility can be assessed readily. Unfortunately, biologic measures of exposure are not always available, such as in the case of social integration. In these situations, the investigator may have to rely on information recorded in other sources (e.g., hospital records), or as in the case of the HPFS, on information self-reported by the subjects. The latter sources of information have the advantage of ease of collection but may suffer from limitations in their quality. For example, hospital records may be characterized by incomplete information and inconsistencies in how data are classified and recorded. Self-reports may be distorted by personal perceptions and respondents' beliefs about preferred responses. For example, in self-reports about social integration, respondents may view social isolation as an undesirable circumstance and therefore consciously or unconsciously tend to overestimate their level of social interaction. The impact of this type of misclassification may be difficult to predict, but if it occurs nondifferentially, that is, uniformly without regard to eventual outcome, it will tend to blur distinctions between or among exposure groups and thereby diminish any apparent exposure-disease association.

Regardless of the source of information on exposure, it is desirable to demonstrate that it is reliable. That is, repeated measures on an individual subject tend to provide similar results. It is also desirable to demonstrate that the measure is accurate. That is, that it produces a classification that correctly identifies the true exposure status of individuals. Often, reliability is assessed by a substudy that examines the consistency of repeated measurements among individuals. Similarly, accuracy typically is assessed either within the study or outside of it by comparing the classification obtained with the method of interest used versus some more definitive "gold standard."

OUTCOME STATUS

As indicated earlier, at the outset of a cohort study, it is important to ensure that none of the subjects have the outcome of interest. For a study in which the outcome is suicide, simply enrolling living subjects would avoid this problem, although one might consider additionally excluding subjects who have a history of a precursor condition, such as attempted suicide. For an outcome that is slow in developing and may have a long presymptomatic phase, such as coronary heart disease or cancer, it may be more difficult to exclude affected individuals who have undiagnosed disease. For this reason, a strategy that occasionally is deployed is to exclude from consideration any affected persons who are diagnosed within the first few years after enrollment.

To reach valid conclusions, it is important that the level and methods of surveillance for the outcomes are comparable between exposed and nonexposed subjects. This point is well illustrated in the HPFS, in which all subjects received the same follow-up questionnaire every 2 years, there were uniform numbers of attempts (seven) to solicit responses from non-responders, and record linkage to external death information was deployed to determine outcomes for all subjects.

An important issue is the duration of time for which subjects should be followed. The appropriate duration of follow-up is driven by several factors, including most important, the time course from exposure to disease occurrence, as well as the size of the study population and the frequency of the outcome.

In terms of the time period from exposure to outcome, this can range from a matter of days for infectious diseases to decades for chronic illnesses such as cancer and heart disease. Beyond the considerations of disease time course, study duration is affected by the pragmatic concerns of having a sufficient number of outcomes to identify differences between exposed and nonexposed persons. Everything else being equal, a smaller sample size may require a longer observation period to accrue sufficient outcomes. Similarly, a less frequent outcome may require more observation time to accrue an adequate number of outcomes.

The duration of follow-up (24 years) in the HPFS illustrates these issues well. Even though the study was quite large (nearly 35,000 subjects), the outcome (suicide) was quite rare (with 147 events in total). A shorter duration of follow-up would have resulted in proportionately fewer outcomes and may have made it more difficult to detect an effect of social integration on suicide risk.

Information about the outcome of interest may derive from a variety of sources, including direct observation by the investigators; self-report from the subjects; or access to other record sources, such as hospital or workplace data, or as in the HPFS, from death registration information. The accuracy of cause of death information on death certificates has been questioned by multiple studies, which have found error rates exceeding one quarter of all deaths. For suicide, in particular, there may be challenges in distinguishing whether the cause of death was intentional or accidental, and if intentional, whether homicide could be ruled out. The physician, coroner, or medical examiner who certifies a death as suicide often must rely on ancillary information, such as knowledge of prior attempts, finding a note specifying intent, awareness of the presence of mental illness, and other circumstantial evidence. There also may be a hesitancy to classify a death as a suicide because of social stigmatization or legal or financial reasons. To the extent that errors are made in classifying suicides, it is likely that these events are underreported rather than overreported. As long as such errors are not differential according to social integration status, the impact on the exposure–disease association should be to blur distinctions and make it more difficult to identify a link. That is, the true low social integration–suicide association should be as strong or stronger than that observed if outcomes are misclassified nondifferentially.

ANALYSIS

One approach to analysis of a cohort study is illustrated in **Table 8-1**. This format involves a simple binary classification of exposure (yes vs. no) and outcome

Table 8-1. Summary presentation of risk data from a cohort study.

Outcome	Exposed	Unexposed	Total
Yes	A	B	A + B
No	C	D	C + D
Total	A + C	B + D	A + B + C + D

(yes vs. no). More complicated data arrays can be constructed for multiple levels of exposure or outcome, but the basic principles of analysis are readily apparent in this basic format.

There are four possible combinations of exposure and outcome status, as represented in the table:

A: Exposed persons who develop the outcome

B: Unexposed persons who develop the outcome

C: Exposed persons who do not develop the outcome

D: Unexposed persons who do not develop the outcome

The risk (or cumulative incidence) of developing the outcome among the exposed persons is given by:

$$R_{exposed} = \frac{\text{Exposed persons with outcome}}{\text{All exposed persons}}$$

$$= \frac{A}{A + C}$$

As a reminder, risk requires a specific timeframe as a reference, such as 1 year, 10 year, and so on. Also, risk can vary between 0 (A = 0, no exposed persons develop the outcome) and 1 (C = 0, all exposed persons develop the disease of interest).

We can calculate the risk among unexposed persons in the same manner:

$$R_{unexposed} = \frac{\text{Unexposed persons with outcome}}{\text{All unexposed persons}}$$

$$= \frac{B}{B + D}$$

Risk Ratio

We can contrast the risk among exposed and unexposed persons by dividing the former by the latter. This measure is referred to as the **risk ratio (RR)** and can be calculated as:

$$RR = \frac{R_{exposed}}{R_{unexposed}} = \frac{A/(A + C)}{B/(B + D)}$$

A critical value of the RR is 1, where the risk of the outcome is identical for exposed and unexposed persons. That is, exposure has no effect on the likelihood of the outcome, or equivalently expressed, there is no association between exposure and outcome. Values of the RR above 1 correspond to situations in which the risk among exposed persons exceeds that among unexposed persons. In other words, exposure appears to increase risk or hazard to those involved. The reverse is true for situations in which the RR has a value less than 1. Here, risk among exposed persons is less than that among unexposed persons. This is equivalent to saying that exposure appears to lower risk and therefore is protective for those involved.

The calculation of RR can be illustrated from the HPFS study of suicide. A summary of the study results is shown in **Table 8-2**. The risk among exposed (defined here as the highest level of social integration) is:

$$R_{exposed} = \frac{41}{14,476} = 0.0028 = 0.28\%$$

That is, the 24-year risk of suicide among middle-aged men in the health professions with the highest social integration was about almost one third of 1%. The corresponding risk among unexposed (defined here as the lowest level of social integration) is:

$$R_{unexposed} = \frac{23}{2937} = 0.0078 = 0.78\%$$

In other words, the 24-year risk of suicide among middle-aged men in the health professions with the lowest social integration was slightly more than

Table 8-2. Summary of results from Health Professionals Follow-up Study showing the suicide risk among men with the highest level of social integration compared with the corresponding risk among men with the lowest levels of social integration.

| Suicide | Social Integration | | |
	Highest	Lowest	Total
Yes	41	23	64
No	14,435	2914	17,349
Total	14,476	2937	17,413

Data from Tsai AC, Lucas M, Sania A, Kim D, Kawachi I. Social integration and suicide mortality among men: 24-year study of U.S. Health Professionals. *Ann Intern Med.* 2014;161:85-95.

three quarters of 1%. The RR, therefore, is calculated as:

$$RR = \frac{41}{14,476} \Big/ \frac{23}{2937} = 0.36$$

In other words, in this population of middle-aged men in the health professions, those with the highest level of social integration had about one third the 24-year risk of suicide than those with the lowest levels of social integration. Increasing social integration, therefore, appears to be protective against risk of suicide in this population. The magnitude of this association is assessed by how far the observed RR is away from the null value of one (no association). An RR of 0.36 is consistent with a moderate to strong protective effect.

To characterize the statistical precision of this estimate, we can calculate approximate 95% confidence intervals (CIs) around it. If we perform that calculation, the interval ranges from 0.26 to 0.50. That is, at the 95% level of confidence, the range of RR values consistent with the data observed falls between 0.26 and 0.50. The HPFS data are compatible, therefore, with an effect of high social integration on suicide risk that ranges from one quarter to half of the corresponding risk among those with the lowest level of social integration. It is worth noting that the null value of the RR (=1) is excluded from the range of values in this 95% CI. This is equivalent to stating that the association is statistically significant (at the 5% level or $P < 0.05$). We can conclude, therefore, that an association as strong or stronger than the one observed in a sample of this size would be unlikely to arise from chance alone.

As indicated earlier, for exposures that can be categorized in multiple ordered categories, it is possible to evaluate dose-response gradients of effect. In the HPFS of suicide, the social integration measure actually had four ordered categories. To this point, we have considered only the most extreme contrast of risk among the highest level of social integration compared at the corresponding risk for the lowest level. To examine a dose-response gradient, we can calculate an RR for each of the two intermediate levels of social integration. For purposes of consistency, we always use the same referent or baseline group as the unexposed (in this example, men with the lowest level of social integration). **Table 8-3** provides a summary of the comparison of the suicide risk for the men in the second highest level of social integration compared with those in the lowest social integration category. Here, the RR is:

$$RR = \frac{28}{7508} \Big/ \frac{23}{2937} = 0.48$$

Table 8-3. Summary of results from Health Professionals Follow-up Study showing the suicide risk among men with the second highest level of social integration compared with the corresponding risk among men with the lowest levels of social integration.

Suicide	Social Integration		
	Second Highest	Lowest	Total
Yes	28	23	51
No	7480	2914	10,394
Total	7508	2937	10,445

Data from Tsai AC, Lucas M, Sania A, Kim D, Kawachi I. Social integration and suicide mortality among men: 24-year study of U.S. Health Professionals. *Ann Intern Med.* 2014;161:85-95.

Table 8-4. Summary of results from Health Professionals Follow-up Study showing the suicide risk among men with the third highest level of social integration compared with the corresponding risk among men with the lowest levels of social integration.

Suicide	Social Integration		
	Third Highest	Lowest	Total
Yes	55	23	78
No	9925	2914	12,839
Total	9980	2937	12,917

Data from Tsai AC, Lucas M, Sania A, Kim D, Kawachi I. Social integration and suicide mortality among men: 24-year study of U.S. Health Professionals. *Ann Intern Med.* 2014;161:85-95.

Next we calculate the suicide RR for men in the third highest level of social integration compared with those in the lowest level of social integration from the data shown in **Table 8-4**.

$$RR = \frac{55}{9980} \bigg/ \frac{23}{2937} = 0.70$$

Now we have the data necessary to calculate a dose-response curve. **Figure 8-2** provides a graphical summary of suicide RRs by level of social integration, with the lowest level of social integration used as the referent (RR = 1). Here we can see a progressive

decline in suicide risk as social integration increases. This dose (of social integration) response (suicide risk) provides evidence to support an inference that the association is one of cause and effect.

Attributable Risk Percent

The difference in risk of the outcome of interest in relation to exposure level can be quantified in ways other than a ratio. One alternative is to subtract the risk among unexposed persons from the risk among the exposed. This measure is referred to as **risk difference (RD)** (sometimes also called the **attributable risk**).

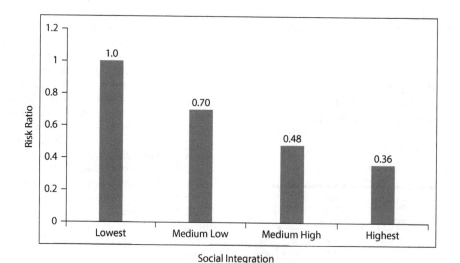

Figure 8-2. Dose-response relationship of suicide risk as a function of increasing levels of social integration among men. (Data from Tsai AC, Lucas M, Sania A, Kim D, Kawachi I. Social integration and suicide mortality among men: 24-year study of U.S. Health Professionals. *Ann Intern Med.* 2014;161:85-95.)

Referring to the notation introduced in **Table 8-1**, the RD is calculated as:

$$RD = R_{exposed} - R_{unexposed} \frac{A}{A + C} - \frac{B}{B + D}$$

Using the data from **Table 8-2**, the **RD** for suicide comparing the highest level of social integration to the lowest is:

$$RD = \frac{41}{14,476} - \frac{23}{2937} = 0.0028 - 0.0078$$

$$= -0.005$$

This means that the suicide risk among men in the highest category of social interaction is 0.005 lower than that for those in the lowest category. To place this difference in risk into perspective, it is useful to scale it to the total risk (from exposure and other contributors). For exposures that increase risk, we use the total risk among the exposed as the scaling factor. This scaled measure is referred to as **attributable risk percent (ARP)** and is calculated as:

$$ARP = \frac{R_{exposed} - R_{unexposed}}{R_{exposed}} \times 100$$

$$= \frac{A/(A + C) - B/(B + D)}{A/(A + C)} \times 100$$

When the exposure reduces risk, it makes more sense to scale the apparent protective effect against the total risk among the unprotected (or unexposed) group as:

$$ARP_{prot} = \frac{R_{exposed} - R_{unexposed}}{R_{unexposed}} \times 100$$

For the social integration–suicide example, this corresponds to:

$$ARP_{prot} = \frac{0.0028 - 0.0078}{0.0078} \times 100 = \frac{-0.005}{0.0078} \times 100$$

$$= -64\%$$

That is to say, the highest level of social integration is associated with a reduction in the risk of suicide of 64% compared with men with the lowest level of social integration.

Rate Ratio

Thus far, we have focused on a comparison of risks, or cumulative incidence, in contrasting the experience of

Table 8-5. Summary of incidence (or mortality) rate data from a cohort study.

	Exposed Persons	Unexposed Persons	Total
Number of outcomes	A	B	A + B
Person-time (PT)	$PT_{exposed}$	$PT_{unexposed}$	PT_{Total}

exposed and unexposed persons. Alternately, one can use a contrast of incidence rates (or mortality rates) for this purpose. Data for a rate comparison would appear in the format shown in **Table 8-5**. The **rate ratio** is calculated as:

$$Rate\ ratio = \frac{Rate\ of\ outcome\ among\ exposed}{Rate\ of\ outcome\ among\ unexposed}$$

$$= \frac{A/PT_{exposed}}{B/PT_{unexposed}}$$

where PT is person-time. As a ratio measure of comparison, the value of the rate ratio has an analogous interpretation to that of the RR. Specifically, an exposure associated with a lowered rate of the outcome has a rate ratio less than 1. An exposure that is associated with an increased rate of the outcome has a value greater than 1. When the exposure has no association with the outcome, the rate ratio is 1. The further away the rate ratio lies from 1 (the null value), the stronger the apparent association.

The calculation of a rate ratio can be illustrated from data reported from the HPFS of suicide. In that study, the contrast of men with the highest level of social integration compared with the men with the lowest level is summarized in **Table 8-6**. The rate ratio is calculated as:

$$Rate\ ratio = \frac{41/297,146}{23/58,634} = 0.35$$

That is, the suicide rate among men with the highest level of social integration was about one third of that for men with the lowest level of social integration. This association was unchanged by mathematical adjustment for the effect of age on the suicide rate. The investigators then went on to conduct a statistical analysis adjusting for the effects of hypertension, elevated cholesterol levels, diabetes, renal failure, employment status, smoking, alcohol use, caffeine consumption, use of antidepressants, physical activity, obesity, and having had a physical examination

Table 8-6. Summary of results from the Health Professions Follow-up Study showing the suicide rate among men with the highest level of social integration compared with the corresponding rate among men with the lowest level of social integration.

	Social Integration		
	Highest	Lowest	Total
Suicides	41	23	64
Person-time	297,146	58,634	355,780

Data from Tsai AC, Lucas M, Sania A, Kim D, Kawachi I. Social integration and suicide mortality among men: 24-year study of U.S. Health Professionals. *Ann Intern Med.* 2014;161:85-95.

within 2 years. Even after all of these other characteristics were considered, the rate ratio comparing the highest to lowest levels of social integration remained 0.41. The 95% CI ranged from 0.24 to 0.69. The investigators could conclude, therefore, that increasing social integration had a moderately strong association with a lower suicide rate among men and that this association was not attributable to a large number of other characteristics, nor was it likely to have arisen by chance alone.

The analysis of cohort studies, while following the basic principles outlined above, often involves more sophisticated statistical modeling techniques. These methods allow the treatment of the exposure (as well as the outcome) in multiple categories or as a continuous variable. In addition, mathematical models can account for the potential influence of other prognostic factors that are measured. When there are multiple variables that could affect the outcome of interest and may be differentially distributed between exposed and unexposed persons, it is important to ensure that the effects of these other variables are considered in the analysis. The approach to mathematical modeling is beyond the scope of the present discussion. For those interested in conducting analyses of cohort studies, Epi Info, a free, easy-to-use software package developed by the Centers for Disease Control and Prevention, is available at wwww.cdc.gov/epiinfo.

SUMMARY

In this chapter, we introduced the basic principles of the conduct of cohort studies, using research on levels of social integration and suicide risk to illustrate the concepts. A cohort study is an observational (as opposed to experimental) research design in which the investigator observes the natural occurrence of

exposures and disease. Sampling for a cohort study is based on exposure status, and subjects are followed over time to determine their respective risk or rate of disease development. Some cohort studies are **prospective** in approach. That is, all events—exposure and disease occurrence—happen after the onset of the study. Other cohort studies are **retrospective** in design, meaning that all of the events in question—both exposure and disease occurrence—have occurred before the onset of the study. The retrospective approach may be advantageous for diseases that are slowly developing over many years or decades by allowing faster answers, generally at much lower expense. However, retrospective studies typically rely on already available data sources, which can be incomplete or inaccurate, thereby potentially affecting the validity of inferences that can be drawn.

Cohort studies are useful for the study of rare exposures because sampling can be based on the selective inclusion of exposed persons. In contrast, for disease outcomes that are rare, the cohort study design can be inefficient because very large study populations may be required for researchers to observe a sufficient number of outcome events. Suicide is an example of a relatively infrequent event, necessitating the study of tens of thousands of subjects.

The analysis of a cohort study is based on a comparison of disease occurrence among exposed persons in relation to that among unexposed persons. Most often, this is expressed as a ratio measure. If the contrast is based on the risk (or cumulative incidence) of disease occurrence over a specified period of time, the measure of effect is the **RR** (the risk of disease among exposed divided by the corresponding risk among unexposed). The null value of the RR is 1—that is, risk of disease is not affected by exposure of interest. Values of the RR between 0 and 1 reflect lowered risk associated with exposure, with further distance from the null value indicating stronger association. Conversely, values of the RR greater than 1 correspond to increased risk associated with exposure, and again, stronger relationships are indicated by greater distance from 1. Typically, 95% CIs are calculated around the point estimate of the association to demonstrate the range of values that are statistically consistent with the observed data.

The **rate ratio** is an alternate summary measure of association in a cohort study and is preferred when the focus is on the rate (either incidence or mortality or both) of disease occurrence and contrasted between exposed and unexposed persons. The interpretation of the rate ratio values is analogous to that of the RR, with a null value of 1, lowered rate among exposed indicated by values less than 1, and increased rate among exposed indicated by values greater than 1. In addition, we introduced the concept of **RD** and **ARP** as alternative ways to quantify the association of exposure and disease occurrence.

Throughout this chapter, we illustrated basic concepts with data from the HPFS, which studied social integration level and subsequent suicide risk. For this study, a large cohort of middle-aged men in the health professions was identified in 1986, and 2 years later, nearly 35,000 of them completed a self-administered survey that allowed classification into four levels of social integration. The men were followed for 24 years to determine subsequent occurrence of suicide, of which 147 were identified. The suicide RR (95% CI) comparing men with the highest level of social integration to those with the lowest level was 0.36 (0.26, 0.50). In other words, men with the highest level of social integration had only about one third the risk of subsequent suicide as did men in the lowest level of social integration. The exclusion of the null value from the CI indicated that this association was unlikely a result of chance alone. Moreover, when graded levels of increasing social integration were each assessed against the baseline lowest level, a dose-response relationship with suicide risk was observed, falling progressively from 1 to 0.70 to 0.48 to 0.36. A similar set of findings was obtained if suicide rates were contrasted with a **rate ratio** measure (0.35 for the most extreme contrast of social integration levels), and mathematical adjustment for a wide range of other suspected predictors of suicide risk had minimal impact on the observed association with social integration. The HPFS, therefore, provides support for the notion that social factors are influential in determining suicide risk, at least among middle-aged male health professionals.

STUDY QUESTIONS

1. Which of the following is NOT a feature of a cohort study?
   A. Exposure is determined by randomization.
   B. Exposure level must be assessed.
   C. Subjects are followed for the development of disease.
   D. Risk ratio is a commonly used measure of effect.
   E. It can be used to study either protective or harmful exposures.

2. A rate ratio (95% CI) calculated from a cohort study is 1.7 (0.8, 3.4). The most appropriate interpretation is
   A. the exposure is associated with a lower rate and the result is statistically significant.

   B. the exposure is associated with a lower rate, but the result is not statistically significant.
   C. the exposure is associated with increased rate, and the result is statistically significant.
   D. the exposure is associated with increased rate, but the result is not statistically significant.
   E. none of the above.

3. Each of the following is a feature of a retrospective cohort study EXCEPT
   A. it is efficient for the study of rare exposures.
   B. information on exposures typically is accurate and complete.
   C. it is efficient for the study of slowly developing diseases.
   D. it typically can be completed more quickly than a prospective cohort study.
   E. it may rely on already collected information.

4. Misclassification of disease status, if it is unrelated to exposure, is expected to have what impact on the results of a cohort study?
   A. Result in a reversal of the association of interest
   B. Increase the apparent strength of association
   C. Decrease the apparent strength of association
   D. Impact cannot be predicted

5. The null value of the rate ratio is
   A. 0.
   B. 0.1.
   C. 1.
   D. 10.
   E. infinity.

6. If initial exposure status changes during the course of a cohort study, but this is not related to disease status, the likely impact on the strength of the apparent exposure–disease association is to
   A. increase it.
   B. decrease it.
   C. not change it.
   D. not be predictable.

7. Cohort studies are efficient for the study of the following EXCEPT
   A. diseases that are rare.
   B. diseases with short incubation periods.
   C. exposures that are rare.
   D. exposures that are common.

8. A dose-response relationship in a cohort study helps to support the conclusion that an association is

   A. therapeutic.

   B. statistically significant.

   C. clinically significant.

   D. biologically significant.

   E. cause and effect.

9. Compared with a retrospective cohort study, a prospective cohort study of a particular question has what advantage?

   A. Can be completed more quickly

   B. Can be used to study exposures that no longer occur

   C. Typically is less expensive

   D. Is sufficient for studying slowly developing diseases

   E. Allows more complete and accurate information on exposures

10. To reduce any impact in a cohort study from a clinically unrecognized disease at the outset of the study, the investigator may

   A. perform autopsies on all persons with a diagnosis of the disease of interest.

   B. eliminate from analysis all disease diagnosed in the first few years of the study.

   C. review all prior medical records and laboratory reports for exposed and unexposed subjects.

   D. consult a panel of experts in the disease of interest.

   E. blind the subjects to the exposure of interest.

FURTHER READING

Goldberg RJ, McManus DD, Allison J. Greater knowledge and appreciation of commonly used research study designs. *Am J Med*. 2013;126:169e1-e8.

Thiese MS. Observational and interventional study design types; an overview. *Biochmia Medica*. 2014;24:199-210.

REFERENCES

Clinical Background

du Roscoät E, Beck F. Efficient interventions on suicide prevention: a literature review. *Rev d'Epidemiol Santé Publique*. 2013;61:363-374.

Morriss R, Kapur N, Byng R. Assessing risk of suicide or self harm in adults. *BMJ*. 2013;347:f4571.

Nock MK, Deming CA, Fullerton CS, et al. Suicide among soldiers: a review of psychosocial risk and protective factors. *Psychiatry*. 2013;76:97-125.

O'Connor E, Gaynes BN, Burda BU, Soh C, Whitlock EP. Screening for and treatment of suicide risk relevant to primary care: a systematic review for the U. S. Preventive Services Task Force. *Ann Intern Med*. 2013;158:741-754.

Pandey GN. Biological basis of suicide and suicide behavior. *Bipolar Disord*. 2013;15:524-541.

Observational Studies

Alspach AG. Make time to make nursing history in the Nurses' Health Study. *Crit Care Nurse*. 2011;31:9-11.

Concato J. Study design and "evidence" in patient-oriented research. *Am J Respir Crit Care Med*. 2013;187:1167-1172.

Tsai AC, Lucas M, Sania A, Kim D, Kawachi I. Social integration and suicide mortality among men: 24-year study of U.S. Health Professionals. *Ann Intern Med*. 2014;161:85-95.

Analysis

Tsai AC, Lucas M, Sania A, Kim D, Kawachi I. Social integration and suicide mortality among men: 24-year study of U. S. Health Professionals. *Ann Intern Med*. 2014;161:85-95.

Case-Control Studies

Raymond S. Greenberg and Daniel T. Lackland

HEALTH SCENARIO

In 1986, Barker and Osmond published a study that examined patterns of death related to coronary heart disease in England and Wales between 1968 and 1978. These investigators found that the death rates in the northern industrial towns were about 20% above the national average. In contrast, the more affluent areas in the rural south and east had heart disease death rates that were 20% below the national average. The pattern of death rates from coronary heart disease among adults paralleled that for infant mortality a half century earlier. One in 10 newborns died in the first year of life in the industrial north compared with one in 20 in the rural south and east.

This ecological association between infant mortality and adult heart disease led these investigators to conduct a subsequent study of men born between 1911 and 1930 in Hertfordshire, England and followed them for subsequent risk of death from coronary heart disease. They found that low-birth-weight (LBW) infants had a 50% increased death rate from heart disease as adults. The results were even more striking with weight at 1 year of age—those in the lowest weight category (≤18 lb) had a twofold increase in risk of death from adult heart disease.

The observation that events before birth and shortly thereafter could affect the risk of disease five or more decades later became known variously as the "Barker Hypothesis," "The Thrifty Phenotype Hypothesis," or the "Fetal Origins Hypothesis." The basic premise of this theory is that adult heart disease (and related conditions such as diabetes mellitus, obesity, and hypertension) may arise because of the body's response to undernutrition early in life. A number of mechanisms have been suggested, including metabolic responses to undernutrition in utero leading to decreased insulin secretion from the pancreas, diminished insulin sensitivity in muscles in order to conserve glucose, increased cortisol secretion, reduced number of nephrons, diminished myocytes, and impaired endothelial function.

The association between low birth weight and chronic diseases in adulthood has been demonstrated in many populations for heart disease, diabetes mellitus, hypertension, and obesity. Less clear is whether other chronic conditions, such as renal insufficiency, may have a link to LBW. In this chapter, we will explore how the LBW association with adult renal insufficiency can be explored using the case-control research approach.

CLINICAL BACKGROUND

Low birth weight is defined as a weight at birth of less than 2500 g (5 lb, 8 oz). Further distinctions, such as very low birth weight (VLBW) at less than 1500 g and extremely low birth weight (ELBW) at less than 1000 g, can be made, but our focus here is on LBW. At present, approximately 1 in 12 newborns in the United States falls with the LBW classification, which represents nearly a quarter of a million affected births in the United States each year. There are two major contributors to LBW: prematurity (<37 weeks' gestation), which accounts for about 70% of LBW, and fetal growth restriction, which can occur at any gestational age. The maternal characteristics associated with pregnancies resulting in LBW infants include low socioeconomic status (as indicated by either income or education level), being African American, or being young (younger than 17 years of age).

A number of specific risk factors are associated with the likelihood of delivering an LBW infant, including multiple fetus pregnancies; use of cigarettes, alcohol, or street drugs; placental problems; cervical incompetence; insufficient maternal weight gain; and various infections (e.g., rubella, cytomegalovirus, toxoplasmosis, syphilis). LBW newborns are at risk of a variety of adverse events during infancy, including, but not limited to, infection, developmental delay, and death.

Turning now to chronic kidney disease (CKD), this condition may be defined as the progressive loss of renal function over a period of at least 3 months. Five stages of CKD have been delineated on the basis of level of impairment from 1 (often asymptomatic and undetected but possibly discovered by the presence of either blood cells or protein in the urine) through 5 (end-stage renal disease requiring replaced kidney function either through dialysis or transplantation). Globally, CKD is the 18th leading cause of death, with the highest incidence and prevalence in Taiwan; the second highest incidence and third highest prevalence occur in the United States. Approximately 10% of the adult population of the United States—in excess of 20 million persons—has CKD. The occurrence is elevated among African Americans and Mexican Americans compared with non-Hispanic whites. An estimate of the cost of care through the Medicare program is about $75,000 per affected person, or more than $50 billion per year in aggregate.

There are two leading risk factors for the development of CKD, which together account for nearly three fourths of all affected individuals. These risk factors are diabetes mellitus (about one third of individuals with diabetes have CKD) and high blood pressure (about one fifth of individuals with hypertension have CKD). Other risk factors include cardiovascular disease, hyperlipidemia, obesity, systemic lupus erythematosus, and a positive family history. CKD, in turn, can increase the risk of cardiovascular disease, myocardial infarction, and stroke. Other complications include pulmonary edema, anemia, immune compromise, and protein malnutrition. The management of CKD is targeted at addressing its many manifestations, typically involving dietary phosphate restriction and calcium supplementation; oral alkali agents; loop diuretics; and if necessary, erythropoietin for anemia. When the disease progresses to stage 5, either dialysis or organ transplantation is indicated. Obviously, it is far preferable to either prevent the disease in the first place or manage it effectively at its early phases than to try to treat it when it has reached the end stage.

INTRODUCTION

The question of whether LBW is associated with the risk of CKD in adulthood illustrates the challenges of using either clinical trials (see Chapter 7) or cohort studies (see Chapter 8) to address the hypothesis. For a clinical trial, one has the obvious prohibition on ethical grounds of exposing subject to an intervention (LBW) that one knows to be harmful. Whether or not it causes CKD in adults, LBW is known to lead to many adverse health outcomes in childhood. Even if the ethical constraint did not exist, it is unclear how one could randomly allocate subjects to having LBW, short of intentionally malnourishing pregnant women or delivering their babies prematurely, each of which

is associated with its own set of near-term adverse consequences.

A cohort study design would avoid the ethical problems of a clinical trial, but it would come with its own set of pragmatic constraints. Most obvious is the fact that the exposure (LBW) occurs a half century or more before the occurrence of the outcome (CKD). To identify and follow a cohort for such a lengthy period of time in a prospective manner would be a protracted and expensive process, with a high likelihood of subjects being lost to follow-up. Moreover, for either a clinical trial or a prospective cohort study, one would not be able to obtain an answer to the research question for 50 or more years.

By using a retrospective cohort design, one can essentially "compress time" by using historical information on exposure (LBW), with either historical or current information on the outcome (CKD). In fact, a number of retrospective cohort studies of this question have been performed. Settings in which relatively complete and accurate historical data are available on exposure, other comorbid conditions, and outcome status would be particularly well suited to this kind of investigation. Even in those settings, however, the completeness of ascertainment of the outcome may be questioned because CKD typically is asymptomatic in its early stages and may be discovered only as an incidental finding or because of heightened suspicion because of the presence of other predisposing conditions, such as hypertension or diabetes mellitus.

The long latent period between exposure and disease occurrence, although somewhat extreme for the LBW–CKD example, is not uncommon for chronic diseases. The development of many conditions, such as coronary heart disease, cancer, and stroke, among others, typically spans many years, if not decades. This presents a challenge for reaching timely and cost-effective conclusions. In addition to the retrospective cohort study, one might consider the use of another research design—the case-control study—to address an exposure–disease relationship with a long latent period.

CASE-CONTROL STUDIES

Chapter 8 discussed that the basic design of a cohort study is to sample subjects based on their being exposed or not and then to follow them for subsequent development of the outcome. A case-control study starts at the end of the process, when the outcome is already determined. Instead of sampling exposed and nonexposed persons, the investigator of a case-control study samples persons with the outcome of interest (cases) and constructs a comparison group (controls) of individuals who do not have the outcome of interest. The design of the case-control study is illustrated in

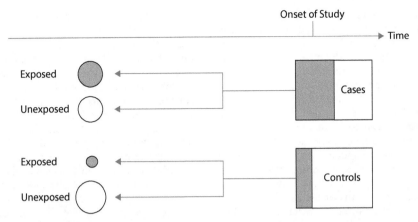

Figure 9-1. Illustration of the design of a case-control study. Shaded areas represent exposed persons, and unshaded areas represent unexposed persons.

Figure 9-1. In essence, the study starts on the right-hand side of the diagram with the identification of cases and controls. It then "looks backward in time" to identify earlier exposure patterns among the subjects. If it turns out that more cases than controls had an exposure of interest, it may be evidence that exposure is associated positively with outcome (i.e., exposure increases the risk of disease development). However, if cases are less likely than controls to have had the exposure of interest, it may constitute evidence that exposure is associated inversely with outcome (i.e., exposure decreases the risk of disease development).

The general design of a case-control study shown in **Figure 9-1** can be illustrated by a study of LBW and CKD. The investigator would initiate such a study by identifying either newly diagnosed (**incident**) or existing (**prevalent**) cases of CKD. She would then proceed to collect information on exposure (LBW) from subject recall, or preferably, birth records or registration data, if available. In the next sections, we will consider each of these steps in greater detail.

Cases

The sampling of cases is one of the first steps in conducting a case-control study. The investigator must begin by defining the criteria for establishing what constitutes an affected individual. In some instances, it may be relatively clear how to diagnose the condition of interest. For example, many forms of cancer require a histologic confirmation of diagnosis to establish the presence of the disease of interest. As already mentioned, CKD is a spectrum of illness that stretches from asymptomatic mild impairment to severe, end-stage disease. Fortunately, there are standardized criteria for establishing a diagnosis and further categorizing the stages of illness. It should be evident that patients with more severe manifestations of illness are more likely to come to clinical recognition. This may not be a concern for a case-control study if the exposure is equally linked to all stages of illness. In some situations, however, there may be reason to believe that the disease associated with a particular exposure is either very mild or very severe. In such a circumstance, studying a limited range of disease severity in a case-control study may either miss or overstate the magnitude of the association between exposure and disease. To avoid such a problem, the investigator in a study of CKD may need to find affected individuals who have not otherwise come to medical attention already. For example, one might identify individuals in stage 1 CKD through a community-based screening program.

When affected individuals become symptomatic and seek medical care, the process of identifying them becomes more straightforward. Traditional sources of information for finding cases include medical records in hospitals and outpatient clinics, laboratories and other diagnostic facilities, reimbursement data, and other registration systems.

Equally important to establishing the definition of a case is to identify the sampling frame from which cases will be selected. At least two different general approaches warrant further discussion. One is to choose a **hospital-based** sample, which generally means finding the cases from the records of one or more treating facility. The advantages of this approach are that it is efficient, cost effective, and fast. It can also simplify the selection of controls if they are sampled from other patients (without CKD) who are treated at those same facilities.

These pragmatic advantages of a hospital-based case-control study must be weighed against several disadvantages. First, as already mentioned, it tends to select a sample of affected individuals who are symptomatic and have sought care. Those who are either asymptomatic or symptomatic but have poor access to care (generally associated with lower socioeconomic status) are less likely to be included. Second referral patterns to hospitals can be quite selective and could result in a skewed sample of patients at any particular facility. For example, public hospitals may tend to treat more low-income or uninsured patients. Teaching hospitals may tend to have more patients with unusual or severe forms of disease. These selection factors can be minimized somewhat by including multiple hospitals with differing referral patterns. Ideally, the inclusion of all hospitals in a region would tend to minimize selective inclusion of affected patients. Choosing controls from the same hospitals tends to control for differential referral patterns because, presumably, they would be similar for cases and controls admitted to the same hospitals. Choosing controls in a hospital-based case-control study has its own issues, which will be discussed in the next section.

The counterpart to a hospital-based case-control study is a **population-based** case-control study. Here, the intent is to identify all of the cases that arise within a population. Typically, the population is defined by place of residence, such as within a particular city, region, or state. The population could be defined by other parameters, however. For example, one could select the population of interest on the basis of occupation or participation in a particular health insurance plan. A population-based study has the advantage of potentially more complete case finding and avoiding potential pitfalls of referral patterns. Because controls can be selected from the same well-defined source population, they may constitute a more representative and unbiased comparison group. The challenges of a population-based study are pragmatic concerns, such as potentially greater time and expense to complete.

Controls

Although the selection of cases may seem to be the complicated sampling issue in a case-control study, it turns out that there are at least as many considerations in the selection of controls. The guiding principle for control selection is that they should come from the same population as gave rise to the cases. Another way of expressing this concept is to choose controls who would have been included as cases, had they developed the disease of interest. For population-based studies, there are a variety of methods to choose controls at random from the general population. One can use census data, or alternatively, tax records, driver's license registration, random telephone calling, or a variety of other methods. The key issues are to use a source that has complete or nearly complete enumeration of the population and a sampling strategy that gives all eligible persons an equal chance to be selected.

For hospital-based studies, as already indicated, controls can be selected from among other patients treated at the same facilities. This tends to reduce or eliminate any distortion that might arise from selective referral patterns to the facilities of interest. Among the many patients treated at the hospital(s) included, however, how does one choose which individuals to enroll as controls? One wants to avoid any diagnosis that shares risk factors with the disease of interest. So, for example, in a hospital-based case-control study of LBW and CKD, one would want to avoid sampling controls from patients who have risk factors for CKD, such as hypertension or diabetes, or conditions related to them, such as coronary heart disease, stroke, peripheral vascular disease, retinopathy, or neuropathy. In a study of LBW as the exposure, it also would be important to avoid sampling controls from conditions known to be related to LBW (hypertension, diabetes mellitus, heart disease, and lipid abnormalities). These many exclusions may greatly limit the pool of eligible hospitalized patients. One often used guideline is to sample controls from patients admitted with a number of different diagnoses so that the controls are not unduly weighted by a risk factor profile of one or a few conditions. Another frequent guideline is to sample controls preferentially from patients with acute diagnoses so that they do not have a long-standing condition that could distort their exposure history. Examples of conditions that would meet such a criterion would be trauma, acute appendicitis, pneumonia, sepsis, urinary infections, and skin infections. It should be emphasized that although these guidelines may be helpful in selecting a comparison group, there is not a guarantee that bias will be eliminated.

Determination of Exposure

After the cases and controls have been selected, the next task is to collect information on the exposure of interest. Because the exposures all occurred in the past, there may be real constraints in terms of the sources of information, as well as the level of completeness and accuracy. A variety of methods may be considered for collecting exposure information.

One of the most common strategies is to conduct interviews with cases and controls or ask them to complete questionnaires. Interviews and questionnaires generally involve minimal burden on the subjects and can be completed relatively quickly and inexpensively. At the same time, interview data are imperfect at best because the ability of subjects to recall exposures can be highly variable, especially for exposures that occurred many years earlier. In addition, often there is concern that the recall of earlier events will differ systematically between cases and controls. Specifically, persons with serious illnesses have a high level of motivation to recall events that might have contributed to their illnesses. Controls, especially if they are healthy or have only an acute illness, have a different mindset and may not be as thorough in their recall. It is also possible that cases may tend to overreport actual exposures, especially if they have done research on their illnesses and are aware of suspected risk factors, including the focus of the study. To the extent possible, one would like to blind the interviewers and respondents to the exposure of interest and to ask about a variety of exposures so that the exposure of interest is not obvious.

Whenever possible, it also is beneficial to validate reported exposure histories through other data sources. It is also desirable to assess the reliability of the questionnaire or interview by asking a sample of subjects the same questions at different points in time and looking for consistency across the responses.

Another common approach to collecting information on exposure is to access medical, education, work, or other record sources. This is particularly relevant for a study of LBW because birth weights have been recorded on birth certificates and in hospital records for many years, and this information tends to be fairly accurate and complete. Total reliance on historical records, however, can be difficult or impossible depending on their quality and thoroughness. Because the information was not originally recorded for scientific purposes, it often lacks the kind of rigor one expects and requires in a research study. The level of missing or incomplete information can be substantial. Statistical methods can be used to impute missing values, but this is sophisticated guesswork and has uncertainty associated with it. Inaccurate information, whether from records or recall, if it arises similarly for cases and controls, will serve to make it more difficult to detect a true exposure–disease association. That is, any bias will be a conservative one. If an association is still observed despite the misclassified exposure information, the true association is expected to be as large as or larger than the magnitude observed. The same cannot be said if the misclassification of exposure is differential for cases and controls. If cases preferentially tend to overreport a putative harmful exposure, the observed association may be stronger than the true effect. If cases preferentially tend to underreport a putative harmful exposure, it could produce an underestimate of the true effect.

A third approach to collecting information on exposure is to have some direct or indirect measurement of it. For example, one might be able to measure blood levels of certain agents. This is particularly helpful if there are appropriately stored specimens (e.g., umbilical cord blood) that can be assessed for cases and controls. The problem is that such banks of stored specimens are not widely available. Even if they were, for many case-control studies, the specimens would have to be stored without degradation or compromise for many years or decades. Even if blood specimens are available, for many exposures, there is not an appropriate biological marker available. In other instances, a marker may be available, but it is only measurable for a short period of time, making it impossible to use in a study that spans many years.

Analysis

In the most basic form of analysis, for a case-control study, both disease status (case vs. control) and exposure status (exposed vs. unexposed) are treated as simple dichotomous variables. In such a situation, there are four possible classifications of individual subjects:

A. Cases who were exposed

B. Cases who were not exposed

C. Controls who were exposed

D. Controls who were not exposed

We can summarize these four groups in a tabular format as illustrated in **Table 9-1**. This display appears identical to the 2 × 2 (or fourfold) table introduced in the analysis of cohort studies (see Chapter 8). Nevertheless, the approach to sampling in cohort studies (based on exposure status) is fundamentally different from that in case-control studies (based on disease status). As a result, in a cohort study, the investigator determines the ratio of exposed (A + C) to unexposed (B + D) persons and determines the risk of disease development in each group. In contrast, in a case-control study, the investigator determines the ratio of cases (A + B) to controls (C + D) and thereby sets the proportion of individuals in the study who are affected by the disease. For example, if there are equal numbers of cases and controls, half of the study subjects will have the disease of interest. Typically, in a case-control study,

Table 9-1. Summary format for data collected in a case-control study.

	Exposed	Unexposed	Total
Case	A	B	A + B
Control	C	D	C + D
Total	A + C	B + D	A + B + C + D

the investigator will oversample affected individuals in the source population, especially if the disease of interest is rare. In such a setting, it no longer makes sense to consider risk of disease development as the outcome of interest. If calculating risk no longer makes sense, then the risk ratio is not an appropriate measure of association. We can, nevertheless, calculate another measure of association in the case-control study design.

We begin by considering the exposure probability among cases, or the proportion of cases who were exposed previously. Using the notation introduced in **Table 9-1**, we calculate this probability as:

$$\text{Case exposure probability} = \frac{\text{Exposed cases}}{\text{All cases}}$$

$$= \frac{A}{A + B}$$

The odds of a case being exposed are estimated by the probability of a case being exposed divided by the probability of a case being unexposed. This measure is calculated as:

$$\text{Odds of case exposure} = \frac{\text{Exposed cases}}{\text{All cases}} \Big/ \frac{\text{Unexposed cases}}{\text{All cases}}$$

$$= \frac{A}{A + B} \Big/ \frac{B}{A + B} = \frac{A}{B}$$

Using a comparable calculation, the odds of exposure among controls can be shown to be estimated by:

$$\text{Odds of control exposure} = \frac{C}{D}$$

The ratio of these two odds (odds of exposure among cases divided by odds of exposure among controls) is referred to as the **odds ratio** (**OR**). The OR is calculated as:

$$\text{OR} = \frac{\text{Odds of case exposure}}{\text{Odds of control exposure}}$$

$$= \frac{A}{B} \Big/ \frac{C}{D} = \frac{A \times D}{B \times C}$$

When newly diagnosed (incident) cases are sampled from the same source population as controls, and sampling is independent of exposure history (all features of a well-designed case-control study), it can be shown that the OR gives an approximation to the incidence rate ratio. So, although the OR is a distinct

measure of association and the preferred measure in a case-control study, it has an interpretation analogous to the rate ratio or risk ratio. The null value (no association) of the OR is 1. Values of the OR greater than 1 indicate a positive association between exposure and disease. Values of the OR below 1 indicate an inverse association between exposure and disease.

To illustrate the calculation of an OR, let us consider a case-control study of LBW and end-stage renal disease (ESRD) conducted by Lackland and colleagues (2000). The investigators identified patients with ESRD from a regional registry of all persons undergoing dialysis for chronic renal failure. The birth certificates of these individuals were then located through a search of vital records information. From the birth certificates, information was extracted on LBW and other characteristics. Two controls of the same sex and race were selected for each case from the next registered birth certificates, which were filed in order of receipt, thereby tightly linking the respective birthdates of cases and controls. For the purposes of analysis, birth weights were classified into five ordered categories, with LBW defined, following convention, as less than 2500 g. The middle birth weight category of 3000 to 3499 g chosen as the referent (unexposed) group. A summary of the data that were observed is shown in **Table 9-2**. The OR calculated from these data would be:

$$\text{OR} = \frac{A \times D}{B \times C} = \frac{147 \times 882}{435 \times 222} = 1.34$$

In other words, the odds of having been LBW were 34% higher among cases of ESRD than among controls. As with risk ratios, 95% confidence intervals (CIs) can be calculated around the point estimate of the OR. The approximate 95% CI for this OR is (1.06, 1.70). Because it excludes the null value (OR = 1), we can conclude that the observed association is unlikely to have arisen from chance alone. The strength of the association, as judged by the distance from the null value, nevertheless, may be characterized

Table 9-2. Summary of data on the association of low birth weight (LBW) with end-stage renal disease (ESRD).

	LBW	Not LBW	Total
Case	147	435	582
Control	222	882	1104
Total	369	1317	1686

Data from Lackland DT, Bendall HE, Osmond C, Egan BM, Barker DJ. Low birth weights contribute to the high rates of early-onset chronic renal failure in the Southeastern United States. *Arch Intern Med.* 2000;160:1472-1476.

as relatively weak. As a rough guideline for interpretation, a moderate association would correspond to an OR approaching 2, and a relatively strong association would correspond to an OR of 3 or greater. These are somewhat subjective interpretations; however, a relatively weak strength of association may still have public health importance if the exposure is common and the disease involves appreciable morbidity and mortality.

Matching

A commonly used approach to selecting controls is to choose them in a direct pairing with individual cases. So, for example, we might choose for a white, male case who is age 65 years a white, male control of similar age (± a few years). We refer to this person-to-person alignment of cases and controls as **matching**. Another way of expressing this process is that controls are selected to parallel selected attributes of cases, such as demographic characteristics. The motivation for matching usually is to remove any disparity in these characteristics between the groups under comparison. There are two reasons for wanting to remove the influences of these other variables. The first is to reduce the potential for **confounding**. Confounding is a distorted exposure–disease association that is attributable in part or in whole to the influence of factors other than the exposure of interest. Confounding may be present when the persons who have the exposure of interest also have other risk factors that are less common in nonexposed persons. By matching, we remove any association of these matched factors with disease status (case vs. control) in the study population. This intent is achieved if matching is considered appropriately in the analysis.

A second motivation for matching is to obtain a more statistically precise estimate of effect, as might be reflected in narrower CIs around the point estimate. Again, this benefit requires an appropriate analysis for the matched design. From a purely pragmatic point of view, matching can help direct and simplify the process of selecting controls. For example, in the cited study of LBW and ESRD, after the cases were selected, a variety of methods could have been used to select controls, including using random digit telephone dialing, tax records, motor vehicle registrations, and so on. Because the information on LBW was going to be extracted from birth records, it made sense to use this source of information for selecting controls. By doing so, one could ensure that exposure information was available on controls and would be of similar quality and completeness to that of cases. The subjects were easily, quickly, and inexpensively sampled on the basis of sex, race, and date of birth. Here, then, the matching factors were three commonly used demographic characteristics. One often sees matching

performed on the basis of these (or other) demographic attributes because often they are related to exposure likelihood as well as disease occurrence.

Matching can be performed on a one case-to-one control basis (pair matching). Alternatively, one often sees two, three, or more controls matched for each case. Enlarging the number of controls per case increases the statistical power of the study. This may be an important consideration for rare diseases where the number of eligible cases is limited. However, one reaches the point of diminishing returns in terms of statistical power by increasing the size of the control group. Typically, there is minimal gain in precision beyond a ratio of four controls per case. In the instance of the cited study of LBW and ESRD, for example, the matching ratio was two controls for every case.

It should be emphasized that the format for analysis described earlier and illustrated in **Table 9-1** is for data in an unmatched study. If matching is performed, a slightly different tabular summary and analysis must be performed taking into account the matching in the design. The results of a matched and an unmatched analysis may give similar results, but this is not guaranteed, and the preferred approach on both validity and precision grounds is to consider the matching in the analysis. In fact, the analysis presented in **Table 9-2** is an unmatched analysis and therefore not the preferred one for the manner in which the study was designed. As reported in the original publication, the analysis taking into account matching on sex, race and date of birth yielded an OR (95% CI) of 1.4 (1.1–1.8). The unmatched analysis yielded a similar but not identical OR of 1.3 (1.1–1.7). Such similarity is not a certainty, so ideally, the matched analysis is performed often using mathematical modeling to adjust for yet other factors. Mathematical modeling is beyond the scope of the present discussion. For those interested in conducting analyses of matched or unmatched case-control studies, Epi Info, a free, easy-to-use software package that has been developed by the Centers for Disease Control and Prevention, is available at wwwn.cdc.gov/epiinfo.

SUMMARY

In this chapter, we introduced another important type of observational research design referred to as a case-control study. This type of research approach is particularly well suited to the study of rare diseases and those with long developmental (latent) periods. The case-control study begins with the sampling of cases (persons with the disease of interest). A comparison group (controls) without the disease of interest then is selected. Information on earlier exposure histories of both cases and controls then is collected and contrasted between cases and controls.

Cases often are sampled from one or more hospital or other clinical facilities (a **hospital-based sample**). In other settings, an attempt is made to identify all cases within a community, region, workforce, or other group (**population-based sample**). Whereas some sampling schemes limit eligibility to newly diagnosed (**incident**) cases, other studies allow already existing (**prevalent**) cases to be included. A clear definition of diagnostic criteria is essential in order to select affected subjects appropriately.

Controls are sampled from the same source population that gave rise to the cases. This can be accomplished through a variety of sampling strategies from the same community or other group in a population-based study. Alternatively, in a hospital-based study, the controls tend to be selected from the same clinical facilities used to identify cases. Sampling controls from a hospital or outpatient facility is logistically advantageous, but it could lead to distorted exposure patterns if the illnesses of controls are long standing. To minimize the risk of a distorted conclusion, general guidelines for selecting hospital-based controls include choosing them from among multiple diagnostic categories and focusing on acute conditions such as trauma, infectious diseases, or other short-term illnesses.

The collection of information on exposure often is done through questionnaires or interviews with patients. This is a simple and quick technique, but it may be adversely affected by the ability of subjects to recall historical exposures. Even more concerning is the possibility that cases will recall exposures differently from controls, thereby distorting the results observed. Other approaches to collecting information on exposure include extracting data from historical records or, when possible, to collect biological markers of exposure.

The analysis of a case-control study involves comparing the odds of exposure among cases to the odds of exposure among controls. This contrast typically is presented as an OR, and it has a scale of measurement analogous to that of a risk ratio or rate ratio, with the null value of 1 and risk increasing exposures having values greater than 1 and risk lowering exposures having values less than 1. The further the point estimate of the OR is from 1, the stronger the association. Statistical precision of the estimate is reflected in the width of CIs around the point estimate.

Matching is a strategy for sampling control subjects in which key attributes (e.g., age, race, and sex) are linked on a person-to-person basis between cases and controls. Matching can be done on a one-to-one basis (pair matched) or with two or more controls per case. There may be some gain in statistical power by increasing the number of controls per case, but there usually is a diminishing return beyond

four controls per case. The intent of matching is to control the influence of the matching factors on any observed association between the exposure and disease (confounding), as well as to improve the statistical precision of the study. To achieve these benefits, the matched sampling needs to be accompanied by a matched analysis. Data analysis software for both matched and unmatched analyses are widely available and easily used.

 STUDY QUESTIONS

1. In a case-control study, the individuals with the disease of interest are limited to those who are newly diagnosed. We may describe these cases as
A. hospital based.
B. prevalent.
C. incident.
D. population based.
E. none of the above.

2. In a hospital-based case-control study, which of the following guidelines may be useful in sampling controls?
A. Choose them from a single diagnostic category
B. Choose them from a variety of diagnostic groups
C. Choose them from chronic conditions
D. Choose them from acute conditions
E. A and C
F. B and D

3. In a case-control study, matching may be performed to select controls in order to
A. control confounding.
B. control selection bias.
C. improve statistical precision.
D. increase the strength of association.
E. A and C.
F. B and D.

4. In contrast to a prospective cohort study, a case-control design may be preferred for the study of
A. rare exposures.
B. rare diseases.
C. shorter latent periods.
D. long latent periods.
E. A and C.
F. B and D.

5. The preferred measure of association in a case-control study is the

A. risk ratio.

B. rate ratio.

C. odds ratio.

D. attributable risk.

E. attributable risk percent.

6. Increasing the number of controls per case in a case-control study tends to reach diminishing returns in terms of increasing statistical power beyond what ratio?

A. 0.5 controls per case

B. 1.0 control per case

C. 2.0 controls per case

D. 3.0 controls per case

E. 4.0 controls per case

7. Which of the following are potential limitations of the use of historical records to determine exposure status in a case-control study?

A. Incomplete information

B. Missing records

C. Inaccurate information

D. All of the above

8. In a case-control study, the exposure of interest appears to be occurring more frequently among controls than among case, and the results appear to be unlikely to have occurred by chance alone. The corresponding OR (95% CI) is most likely to be

A. 0.5 (0.1, 1.1).

B. 0.7 (0.5, 0.9).

C. 1.0 (0.5, 2.0).

D. 1.5 (1.1, 2.3).

E. 2.0 (0.9, 3.5).

9. In a case-control study, if cases have a greater propensity than controls to remember earlier exposure histories, the study findings may be subject to

A. recall bias.

B. selection bias.

C. confounding.

D. length-biased sampling.

E. lead time bias.

10. Which of the following study types generally is considered to be most susceptible to bias?

A. Randomized controlled trial

B. Prospective cohort study

C. Case-control study

D. A cross-over study

FURTHER READING

Boyko EJ. Observational research-opportunities and limitations. *J Diabetes Complications.* 2013;27:642-648.

Goldberg RJ, McManus DD, Allison J. Greater knowledge and appreciation of commonly used research study designs. *Am J Med.* 2013;126:169.el-8.

Thiese MS. Observational and interventional study design types; an overview. *Biochem Med (Zagreb).* 2014;24:199-210.

REFERENCES

Health Scenario

Barker DJ, Osmond C. Infant mortality, childhood nutrition, and ischaemic heart disease in England and Wales. *Lancet.* 1986;1:1077-1081.

Barker DJ, Winter PD, Osmond C, Margetts B, Simmonds SJ. Weight in infancy and death from ischaemic heart disease. *Lancet.* 1989;2:577-580.

Lackland DT. Mechanisms and fetal origins of kidney disease. *J Am Soc Nephrol.* 2005;16:2531-2532.

White SL, Perkovic V, Cass A, et al. Is low birth weight an antecedent of CKD in later life? A systematic review of observational studies. *Am J Kidney Dis.* 2009;54:248-261.

Clinical Background

Collins AJ, Foley RN, Chavers B, et al. US Renal Data System 2013 Annual Data Report. *Am J Kidney Dis.* 2014;63(1 suppl):A7.

Kramer MS. The epidemiology of low birthweight. *Nestle Nutr Inst Workshop Ser.* 2013;74:1-10.

Parzer RE, McClellan WM. Influence of race, ethnicity, and socioeconomic status on kidney disease. *Nat Rev Nephrol.* 2012;8:533-541.

Taal MW. Chronic disease 10 years on: what have we learned. *Curr Opin Nephrol Hypertens.* 2012;21:607-611.

Case-Control Studies

Lackland DT, Bendall HE, Osmond C, Egan BM, Barker DJ. Low birth weights contribute to the high rates of early-onset chronic renal failure in the Southeastern United States. *Arch Intern Med.* 2000;160:1472-1476.

Diagnostic Testing

Raymond S. Greenberg

HEALTH SCENARIO

Mrs. D., a 68-year-old divorced mother of three children and retired grocery store employee, presented to the emergency department with the sudden onset of indigestion, weakness, shortness of breath, and fatigue. The patient was a cigarette smoker with a history of hypertension that was poorly controlled, with intermittent adherence to prescribed medications. Upon examination, the patient was anxious, sweating, and breathing rapidly. Both her heart rate (86 beats/min) and blood pressure (178/112 mm Hg) were increased. Blood was drawn and revealed elevated levels of both troponin and creatine kinase. An electrocardiogram indicated ST segment elevation, and Mrs. D. was diagnosed with an acute ST segment elevation myocardial infarction (STEMI).

Mrs. D. was transported immediately to the cardiac catheterization laboratory, where virtually complete blockages were identified in two coronary arteries. The blockages were treated with balloon angioplasty followed by the placement of stents to keep the vessels open. The patient recovered well from the procedure and was discharged to her home on the third hospital day with prescriptions for aspirin, a diuretic, a beta-blocker, a statin, and an anticoagulant.

One week later, Mrs. D. was seen in follow-up by the cardiologist, who noted that the patient was regaining her strength and that her blood pressure, although still elevated (136/94 mm Hg), was under better control. However, Mrs. D. continued to smoke cigarettes, and the cardiologist encouraged her to participate in a smoking cessation program and to begin a regular exercise program. The cardiologist referred the patient back to her family physician for further follow-up.

Six weeks later, Mrs. D. was seen by her family physician, who noted that her mood was somewhat depressed and that she had not attempted to quit smoking nor start an exercise program. She complained about the number of medications that were prescribed by the cardiologist and admitted taking them only sporadically. Using a brief self-administered screening test for depression, Mrs. D. tested positive. She was encouraged to quit smoking, start exercising, and take her medications regularly. A referral also was made to a psychiatrist for evaluation and treatment of her depression.

Four weeks later, Mrs. D. was seen by a psychiatrist who conducted an interview and concluded that the patient had a major depressive disorder and started her on a selective serotonin reuptake inhibitor (SSRI) and began a course of cognitive behavioral therapy (CBT). Although there was some initial improvement in her depressive symptoms, Mrs. D. continued to have difficulty adhering to the prescribed medications and treatments. She continued to smoke and live an isolated and sedentary lifestyle.

Approximately 9 months after her percutaneous coronary intervention, Mrs. D. experienced an acute myocardial infarction (MI) at home, and attempts at resuscitation were unsuccessful.

CLINICAL BACKGROUND

It has been shown in many different settings that patients with coronary artery disease (CAD) have a comparatively high prevalence of depression. A major depressive disorder is found in about 15% to 20% of MI patients, which is two to three times the corresponding prevalence in the general population.

A major depressive disorder has been defined in the American Psychiatric Association's *Diagnostic and Statistical Manual of Mental Disorders* (DSM) on the basis of persistence of symptoms for at least 2 weeks of (1) depressed mood or (2) loss of interest or pleasure and at least five symptoms in total, including (1) and (2) along with others, such as unintended weight loss, sleep disturbance, altered psychomotor activity, fatigue, feelings of worthlessness, poor concentration, and suicidal ideation.

The coexistence of depression with other medical conditions is understandable and may arise from any of the following reasons:

1. Depression alters the host's response to illness and increases susceptibility to other conditions.
2. Other medical illnesses adversely affect a patient's mood and outlook.
3. Depression shares common risk factors or genetic predisposition with other medical illnesses.
4. Some combination of the above

As it pertains specifically to CAD, a number of biologic and behavioral mechanisms have been suggested to explain the frequent co-occurrence of these conditions. Among the possible biologic processes are an increase in heart rate variability because of altered autonomic nervous system regulation, increased platelet activation leading to clot formation, enhanced coagulation, increased inflammatory responses, and neurohormonal factors. Possible behavioral explanations relate to the higher observed frequency among depressed persons of nonadherence to prescribed medication regimens, cigarette smoking and food and alcohol consumption, physical inactivity, and social isolation and stress. Although the precise mechanism(s) remains unclear, there is little disagreement that cardiac patients have comparatively high rates of depression.

There is equally compelling evidence that depressed patients with CAD tend to have worse outcomes than those without depression. The mortality rate among depressed patients after an acute MI is about three times greater than for nondepressed patients. The effect of depression appears to be independent of age, sex, smoking status, or level of heart function. It also tends to vary according to the severity of depression, with mortality rates rising with an increasing number of depressive symptoms. Whether the worse outcome among depressed patients is a causal effect is not clear. It is possible that the apparent prognostic effect of depression could be attributable in part or in whole to the behaviors attendant to depression, including a decreased ability to quit smoking, participate in cardiac rehabilitation, adhere to prescribed medications, and interact with a wide social network.

In part, the uncertainty about whether depression per se increases adverse outcomes in CAD relates to the lack of compelling evidence from randomized controlled trials that treating depression improves prognosis. The standard treatments for depression among cardiac patients are pharmacotherapy with a SSRI or structured psychotherapy. CBT typically is provided by a therapist in weekly sessions over 4 months with the goal of reducing thoughts and behavioral practices associated with depression. Both CBT and SSRI

medications have been shown to improve depressive symptoms and enhance quality of life among patients with CAD. Nonrandomized studies also have demonstrated more favorable cardiac outcomes among patients treated for depression. The more definitive evidence that one would desire from large randomized controlled clinical trials does not yet exist, however.

Even in the absence of definitive evidence that detection and treatment of depression in cardiac patients can improve their survival, authoritative groups such as the American Heart Association (AHA) have suggested that all patients with coronary heart disease should be screened for depression and that depression should be treated as an adverse prognostic factor among patients with heart disease. The proposed benefits of such a strategy would include improving quality of life, possibly increasing the ability to adhere to treatment recommendations, and ultimately enhancing survival.

The patient in the Health Scenario illustrates the challenges of managing depressed persons with CAD. Although the patient's depression was detected, it was not managed successfully, further complicating the care of her cardiac disease. The haunting question is whether her clinical outcome might have been different if her depression was managed more successfully. Although we cannot know the answer to this question, we can focus on how best to diagnose depression in similar patients and treat their depression effectively.

SCREENING FOR DEPRESSION

A number of instruments have been developed to detect persons with a major depressive disorder. The "gold standard," or most definitive approach, to making a diagnosis of depression is for a qualified clinician to conduct an interview that assesses the extent to which the patient meets the previously cited criteria in the DSM. Because the majority of patients with CAD do not have depression, it would be highly inefficient to have clinicians conduct these detailed interviews with every patient who has cardiac disease. In an environment of limited human and fiscal resources, such a strategy would be time consuming and wasteful. It would be far more efficient to narrow down the pool of patients who undergo these rigorous interviews. For that purpose, several tools have been developed that are quick and easy to administer and can help to identify the subset of patients that warrants further, more definitive evaluations.

One of the simplest instruments used to screen for depression is referred to as the two-item Patient Health Questionnaire (PHQ-2). For this purpose, a two-question mini-survey is either self-administered by the patient or by a clinician. The two questions in the PHQ-2 are shown in **Table 10-1**. It should

Table 10-1. Questions on the yes/no version of the two-item Patient Health Questionnaire (PHQ-2).

	Response	
Question	Yes	No
1. During the past month, have you been bothered by feeling down, depressed, or hopeless?	(1)	(0)
2. During the past month, have you often been bothered by little interest or pleasure in doing things?	(1)	(0)

Reproduced with permission from Elderon L, Smolderen KG, Na B, Whooley MA. Accuracy and prognostic value of American Heart Association—recommended depression screening in patients with coronary heart disease: data from the Heart and Soul Study. *Circ Cardiovasc Qual Outcomes.* 2011;4:533-540.

be evident that these questions are targeted at two of the necessary components of the DSM definition of a major depressive disorder. Moreover, this information can be collected quickly and inexpensively.

A slightly more detailed screening instrument for depression is the nine-item Patient Health Questionnaire (PHQ-9). The questions that are included in this instrument are shown in **Table 10-2**. The nine-item version collects basic information on each of the potential manifestations of major depressive disorder

cited in the DSM definition. Clearly, it requires longer than the two-item version, but it still can be self-administered or conducted by a clinician relatively quickly and inexpensively compared with a much more detailed clinical interview. The obvious question is whether such a condensed and concise screening instrument can provide an accurate characterization of depression status. The savings in time, money, and burden on patients and staff would not be justified if the PHQ-2 and PHQ-9 led to incorrect conclusions about which patients are experiencing depression. In the following sections, we will explore how one can assess the performance of a screening test. These methods can be applied to screening and diagnostic tests regardless of whether they are obtained from a questionnaire, a blood test, a radiologic examination, or a surgical biopsy.

SENSITIVITY AND SPECIFICITY

To characterize the ability of the PHQ-2 to identify patients with a major depressive disorder and separate them from those without such a disorder, Elderon and colleagues (2011) conducted a study of more than 1000 patients with heart disease. Every patient completed the screening instrument and that same day separately underwent a structured computerized, diagnostic interview, which represented the "gold standard" for making a diagnosis of a major depressive

Table 10-2. Questions on the nine-item Patient Health Questionnaire (PHQ-9).

	Response Options			
Over the past 2 weeks, how often have you been bothered by any of the following problems:	Not at all	Several days	More than half the day	Nearly every day
1. Little interest or pleasure in doing things	(0)	(1)	(2)	(3)
2. Feeling down, depressed, or hopeless	(0)	(1)	(2)	(3)
3. Trouble falling or staying asleep or sleeping too much	(0)	(1)	(2)	(3)
4. Feeling tired or having little energy	(0)	(1)	(2)	(3)
5. Poor appetite or overeating	(0)	(1)	(2)	(3)
6. Feeling bad about yourself, or that you are a failure or have let yourself or your family down	(0)	(1)	(2)	(3)
7. Trouble concentrating on things such as reading the newspaper or watching television	(0)	(1)	(2)	(3)
8. Moving or speaking so slowly that other people could have noticed. Or the opposite, being so fidgety or restless that you have been moving around a lot more than usual.	(0)	(1)	(2)	(3)
9. Thoughts that you would be better off dead or hurting yourself in some way	(0)	(1)	(2)	(3)

Reproduced with permission from Elderon L, Smolderen KG, Na B, Whooley MA. Accuracy and prognostic value of American Heart Association—recommended depression screening in patients with coronary heart disease: data from the Heart and Soul Study. *Circ Cardiovasc Qual Outcomes.* 2011;4:533-540.

order according to the criteria of the DSM. For simplicity, patients were classified in a simple dichotomous manner (screen positive vs. screen negative and depression present or absent). For each patient, one can imagine four possible combinations of screening test results and depression diagnoses:

a. Screening test positive; depression present
b. Screening test positive; depression absent
c. Screening test negative; depression present
d. Screening test negative; depression absent

As the results accumulate within the patient population, one can summarize the findings in a simple tabular format, as shown in **Table 10-3**. Here, the "true" disease status is defined by the gold standard method, in our example, the computerized, structure diagnostic interview. In the cell labeled **a** in **Table 10-3**, we include all patients who had a positive screening test result (e.g., PHQ-2) and had the disease of interest (e.g., major depressive disorder) according to the gold standard diagnostic method. For these patients, the screening test identified their disease status correctly, so we refer to these individuals as "true positives." If we consider the group diagonally opposite—those who had negative screening results and did not have the disease of interest—again, the screening test performed correctly, and we refer to these individuals as "true negatives."

In the remaining two cells of **Table 10-3**, we have the situations, where the screening test incorrectly classified persons. For example, in cell **b**, the patients had positive test results but did not have the disease of interest. We refer to these individuals as "false positives" because the screening test falsely indicated the presence of disease. In the final cell, **c**, we have the individuals who had negative test results but truly had the disease of interest. We refer to these individuals as "false negatives" because the screening test falsely indicated the absence of disease.

It should be readily apparent that a screening test that is highly accurate in classifying persons with regard to disease status will tend to place subjects into cells **a** and **d**, where disease status is classified

correctly. This also implies that errors are being made less often, so cells **b** and **c** will tend to have fewer occupants. Indeed, if the test was perfect at discriminating between truly affected and unaffected individuals, all of the results would fall into cells **a** and **d**, with none in **b** and **c**. Unfortunately, even the best screening tests occasionally make mistakes, so we need a way to quantify the extent to which the test is classifying subjects correctly. We begin with two basic measures that are commonly used to describe test performance—**sensitivity** and **specificity**.

The sensitivity of a test is the percentage of persons with the disease of interest who have positive test results. We might express this concept mathematically as:

$$\text{Sensitivity} = \frac{\text{True positives}}{\text{True positives} + \text{False negatives}} \times 100$$

$$= \frac{a}{a+c} \times 100$$

The specificity of a test is the percentage of persons without the disease of interest who have negative test results. The formula for calculating specificity is:

$$\text{Sensitivity} = \frac{\text{True negatives}}{\text{True negatives} + \text{False positives}} \times 100$$

$$= \frac{d}{d+b} \times 100$$

Example: The previously mentioned study of Elderon and colleagues (2011) was designed to explore the relationship between depression and cardiovascular disease among patients. They included more than 1000 patients from two U.S. Department of Veterans Affairs hospitals, a university hospital, and nine public health clinics. The enrolled patients underwent an initial examination and were followed annually thereafter through telephone interviews.

Several instruments were used to screen for depression, including the previously cited PHQ-2 and PHQ-9. As the "gold standard" for making a diagnosis of major depressive disorder, the investigators used a structured Computerized Diagnostic Interview Schedule (C-DIS), which requires trained personnel to administer and can take 1 hour or longer to complete.

When compared against the "gold standard" C-DIS, the quick screen PHQ-2 yielded the results shown in **Table 10-4**. From these data, we can see that sensitivity is:

$$\text{Sensitivity} = \frac{201}{201 + 22} \times 100 = 90\%$$

Table 10-3. Tabular summary of the findings of a comparison of screening test results with the "true" status of disease.

Test Result		Disease	No Disease
	Positive	True Positive **a**	False Positive **b**
	Negative	False Negative **c**	True Negative **d**

Table 10-4. Tabular summary of the findings of a two-item Patient Health Questionnaire (PHQ-2) screening test versus a diagnostic interview (Computerized Diagnostic Interview Schedule [C-DIS]).

		Positive	Negative	Total
PHQ-2	Positive	201	244	445
	Negative	22	555	577
	Total	223	799	1022

Data from Elderon L, Smolderen KG, Na B, Whooley MA. Accuracy and prognostic value of American Heart Association—recommended depression screening in patients with coronary heart disease: data from the Heart and Soul Study. *Circ Cardiovasc Qual Outcomes.* 2011;4:533-540.

This is relatively high sensitivity, meaning that the PHQ-2 is reasonably good at detecting persons with major depressive symptoms. Because the test identifies most depressed persons, a negative test result helps to "rule out" or lower the suspicion that the individual in question truly is depressed.

The specificity of the PHQ-2 is calculated as:

$$Specificity = \frac{555}{555 + 224} \times 100 = 69\%$$

This specificity is not particularly high, meaning that a positive test result does not allow us to "rule in" or conclude with high confidence that the person in question truly is depressed.

Elderon and colleagues (2011) also evaluated the sensitivity and specificity of the PHQ-9, again using the C-DIS as the "gold standard." The results of this comparison are summarized in **Table 10-5**. Here, the sensitivity is:

$$Sensitivity = \frac{120}{120 + 103} \times 100 = 54\%$$

This sensitivity is not nearly as high as that previously noted for the PHQ-2. In other words, the PHQ-9 is more likely than the PHQ-2 to miss some persons who truly are depressed. A negative test result, therefore, would not be as helpful in ruling out depression.

The specificity of the PHQ-9 was:

$$Specificity = \frac{721}{721 + 78} \times 100 = 90\%$$

When compared against the PHQ-2, the PHQ-9 had a much higher specificity, meaning that it is more helpful in "ruling in" depression in a person with a positive test result.

Table 10-5. Tabular summary of the findings of the a two-item Patient Health Questionnaire (PHQ-2) screening test versus a diagnostic interview (Computerized Diagnostic Interview Schedule [C-DIS]).

		Positive	Negative	Total
PHQ-9	Positive	120	78	198
	Negative	103	721	824
	Total	223	799	1022

Data from Elderon L, Smolderen KG, Na B, Whooley MA. Accuracy and prognostic value of American Heart Association—recommended depression screening in patients with coronary heart disease: data from the Heart and Soul Study. *Circ Cardiovasc Qual Outcomes.* 2011;4:533-540.

Given the differing characteristics of the PHQ-2 and the PHQ-9, it is reasonable to ask which screening test is preferred. On one hand, the PHQ-2 does a better job at detecting depressed persons than does the PHQ-9. The price for missing fewer affected persons is that the PHQ-2 also has a greater tendency than the PHQ-9 to falsely label nondepressed people as having depression. When the condition of interest is serious, and if undetected, leads to life-threatening consequences, one might prefer to err on the side of overdiagnosis. However, when falsely labeling someone as affected can lead to a serious emotional toll on the patient or treatment that has significant cost and potential side effects, one might prefer to err on the side of underdiagnosis. In the case of depression and cardiovascular disease, the AHA recommends a two-step screening process. First, the PHQ-2 is used, picking up most persons who are truly depressed. The persons who test positive on the PHQ-2 then are screened with the PHQ-9, and those who are positive are treated for depression.

POSITIVE AND NEGATIVE PREDICTIVE VALUE

Sensitivity and specificity are characteristics of screening or diagnostic tests, such as the PHQ-2 and the PHQ-9. Two other measures are helpful in assessing how a test performs within a specific population, such as patients with CAD. These two measures are, respectively, **positive predictive value** (PV+) and **negative predictive value** (PV−).

The PV+ is defined as the percentage of persons with positive test results who actually have the disease of interest. In other words, PV+ tells us the implications of a positive test in terms of the likelihood of having disease (e.g., depression). The PV+ is calculated as follows, using the same symbolic notation found in **Table 10-3**.

$$PV+ = \frac{\text{True positives}}{\text{True positives} + \text{False positives}} \times 100$$

$$= \frac{a}{a+b} \times 100$$

Using the findings of Elderon and colleagues (2011), for PHQ-2 as an example (see **Table 10-4**), the PV+ is calculated as:

$$PV+ = \frac{201}{201+244} \times 100 = 45\%$$

In other words, slightly less than half of the persons who had a positive PHQ-2 in the population studied by Elderon and colleagues (2011) actually had depression. At first impression, getting a positive result on a PHQ-2 screen may seem no more predictive than flipping a coin. It is worth considering, however, what our baseline expectations was for depression in this population before conducting the PHQ-2.

In the patients that Elderon and colleagues (2011) studied, the prevalence of depression as identified by the "gold standard" C-DIS was:

$$\frac{\text{Depressed patients}}{\text{Depressed patients} + \text{Nondepressed patients}} \times 100$$

$$= \frac{223}{223 + 799} \times 100 = 22\%$$

So, for patients who have positive results on the PHQ-2, the likelihood of being depressed rises from the pretest likelihood of 22% to 45%. That is, a positive test result raises the likelihood that depression is present twofold. So, even though the test is making a lot of mistakes, it is still improving one's ability to identify depressed patients.

The PV− is defined as the percentage of persons with negative test results who do not have the disease of interest (e.g., depression). One can calculate the PV− using the symbolic notation introduced in **Table 10-3** as:

$$PV- = \frac{\text{True negatives}}{\text{True negatives} + \text{False negatives}} \times 100$$

$$= \frac{d}{d+c} \times 100$$

We can illustrate the calculation of the PV− using the data for PHQ-2 from Elderon and colleagues (2011), as shown in **Table 10-4**:

$$PV- = \frac{555}{555 + 22} \times 100 = 96\%$$

In other words, in this patient population, a negative test result for a patient makes it very unlikely that he or she is depressed. Another way of looking at this is that the pretest probability of not being depressed (799 of 1022) rises from 78% to the posttest probability of 96% if a patient has a negative PHQ-2 result.

The PV+ and PV− vary according to the baseline risk (prevalence) of the condition of interest in the population being studied. Patients with cardiac disease are at relatively high risk for depression, as reflected by the 20% prevalence of depression in the heart disease patients studied by Elderon and colleagues (2011). Surveys of the general adult population typically reveal a prevalence of 10% or less. To explore how PV+ and PV− vary as a function of prevalence, we can consider a study analogous to the one presented by Elderon and colleagues (2011), but instead of studying heart patients, the focus was on adults in the general population. For this exercise, let us assume that the same number of subjects ($n = 1022$) was studied, the PHQ-2 had the same sensitivity (90%) and specificity (69%), and the prevalence of depression according to the C-DIS is 10%. We can use this information to complete a display of hypothetical test results (**Table 10-6**) in the following manner.

With a prevalence of 10%, the total number of C-DIS positive individuals is 102 (1022 × 0.10), and the remainder (1022 − 102 = 920) are C-DIS negative. Applying a sensitivity of 90% to the 102 C-DIS positive persons yields a true positive number of 90, with the balance (102 − 90 = 12) being false negatives. Applying the specificity of 69% to the total of 920 C-DIS negative persons yields a number of true negatives of 635, with the balance (920 − 635 = 285) being false positives.

From the hypothetical data calculated and displayed in **Table 10-6**, we can now calculate a PV+ and PV−. The PV+ is:

$$PV+ = \frac{90}{90 + 285} \times 100 = 24\%$$

The PV− can be calculated as:

$$PV- = \frac{635}{635 + 12} \times 100 = 98\%$$

If these results are compared with those obtained by Elderon and colleagues (2011) among cardiac patients, one can see the impact of lowering disease prevalence (or alternately expressed, disease risk) on PV+ and PV−. The PV+ dropped from the original 45% among heart patients to 24% in the hypothetical

Table 10-6 Hypothetical data for a study of the Patient Health Questionnaire (PHQ-2) screening test for depression in the general population (prevalence of depression = 10%; sensitivity = 90%; specificity = 69%).

		Positive	Negative	Total
PHQ-2	Positive	90	285	375
	Negative	12	635	647
	Total	102	920	1022

C-DIS, Computerized Diagnostic Interview Schedule.

general population because prevalence declined from 20% to 10%. In contrast, PV− rose from the original 96% among cardiac patients to 98% within the hypothetical general population.

However, if we studied an even higher risk group for depression than cardiac patients in general, we would expect to see PV+ and PV− move in the opposite directions. For example, suppose we identified a subset of heart patients who were either older or had more extensive disease; we might expect such a group to have a higher prevalence (e.g., 30%) of depression than among heart patients in general. If one goes through the same sort of hypothetical exercise, a study of 1022 total subjects would yield 307 depressed persons (1022 × 0.30 = 307), 276 true positives (307 × 0.90 = 276), 31 false negatives (307 − 276 = 31), 715 nondepressed persons (1022 − 307 = 715), 493 true negatives (715 × 0.69 = 493), and 222 false positives (715 − 493 = 222). The PV+ would be calculated as:

$$PV+ \ = \ \frac{276}{276 + 222} \times 100 = 55\%$$

The PV− would be calculated as:

$$PV- \ = \ \frac{493}{493 + 31} \times 100 = 94\%$$

So, we see that as prevalence rises (i.e., we examine higher risk persons), the PV+ increases, and the PV− decreases.

CUTOFF POINTS

Thus far, we have presented the concepts of screening and diagnostic tests as simple positive or negative results. In medicine, it is common practice to measure attributes in a simple dichotomous fashion, such as normal versus abnormal. Advantages of a binary classification (e.g., yes/no, or present/absent) include that

it is easy to communicate and understand. However, it may lack some of the detail that can be found in measures of progressive ordered categories or continuous results. For characteristics that have multiple levels, such as questionnaires about depressive symptoms, an interesting question arises around where one should draw the cutoff point or dividing line between normal and abnormal results.

To illustrate the impact of changing cutoff points for defining an abnormal test result, consider a study published by Zuithoff and colleagues (2010). This investigation involved more than 1300 patients older than age 18 years who were sampled from seven large primary care practices in the Netherlands. Patients were enrolled regardless of their reasons for seeking medical care. Each patient completed the PHQ-9, and the "gold standard" was the Composite International Diagnostic Interview, a standardized, structured interview administered by trained researchers. The PHQ-9 was scored according to the numerical method shown in **Table 10-2**, with each of the nine questions scored from 0 to 3 depending on symptom frequency. Aggregate scores, therefore, could range from a minimum of zero (no depressive symptoms) to a maximum of 27 (all nine symptom categories experienced nearly every day).

Overall, 13% of the patient population had a major depressive disorder according to the reference standardized structured interview. The observed sensitivity and specificity of the PHQ-9 for detecting major depressive disorder are shown in **Figure 10-1** for varying cutoff points. In general, as the cutoff point is raised (more symptoms or greater frequency required to declare a positive test result), the sensitivity falls. That is, as it becomes more difficult to be classified as abnormal, the screening test misses more and more truly depressed persons (i.e., the false-negative rate increases, and the sensitivity falls). However, as the threshold for an abnormal result rises, there is a corresponding progressive increase in specificity. That is, as it becomes more difficult to be classified as abnormal, the screening test produces fewer and fewer false positives.

It can be seen that neither the fall in sensitivity nor the rise in specificity is linear. For the decline in sensitivity, the greatest incremental losses occur between cutoff points of 6 and 10. In contrast, the greatest gains in specificity occur between cutoff points of 4 and 7.

Choosing the optimal cutoff point requires a judgment about the relative consequences of a false-positive and a false-negative error. The kinds of issues that must be considered are whether it is worse to miss a diagnosis of depression (false negative) and thereby have less effective treatment or to mistakenly label a person as depressed (false positive), leading to perceived or real social, employment, or emotional stigma, as well as extra testing and unnecessary treatment. In general, the relative gains in specificity

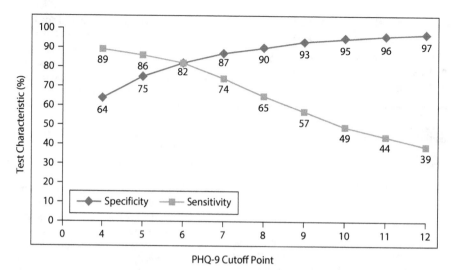

Figure 10-1. Changes in sensitivity and specificity of the nine-item Patient Health Questionnaire (PHQ-9) as a function of changing the cutoff point. (Data from Zuithoff NPA, Vergouwe Y, King M, et al. The Patient Health Questionnaire-9 for detection of major depressive disorder in primary care: consequences of current thresholds in a cross-sectional study. *BMC Family Pract*. 2010;11:98.)

seem to be a reasonable offset to the losses in sensitivity when moving the cutoff point from 4 to 6 or 7. Raising the cutoff point above that level would require a decision that modest reductions in false-positive errors were warranted by greater inflation of false negative errors. It should be noted in this context that a widely recommended and used cutoff point for the PHQ-9 is 10. In deploying this cutoff point, the user should be aware that it entails lower sensitivity than could be achieved with a slightly lower cutoff point.

LIKELIHOOD RATIOS

In addition to the metrics already introduced, screening or diagnostic tests often are assessed with **likelihood ratios (LRs)**. *An LR is the probability for a particular test result for a person with the condition of interest (e.g., depression) divided by the probability of that test result for a person without the condition of interest.* We can further specify an LR for a positive test result (LR+) as the probability of a positive test result for a person with the condition of interest divided by the probability of a positive test result for a person without the condition. The mathematical expression for the LR+, where sensitivity and specificity are expressed as proportions (rather than as percentages) is:

$$LR+ = \frac{Sensitivity}{(1 - Specificity)}$$

Consider the possible range of the LR+. It is minimized when the numerator (sensitivity) is zero. It is maximized when the denominator is zero (specificity = 1). An LR+ = 1 implies that the test does not perform better (i.e., more likely to yield a positive result) among affected persons than among nonaffected persons. In other words, the test is not helpful in sorting out affected persons from unaffected persons. A value greater than one for LR+ implies that a positive test result is more likely when the condition is present, and the larger the LR+, the more a positive test result is indicative of having the condition of interest.

The LR for a negative test result (LR−) is defined as the probability of a negative test result for a person with the condition of interest divided by the probability of a negative test result for a person without the condition. The LR− is calculated as:

$$LR- = \frac{(1 - Sensitivity)}{Specificity}$$

Sensitivity and specificity again are expressed as proportions. The smallest possible value of LR− (= 0) occurs when the numerator is zero, meaning that 1 − sensitivity = 0, so sensitivity = 1. The largest possible value of the LR− occurs when the denominator has its smallest possible value. This occurs when the specificity is zero, resulting in an LR− of positive infinity.

As was the case with the LR+, an LR− with a value of one indicates a test with no discriminatory value. When the LR− is 1, people with and without the condition of interest are equally likely to have a negative test result. A test that is more likely to be negative in the absence of the condition of interest will have an LR− value less than 1, and the further from 1, the stronger the association between a negative test result and the absence of disease.

The calculation of LR+ and LR− can be illustrated for PHQ-2 and PHQ-9 using the data previously cited in **Tables 10-4** and **10-5** based on the study of Elderon and colleagues (2011). For PHQ-2, sensitivity is 0.90, and specificity is 0.69.

The LR+, therefore, is calculated as:

$$LR+ = \frac{\text{Sensitivity}}{(1 - \text{Specificity})} = \frac{0.90}{(1 - 0.69)} = \frac{0.90}{0.31}$$

$$= 2.9$$

The LR− is calculated as:

$$LR- = \frac{(1 - \text{Sensitivity})}{\text{Specificity}} = \frac{(1 - 0.90)}{0.69} = \frac{0.10}{0.69}$$

$$= 0.14$$

For PHQ-9, sensitivity is 0.54, and specificity is 0.90.

Accordingly, LR+ is:

$$LR+ = \frac{\text{Sensitivity}}{(1 - \text{Specificity})} = \frac{0.54}{(1 - 0.90)} = \frac{0.54}{0.10}$$

$$= 5.4$$

LR− is:

$$LR- = \frac{(1 - \text{Sensitivity})}{\text{Specificity}} = \frac{(1 - 0.54)}{0.90} = \frac{0.46}{0.90}$$

$$= 0.51$$

So, how does one interpret these LRs? With an LR+ of 2.9, a positive test result on the PHQ-2 only raises the likelihood of depression a small amount compared with a positive result on the PHQ-9 (LR+ of 5.4), which raises the likelihood of depression a moderate amount. However, a negative test result on the PHQ-2 (LR− = 0.14) conveys a moderate decrease in the likelihood of depression compared with a minimal decrease associated with a negative test result on the PHQ-9 (LR− = 0.51). Neither test has the kind of strong discriminatory power that one would like to see to either confirm a diagnosis of depression or exclude it. To "rule in" or confirm a diagnosis, an LR+ of 10 or greater typically is expected. To "rule out" or exclude a diagnosis, an LR− of 0.10 or less typically is expected. With these criteria in mind, neither the PHQ-2 nor the PHQ-9 is sufficient to rule in depression, but a negative test

result on the PHQ-2 is pretty compelling evidence that depression is unlikely.

RECEIVER OPERATING CHARACTERISTIC CURVES

In the preceding section on cutoff points, we saw how sensitivity and specificity varied inversely as the cutoff point for a positive test result on the PHQ-9 varied. This relationship was illustrated in **Figure 10-1**. Another approach to illustrating this phenomenon is referred to as the **receiver operating characteristic (ROC) curve**. The first use of such a graph, and hence its unusual name, arose in the context of assessing the ability of radar operators to distinguish signals from background noise. In relation to diagnostic or screening tests, we plot sensitivity on the vertical axis against 1 - specificity on the horizontal axis. It may be helpful to think of this graph as depicting the proportion of true positives (sensitivity) as a function of the proportion of false positives (1 − specificity). If a diagnostic test has no discriminating value in helping to make a diagnosis, then the true positive proportion will be identical to the false positive proportion. This line of "no value" would appear as a diagonal at a 45-degree angle and often is depicted in an ROC curve as a reference for comparing against the actual test results. A diagnostic test that helps to separate persons with and without the condition of interest would appear as a departure from this "no value" reference line, and the greater the departure, the better the test performs at distinguishing affected from unaffected persons.

We can construct an ROC curve using the data from Zuithoff and colleagues (2010), as shown in **Figure 10-2**. The solid line in this graph represents the performance of the PHQ-9, and the dotted line corresponds to the reference of a test with no diagnostic value. We can see that the Sensitivity rises rapidly at the far left of the graph, with small increases in 1 − specificity (i.e., with decreases in specificity). The curve begins to flatten out as it moves to the right. In other words, in this region, there are diminishingly small gains in sensitivity for the corresponding losses in specificity.

A summary measure of overall test performance can be calculated as the area under the ROC curve. The minimal value of this measure is 0.5, which corresponds to the area under the dashed diagonal line in **Figure 10-2**, which reflects a test of no value in distinguishing between persons with and without the condition of interest. The maximum value of the area under the ROC curve is 1, which represents a perfect test in which no errors are made. The closer the area under the ROC curve is to 1, the better the test is

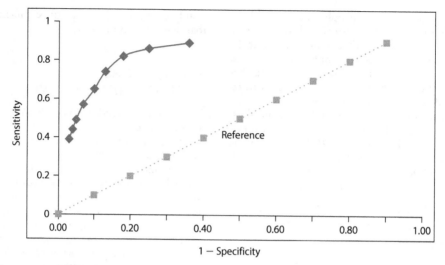

Figure 10-2. Receiver operating characteristic curve for the nine-item Patient Health Questionnaire. (Data from Zuithoff NPA, Vergouwe Y, King M, et al. The Patient Health Questionnaire-9 for detection of major depressive disorder in primary care: consequences of current thresholds in a cross-sectional study. *BMC Family Pract.* 2010;11:98.)

performing. For the PHQ-9, values of the area under the ROC curve have been reported in the range of 0.85 to 0.90 or higher depending on the setting and study population.

The performance of two screening or diagnostic tests can be compared visually, as illustrated with hypothetical data in **Figure 10-3**. Here, test A has a steeper ascent and reaches a higher sensitivity level than does test B. It is readily apparent that the corresponding area under the ROC curve will be greater for test A than for test B, and thus, test A performs better at screening for depression.

EARLY DETECTION BIASES

Screening tests typically are used to detect a condition earlier than it might otherwise come to recognition through clinical manifestations (symptoms) of the disease. The benefit of early detection is that it allows earlier

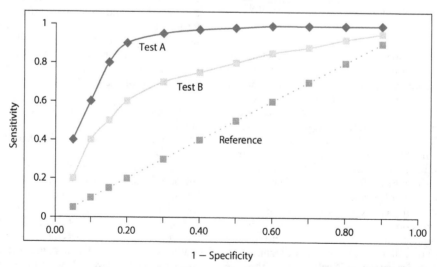

Figure 10-3. Contrast of two different screening tests (A and B) for depression with respective receiver operating characteristic curves, with the dotted line corresponding to a reference test with no diagnostic value.

intervention to either prevent the condition from developing fully or allowing it to be treated at a stage when the condition is more limited and curable. Of course, the benefits will be achieved only if effective treatments are available and if there are therapeutic advantages to early intervention. Examples of screening tests that have been shown to be effective and are widely recommended include the Pap smear for cervical cancer, fecal occult blood screening, sigmoidoscopy and colonoscopy for large bowel cancer, and serum lipid screening for elevated total cholesterol and low density lipoprotein-cholesterol and decreased levels of high density lipoprotein-cholesterol as risk factors for coronary heart disease.

Studies conducted to evaluate the effectiveness of a screening test must take into account several factors that may influence the results. The first of these influences has been referred to as **lead time bias**. *The lead time is the extra amount of time that a condition is recognized by early detection through screening.* For an individual, it begins when the condition is screen-detected and ends when it would be detected in the absence of screening. If one were assessing the effectiveness of a screening test by the extra amount of time that screen-detected persons survive, the lead time would make their survival appear longer than non–screen-detected persons even if there is no prolongation of life. That is, the clock is starting at unequal points in time for screen-detected and non–screen-detected persons, and if an adjustment is not made for this "head start" with screening, the comparison will be unfair.

Yet another type of unfair comparison might arise from so-called **length-biased sampling**. *The length bias arises because slowly progressing forms of a condition are detectable by the screening test for a longer period of time than rapidly progressing forms.* The subset of affected individuals that the screening test detects, therefore, likely will be weighted preferentially to nonaggressive slowly developing forms of the disease. If one assesses the effectiveness of screening by duration of survival, the screen-detected persons will appear to live longer than non–screen-detected persons because they tend to have slower progressing forms of the condition.

To reduce the risk of both lead time bias and length-biased sampling, it is recommended that the evaluation of screening effectiveness should be determined by a comparison of cause-specific mortality rates for the condition of interest. The strongest evidence would derive from a controlled clinical trial in which subjects were randomly assigned to the screening program or no screening.

SUMMARY

In this chapter, we used the example of screening for depression among persons with CAD to present the basic concepts of diagnostic testing. Central to this discussion is the understanding that all clinical information, including information that results from diagnostic tests, is subject to error. We introduced the concept of a **false-negative** result in which a test does not detect the condition of interest when it is present. We also learned about a second type of error, a **false-positive** result, which occurs when the diagnostic test mistakenly indicates that the condition of interest is present when it is not.

Applying these concepts, we learned that **sensitivity** is the proportion of positive test results among all persons with the condition. **Specificity** relates to the proportion of negative test results among persons without the condition. A test is said to be sensitive when it correctly detects a high proportion of truly affected persons. A test may be described as specific when it correctly provides negative results for a high percentage of unaffected persons. Applying these criteria to screening for depression, we saw that the two-question PHQ was sensitive but not very specific, and the nine-question PHQ was specific but not very sensitive.

Positive predictive value (PV+) characterizes the proportion of persons with positive test results who truly are affected with the condition of interest. The companion measure, **negative predictive value (PV−)**, corresponds to the proportion of persons with negative test results who truly lack the condition of interest. We saw that among cardiac patients, in whom the risk of depression is higher than in the general population, the two-question PHQ had a PV+ of 45% and a PV− of 96%. Accordingly, one would expect the PV+ to be lower and the PV− to be higher if the PHQ two-question test for depression was used in a lower risk group (e.g., the general population). The reverse would be true if the PHQ-2 was applied to a higher risk subgroup (e.g., older patients with coronary heart disease or those with greater morbidity).

Next, we examined the impact of changing the cutoff point for declaring a test result to be positive. In general, as one raises the cutoff point, the criteria for a positive result become more difficult to achieve. This will result in a greater proportion of truly affected persons being missed (declared negative) by the test, raising the false-negative rate, or said another way, lowering the sensitivity. Typically, the loss of sensitivity will be accompanied by a drop in false positives, or a rise in specificity. We observed these impacts on the sensitivity and specificity of the nine-question PHQ as a function of raising the cutoff point.

We then considered two further measures, which are termed **likelihood ratios (LRs)**. The LR+ is the probability of a positive test result for a person with the condition of interest divided by the probability of a positive test result for a person without the condition. The LR− is the probability of a negative test result for a person with the condition of interest divided by the probability of a negative test result for a person without the condition. Applied to the PHQ tests, a negative test result on the two-question version conveys a moderate reduction in the likelihood of depression. A positive test result on the nine-question version raises the likelihood of depression to a moderate extent.

The concept of the **ROC** curve was introduced as a way to depict a visual image of the discriminatory ability of a diagnostic test. Furthermore, one can use such an image to compare and contrast the performance of two or more diagnostic tests and a summary measure of performance can be calculated as the area under the ROC curve.

Finally, we saw how the evaluation of a screening test can be distorted by two different types of effects. **Lead time bias** is the apparent increase in survival with screening that is attributable to the time differential related to earlier diagnosis through screening than through nonscreened diagnosis. **Length-biased sampling** relates to the fact that screen-detected disease may be skewed toward slower progressing forms of the condition, resulting in a survival advantage compared with patients diagnosed through nonscreened methods. Both types of distortion can be removed by focusing on cause-specific death rates rather than survival time in a controlled clinical trial where screening is assigned randomly.

STUDY QUESTIONS

1. In raising the cutoff point for a screening test, which of the following is the likely result?
   A. An increase in sensitivity
   B. An increase in specificity
   C. An increase in false positives
   D. An increase in prevalence
   E. An increase in lead time bias

2. If the screening test does not delay the time of death from a condition but makes survival appear longer because of earlier detection of disease, there is evidence of
   A. confounding.
   B. length-biased sampling.
   C. lead time bias.
   D. selection bias.
   E. information bias.

3. A test with an LR+ of 15 can be said to provide evidence to
   A. rule in the condition of interest.
   B. rule out the condition of interest.
   C. make an earlier diagnosis.
   D. prolong survival after diagnosis.
   E. detect slowly progressing forms of the condition of interest.

4. A specific diagnostic test is one that
   A. has a high proportion of false-negative results.
   B. has a low proportion of false-negative results.
   C. has a high proportion of false-positive results.
   D. has a low proportion of false-positive results.
   E. none of the above.

5. A diagnostic test with no discriminatory ability would have an area under the ROC curve of
   A. 0.
   B. 0.25.
   C. 0.5.
   D. 1.
   E. 2.

6. A diagnostic test with an LR- of 0.05 can be said to provide evidence to
   A. rule in the condition of interest.
   B. rule out the condition of interest.
   C. make an earlier diagnosis.
   D. prolong survival after diagnosis.
   E. detect slowly progressing forms of the condition of interest.

7. If a screening test does not delay the time of death from a condition but makes survival appear longer because it is preferentially detecting slowly progressing disease, there is evidence of
   A. confounding.
   B. length-biased sampling.
   C. lead time bias.
   D. selection bias.
   E. information bias.

8. Two screening tests are being compared for a particular disease. Test A has an area under the ROC curve of 0.95. Test B has an area under the ROC curve of 0.83. Which of the following statements is correct?
   A. Neither test has any discriminatory value.
   B. Test A has a total error rate of 5%.
   C. Test B is better than test A at ruling in disease.
   D. The PV+ for test A is 95%.

E. Test A performs better than test B at discriminating the presence of disease.

9. As the prevalence of a condition increases, a screening test for it will tend to have a

A. higher sensitivity.

B. higher specificity.

C. higher predictive value positive.

D. higher predictive value negative.

E. higher length biased sampling.

10. Which of the following measures of diagnostic test performance ideally has a small value?

A. Predictive value positive

B. Predictive value negative

C. Likelihood ratio for a positive test result

D. Likelihood ratio for a negative test result

E. None of the above

FURTHER READING

Lichtman JH, Bigger JT Jr, Blumenthal JA, et al; American Heart Association Prevention Committee of the Council on Cardiovascular Nursing; American Heart Association Council on Clinical Cardiology; American Heart Association Council on Epidemiology and Prevention; American Heart Association Interdisciplinary Council on Quality of Care and Outcomes Research; American Psychiatric Association. Depression and coronary heart disease: recommendations for screening, referral, and treatment. A science advisory from the American Heart Association Prevention Committee of the Council on Cardiovascular Nursing, Council on Clinical Cardiology, Council on Epidemiology and Prevention, and Interdisciplinary Council on Quality of Care and Outcomes Research. *Circulation.* 2008;118:1768-1775.

Lichtman JH, Froelicher ES, Blumenthal JA, et al; American Heart Association Statistics Committee of the Council on Epidemiology and Prevention and the Council on Cardiovascular and Stroke Nursing. Depression as a risk factor for poor prognosis among patients with acute coronary syndrome: systematic review and recommendations: a scientific statement from the American Heart Association. *Circulation.* 2014;129:1350-1369.

Thombs BD, Roseman M, Coyne JC, et al. Does evidence support the American Heart Association's recommendation to screen patients for depression in cardiovascular care? An updated systematic review. *PLoS ONE.* 2013;8:e52654.

REFERENCES

Clinical Background

Burg MM, Edmondson D, Shimbo D, et al. The 'perfect storm' and acute pulmonary syndrome onset: do psychosocial factors play a role? *Prog Cardiovasc Dis.* 2013;55:601-610.

Chauvet-Gélinger JC, Trojak B, Vergès-Patois B, Cottin Y, Bonin B. Review on depression and coronary heart disease. *Arch Cardiovasc Dis.* 2013;106:103-110.

Compare A, Zarbo C, Manzoni GM, et al. Social support, depression, and heart disease: a ten year literature review. *Frontiers Psychol.* 2015;4:384.

Elderon L, Whooley MA. Depression and cardiovascular disease. *Prog Cardiovasc Dis.* 2013;55:511-523.

Hare DL, Toukhsati SR, Johansson P, Jaarsma T. Depression and cardiovascular disease: a clinical review. *Eur Heart J.* 2014;35:1365-1372.

Whooley MA. Depression and cardiovascular disease: healing the broken-hearted. *JAMA.* 2006;295:2874-2881.

Screening for Depression

Maurer DM. Screening for depression. *Am Fam Physician.* 2012;85:139-144.

Sensitivity and Specificity

Elderon L, Smolderen KG, Na B, Whooley MA. Accuracy and prognostic value of American Heart Association—recommended depression screening in patients with coronary heart disease: data from the Heart and Soul Study. *Circ Cardiovasc Qual Outcomes.* 2011;4:533-540.

Positive and Negative Predictive Value

Elderon L, Smolderen KG, Na B, Whooley MA. Accuracy and prognostic value of American Heart Association—recommended depression screening in patients with coronary heart disease: data from the Heart and Soul Study. *Circ Cardiovasc Qual Outcomes.* 2011;4:533-540.

Cutoff Points

Zuithoff NPA, Vergouwe Y, King M, et al. The Patient Health Questionnaire-9 for detection of major depressive disorder in primary care: consequences of current thresholds in a cross-sectional study. *BMC Family Pract.* 2010;11:98.

Likelihood Ratios

Elderon L, Smolderen KG, Na B, Whooley MA. Accuracy and prognostic value of American Heart Association—recommended depression screening in patients with coronary heart disease: data from the Heart and Soul Study. *Circ Cardiovasc Qual Outcomes.* 2011;4:533-540.

ROC Curves

Zuithoff NPA, Vergouwe Y, King M, et al. The Patient Health Questionnaire-9 for detection of major depressive disorder in primary care: consequences of current thresholds in a cross-sectional study. *BMC Family Pract.* 2010;11:98.

SECTION III
Summarizing Evidence for Medical Practice

Comparative Effectiveness

Annie N. Simpson and Kit N. Simpson

HEALTH SCENARIO

Dr. Block was just told by his nurse that Mr. Green had been "squeezed" into his schedule at lunchtime tomorrow. This is Mr. Green's fifth visit in 9 weeks. Mr. Green is a 54-year-old high school football coach who is being treated for major depression. His wife called, very upset, to make the appointment and told the nurse that "his medicine is just not working, and he is really bad." Mr. Green has tried two different types of antidepressant drugs before the currently prescribed medication. One was changed after 14 days because of intolerable side effects, and the second was changed after 3 weeks because of a combination of side effects and lack of improvement. Dr. Block reviewed Mr. Green's record and pondered what to do next. During a previous discussion about potential treatment options, Mr. Green said that he does not believe in counseling because "he tried it when he lived in Michigan and it does not work."

Dr. Block must consider the advantages and disadvantages of the available treatment options for this patient: (1) switch to another antidepressant, (2) augment the current antidepressant with a second agent, (3) try to persuade the patient to get counseling in addition to medication, (4) consider electroconvulsive therapy (ECT), or (5) refer him for repeated transcranial magnetic stimulation (r-TMS) treatment. What to do? Then he remembers having seen some recent reports on advances in depression treatment, and he decides to search for evidence on the comparative effectiveness (CE) of the approaches that he is considering for Mr. Green.

To find a summary of the evidence, he first searches the website of the Agency for Healthcare Research and Quality (AHRQ). He finds a list of Clinician Research Summaries, including one on "Non-pharmacologic Interventions for Treatment-Resistant Depression in Adults" (AHRQ Clinician Research Summaries, 2012). Great, he thinks, my problem is solved. That is until he sees that the summary identifies a number of important gaps in the knowledge in the studies reviewed, including (1) information on quality of life is substantially missing from the studies; (2) few studies compare nonpharmacologic interventions with each other or with pharmacologic interventions or combinations of treatments; (3) there is almost no evidence on how the CE might differ for patient subgroups defined by age or sex; and (4) the studies use inconsistent measures of treatment resistance, clinical outcomes, and adverse events and have short follow-up periods.

When he retrieves the full research report (www.effectivehealthcare.ahrq.gov/trd.cfm), he finds that most of the studies were published before 2008 and thus are 6 or more years old and not clearly relevant to his current patient. Shaking his head at the clear lack of external validity and relevance of these studies to his clinical problem, he gives up and decides he will have to spend some time doing more detailed searches for evidence tonight after dinner.

This physician is a problem solver who is approaching the practice of medicine from the perspective of patient-centered care. He knows that different treatments may work differently in different patients and that the most efficacious treatment for a cohort of patients in a clinical trial may not be the most effective or acceptable therapy for a specific patient. He needs quick information on the CE of the therapies that he thinks will be acceptable to his patient. This very real practice need is the reason for the current focus on comparative effectiveness research (CER).

COMPARATIVE EFFECTIVENESS RESEARCH

The Congressional Budget Office (CBO, 2007) defined CER as: **"rigorous evaluation of the impact of different options that are available for treating a given medical condition for a particular set of patients"** (CBO, 2007 p. 3). A report from the Institute of Medicine (IOM, 2009) that lists CER topics that should be top priorities for funding also identifies four types of research designs that are relevant for CER: (1) systematic reviews and meta-analyses, (2) decision analysis models, (3) observational studies (OSs), and (4) large pragmatic clinical trials.

Performing a systematic review, using a decision analysis model, or analyzing observational data from his own patients or from a large health systems database is clearly not feasible for informing Dr. Block's treatment decisions in the Health Scenario. Furthermore, he knows that these methodological approaches do not provide the level of evidence that would result from a well-designed and executed randomized controlled trial (RCT). It would be ideal if he could find the results of a large pragmatic clinical trial that compared his five treatment choices for middle-aged men who have failed two previous pharmaceutical treatments for depression and who have a history indicating that counseling for depression is not effective. However, such a trial does not exist. Indeed, it may be impossible and unethical to do such a trial because there is substantial evidence available from individual studies to indicate that ECT (Nahas et al., 2013) and r-TMS (Carpenter et al., 2012) are effective in a majority of patients with treatment-resistant depression and that augmentation of antidepressants with additional drugs has only a moderate effect in patients with a history of previous drug failures (Fava et al., 2006). Thus, because Dr. Block will have to rely on reports of effectiveness of treatments that do not use the strongest possible research design to ensure the internal validity of findings and thus may be affected by selection bias, he needs to know how to judge the quality of studies that report results using systematic reviews or meta-analyses, decision analysis models, or observational data analyses.

The objectives of this chapter are to introduce the methods used in CER, illustrate when each specific method is used, and discuss how to (1) avoid selection bias when using observational data to compare effectiveness and (2) integrate evidence to estimate outcomes that patients care about or outcomes expected beyond the observation period using decision analysis modeling. The following chapters will then provide more details on how to plan a review, find and assess the evidence, and address issues involved in doing a meta-analysis.

THE FOUR COMPARATIVE EFFECTIVENESS APPROACHES

The objective of all CER studies is to generate evidence that will help inform day-to-day clinical and health policy decisions. For this reason, CER studies must rely on head-to-head comparisons of active treatments that are used in current practice. These treatments must be used in a study population that is typical of patients with the condition of interest, and outcomes measured must include those that patients care most about. This forges a strong link between CER and the research trend toward measuring patient-related outcomes (PROs), as well as a focus on issues such as cost and quality that are of clear interest to health policymakers. It also ties in recent work on the importance of community engagement for successful research endeavors. The highest quality of evidence clearly will come from CE studies that are designed as large pragmatic clinical trials (LPCTs). However, this design is also the most costly to use as well as the one that takes the longest time to produce new evidence.

The LPCT studies will have to be large because they will compare the effectiveness of two or more treatments used in current clinical practice when we do not know which one is best. Thus, the effect size (treatment difference) is likely to be small, requiring a large number of subjects to be enrolled. Furthermore, the studies will have to measure PRO endpoints that are important to patients and policymakers, limiting the use of surrogate (intermediate) markers for poor clinical outcomes often used in efficacy studies to shorten the time required for patients to be observed in a trial. The most appropriate study design may be a cluster-randomized trial (Campbell and Walters, 2014) in which each practice or hospital is randomized to a different treatment group to prevent cross-contamination between treatment groups. It is clear that LPCTs will be long and costly, so they are likely to be reserved for CE questions that affect a large number of patients and when knowing the "best" treatments to choose may be expected to have a large impact on both population health and total cost of care.

This brings us to the "next best" method for generating evidence of the CE of treatments. We can extract clinical trial reports for the treatments of interest and examine how the efficacy of the treatments compares for patient subgroups or across trials using systematic reviews and meta-analysis. A **systematic review** *is a critical assessment and evaluation of all research studies that address a particular issue* (from the AHRQ, as noted in Chapter 12). Systematic reviews are carefully structured approaches to extract and examine all evidence available for and against a treatment. Authors of a systematic review are very careful to minimize bias in the evidence that they retrieve so their findings describe the body of evidence that exists to date. Classical meta-analysis has been used for many years to identify a mean treatment effect across sets of studies with inconclusive or inconsistent results (Antman et al., 1992). Some of the early work in this area was done to assess the CE of interventions in obstetrics and perinatal care (Chalmers, 1991), which evolved into the large voluntary research group now known as The Cochrane Collaboration (Chalmers and Hayes, 1994).

There are two problems with meta-analysis: (1) we can only use it to examine treatments for which there are published clinical trial results, and (2) most of the data available will be efficacy data, not data on effectiveness, because most clinical trials use stringent inclusion and exclusion criteria for patients and perform treatments in ideal settings, reducing the ability to extrapolate or generalize results to other patients. Thus, meta-analyses are not likely to have outcomes that reflect PROs, nor will they be able to examine effectiveness in "real" practice settings. They also can suffer from **publication bias** *because studies with negative findings may be less likely than those with positive findings to be published.* However, meta-analyses are very important for their role of examining efficacy for population subgroups and for providing data for the third type of CER design type; the decision analysis modeling study.

Decision analysis modeling is becoming a very important part of CER because it was designed originally to integrate evidence and available population and treatment cost data to estimate PROs and cost for competing treatments under routine practice conditions (Simpson, 1995). Decision analysis is a highly evolved specialized discipline that has been used for years to compare the health and economic implications of competing therapies. It has proven especially useful for assessing new drugs and for predicting long-term outcomes for public health interventions, such as screening programs or vaccine use. Very large and complex validated decision analysis models have been constructed to estimate long-term expected outcomes

for diabetes treatments (The Mount Hood Modeling Group, 2007), cancer screening (Eddy et al., 1988), antiretroviral therapy in HIV-disease (Simpson, 2010), vaccine use (Clark et al., 2013), and many other types of interventions. Different structural frameworks and time horizons may be used to organize the available evidence and test the assumptions embedded in a decision model. Options range from simple decision trees to complex statistical models and may use combinations of structures, as well as probabilistic approaches, such as simulation modeling to examine the effects of uncertainty in the evidence on the study outcome.

A well-done complex decision model may require a large team of clinical, statistical, epidemiologic, economic, and computer science experts several years to build and validate it. Many practical but fairly simple CE models simply capture the mean efficacy measures identified in meta-analyses, adjust them to expected effectiveness, and link surrogate outcomes from clinical trials to epidemiologic and health care resource use with data from OSs in relevant patient subgroups. Two separate issues can affect the validity of these CE models: (1) Is the model structure valid? and (2) Are the observational data used to estimate the model drivers affected by selection bias? The issue of selection bias is crucial for the validity of decision analysis modeling or for any CE analysis that uses observational data.

Observational studies use data that are generated from treating patients in routine practice settings. This means that the data have excellent generalizability—they clearly represent the patients that one may expect to see in real practice. When these data are used to compare the effectiveness of competing therapies, however, they are very vulnerable to **confounding by indication**, or **selection bias**. *This bias is injected by the fact that practicing physicians will tend to use the newest or best treatment available for their more severely ill or difficult-to-treat patients.* Thus, if one simply compares the outcomes for patients treated with treatment A with those treated with treatment B, it is very likely one group of patients will have more severe disease, be more difficult to treat, or have many more comorbid conditions that affect their treatment outcome. Thus, one would be comparing "apples to oranges." Indeed, this is the reason patients are randomized in clinical trials. Only if we assign patients to a treatment by chance can we be assured that disease severity, treatment difficulty, comorbidities, demographic characteristics, and any unknown prognostic factors are equally distributed in the treatment groups. However, many important questions in medical care cannot be examined in randomized studies. In some situations, randomized studies may be too expensive to undertake, may be impractical or infeasible, or may be unethical to perform, or there may be some combination of all of these factors. For these situations, the use of prospectively or retrospectively collected observational data offers an alternative. In such situations, it is essential to use study designs that help guard against selection bias. Two "pseudo-randomization" study design approaches have been developed and validated over the past 20 years using either propensity score (PS) methods or instrumental variable design. Although no OS can completely assure the absence of selection bias, the newest methods, when combined with a sensitivity analysis, do a very good job of removing most of the bias and at showing how large the "missed" biasing factor would have to be to nullify the results. These approaches are described in more detail below.

USING OBSERVATIONAL DATA TO COMPARE OUTCOMES

Observational data can be obtained in a number of ways to answer CER questions. One source is national survey data. Some commonly used national surveys are expressly taken for healthcare research or disease surveillance by governmental or private agencies at regular time intervals. Survey data can be inexpensive for the researcher to obtain and often are readily available; however, survey data generally do not allow researchers to follow particular patients over a long period of time and rarely include cost data along with clinical information. These surveys also tend to be limited by patient recall and subjectivity. Some examples of survey data sources are the National Survey on Drug Use and Health (NSDUH), Behavioral Risk Factor Surveillance System (BRFSS), National Health and Nutrition Examination Survey (NHANES), Medical Expenditure Panel Survey (MEPS), National Health Interview Survey (NHIS), National Survey of Sexual Health and Behavior (NSSHB), and Annenberg National Health Communication Survey (ANHCS). These data sources have different associated costs, logistical complications, and feasibility implications (Iezzoni, 1994). More important, each of these main sources of survey data has specific foci that may not include variables needed to answer the questions of interest to the researcher or clinician.

Other sources of archival or observational health data include data sets created using medical record abstraction or patient-derived data, including patient registries (Iezzoni, 1994). Patient-derived data can be collected directly from patients by chart review, interviews, or surveys and may be retrospective or prospective in nature. Collection of these data can be time and cost prohibitive. These data usually are limited to clinical information and may not include information on quality of life, patient-centered outcomes, or costs of care.

Another source of observational data often used in CER studies is billing data. Administrative data, also known as billing data or hospital discharge data, are commonly used in research to examine health-related questions and cost of care. These data are readily available, inexpensive to obtain, available in a computer-readable database format, and cover large populations over long periods of time (Iezzoni, 1994, 1997; Zhan and Miller, 2003).

The utility of administrative claims data for the evaluation of health care services and outcomes has been well established. Over the past 30 years, the analysis of retrospective administrative data has been used to examine practice variation (Shwartz et al., 1994; Wennberg et al., 1989), determine differences in access to care in minority groups (Desch et al., 1996), assess quality of care metrics (Iezzoni, 1997; Lohr, 1990), estimate disease incidence or cost (McBean et al., 1994; Simpson et al., 2013), and compare surgical outcomes and disease related outcomes and costs (Lubitz et al., 1993). Administrative claims data are part of the routine clinical reimbursement of health care services, allowing for availability of longitudinal data sets, with little cost and easy accessibility for the investigator. Medicare and Medicaid billing data are examples of data that often are used to answer CER questions.

The benefits of using these readily available data come with some serious limitations, however, including (1) their lack of representation of certain population groups such as in the case of Medicare (limited to elderly adults) or Medicaid (limited to poor or disabled individuals); (2) constraints based on the use of diagnosis codes to differentiate things such as initial event or repeat event, side of the body, or clinical severity of disease or condition; and (3) whether or not the event is a comorbidity or a complication of the condition or treatment under study. These data also do not contain other important clinical characteristics of care that might influence research results, such as disease severity. These data also do not contain PCOs and health-related quality of life (HRQoL) variables. All of these limitations increase the risk of selection bias in studies that use observational data. Researchers are developing methods to deal with many of these limitations because these data sources also offer considerable strengths including

1. Capacity to provide large samples
2. Capacity to follow patients over very long periods of time that are most often contiguous
3. Their availability at little expense
4. Their representativeness of patient populations that maximizes external validity (generalizability)

5. Their capacity to answer research questions that cannot be answered with randomized studies, such as effects of temporal and substantive trends related to changes in policy or clinical practice

Methods to make observational data behave more like randomized studies have been developed over the years to address the problem of selection bias that results from the lack of random treatment assignment. The objective of randomization in CER is to obtain groups that are balanced, or comparable, in terms of observed and unobserved group characteristics. If this balance is not achieved, it may not be clear whether a difference observed on a certain outcome of interest is due to the "treatment" under study or is the result of underlying differences between or among the groups. Even in randomized studies, balance between groups is analyzed for residual bias caused by unbalanced group characteristics.

However, when using observational data to assess health outcomes, it is not possible to randomize before data collection. Therefore, other methods, often referred to as "pseudo-randomization" methods, must be used to balance groups. One well-developed and largely accepted method to accomplish this task is the use of PS techniques.

Propensity score (PS), as described by the founders of the method, Rosenbaum and Rubin, is "the conditional probability of assignment to a particular treatment given a vector of observed covariates" (Rosenbaum and Rubin, 1983). The first step in using this technique is estimating the likelihood (i.e., the PS) that each individual in the sample would have received the treatment at a baseline time period given a set of their personal characteristics. A mathematical model is used to estimate the probability of inclusion in the group (i.e., receiving rTMS treatment) given a set of covariates, such as age, gender, race, number of failed depression drug regimens, and so on. Application of this model allows researchers to assume that groups of participants with similar PSs can be expected to have similar values of all their background information that is now aggregated into one measurement of probability between zero and one.

After PSs have been estimated for each individual, they can be used to answer the CER question, that is, "comparing treatment group effects," in two different ways: (1) by using the PS to weight individual participant information by the likelihood of their receiving the treatment (PS weighting) (Stuart, 2010) and (2) by matching controls to the cases by similarity in the PS (PS matching). Other methods using PSs to reduce selection bias have been used in the past, but weighting or matching techniques are preferred currently.

The earliest published study using PS matching was published by Gum and colleagues in 2001 (Gum et al., 2001). In this study, researchers examined the effectiveness of aspirin use on mortality in patients undergoing stress echocardiography for the evaluation of known or suspected coronary disease. Researchers matched each aspirin taker to a non–aspirin taker on a large selection of 31 variables likely to influence whether or not a person would be taking aspirin, such as prior cardiac disease, hypertension, heart failure, gender, or use of angiotensin-converting enzyme inhibitors or beta-blockers. So although we can see that this is not a new method, it is relatively recent that computers have allowed us to easily program complex matching algorithms on large samples. After performing the PS matching, these researchers found that there was a significant reduction in all-cause mortality in patients taking aspirin. The intention of PS matching is to match one or more individuals not receiving a certain treatment to a patient who is, based on a large collection of background information that may influence their selection into that particular treatment group (Rosenbaum, 2010).

Although this may sound like mathematical magic, a number of published studies compared results found using PS matching in observational data with results from very similar RCTs. Findings indicate that when the PS studies are done well, they report similar findings (Benson and Hartz, 2000). Thus, as is true in all other research, the key to using observational data to answer CE questions is using good research practices.

Although many methods of instrumental variable design and PS weighting are in current use, these and newer methods continue to be honed and developed, but the details are beyond the scope of the present discussion (Landrum and Ayanian, 2001; Stuart, 2010).

Similar to clinical practice guidelines, observational research methods guidelines have been developed and published by the International Society for Pharmacoeconomics and Outcomes Research (ISPOR) to identify criteria for "rigorous well designed and well executed Observational Studies (OS)" (Berger et al., 2012). The ISPOR outlined recommendations for good OS research, including clarity in specifying hypothesis-driven questions, including clear treatment groups and outcomes; identifying all measured and unmeasured confounders; using large sample sizes that allow studies to increase the number of comparators and subgroups; examining outcomes that are not directly affected by the intervention; understanding the practice patterns that induce bias; and using statistical approaches to better balance groups (e.g., PSs or instrumental variable design). The ISPOR also suggests that when given the opportunity, validity can be greatly improved by prospectively collecting data that would otherwise be unavailable.

As was suggested in an editorial review of the ISPOR OS taskforce findings, readers should be:

> as thoughtful as possible about the choice of an OS, emphasizing the notion that OS can be viewed as RCTs without randomization and that RCTs are OS once the randomization is complete. That kind of thinking moves us to go beyond the rigid definitions and hierarchies of designs and think about inferences, about how systematic review groups will rate the research, how clinical practice guidelines groups will use the research, and how CER can flourish and accomplish its goals (Greenfield and Platt, 2012).

DECISION ANALYSIS MODELING: INTEGRATING WHAT IS KNOWN

The word *modeling* is often confusing to readers of CE studies because modeling is used for two very different approaches to compare outcomes. Multivariable models (often incorrectly called multivariate models), such as regression analyses, are statistical approaches used to analyze data to identify patterns of relationships between variables and to test hypotheses. Stochastic models, usually called decision models, are mathematical structures that are used to link evidence from multiple sources to predict outcomes such as effectiveness, costs, or cost effectiveness. Both methods produce models, which are simplifications of reality. However, whereas the regression model finds patterns in data (a deductive approach), the decision model integrates data from many sources under a set of clearly specified assumptions (an inductive approach).

A decision model can be an extremely useful tool to predict beyond the limits of the data collected by researchers in a clinical trial to attempt to answer important questions facing decision makers (Simpson, 1995). Data from clinical trials or OSs are often limited to surrogate outcomes or have an inadequate time horizon to measure the outcomes that patients and policymakers care most about, such as quality of life and cost. Decision models are frequently used to predict long-term effects and multidimensional outcomes based on actual data on fewer variables observed for a shorter time period (Simpson, 1995). In the absence of direct primary empirical data to assess CE, the use of modeling to estimate effectiveness and cost effectiveness is considered to be a valid form of scientific inquiry (Gold et al., 1996).

Decision models structure a clinical problem mathematically, allowing researchers to enumerate the health outcomes and costs expected from using competing treatments. Decision models integrate data and information from many sources under a

clearly specified set of assumptions and are useful for informing discussions for and against specific treatment choices. Three types of structures are used for linking the data: (1) a decision tree (also called a probability tree), (2) a state-transition model (often called a Markov model), and (3) a discrete event model which is based on a flow chart approach (originally used to answer operations research questions such as how to estimate outcomes in a factory production process).

Decision trees organize data so that patients who traverse similar processes and have similar outcomes are grouped together on "branches." Each branch is linked to the next by probability nodes. Thus, decision trees sort and organize the available data by patients. Decision trees are the simplest decision analysis structures and are well suited for organizing data from many acute care processes and time-limited treatment processes. However, one limitation of decision tree models is that they are not well suited to representing events that recur over time.

Markov models or state-transition models are designed to allow for event recurrence and are used to organize data from chronic diseases such as HIV, depression, or stroke. Markov models capture the disease process by organizing the data into sets of mutually exclusive health states. These health states are assumed to be time limited, and patients' transition between each health state is based on the average rate of progression or cure observed by a clinical trial or an epidemiologic data set. Thus, the data for Markov models are cut into specific time periods based on what is known about the population, the disease, and the effect of interventions to govern the transitions into and out of the various health states (Freedberg et al., 1998).

Discrete event models are relative newcomers to decision analysis in health care. These models use software that was developed originally for manufacturing processes to capture the essence of patients' characteristics as well as the paths and branches that constitute the care process. Thus, each patient (or entity) enters the model and is assigned a "backpack," which contains a random selection of patient characteristics and risk factors. The characteristics for all the entities reflect the characteristics of the study population. Each entity is then moved along the treatment path until it reaches an event "station." These "stations" assign events to each entity. Events have yes or no answers, such as adherence to medication? Gets adverse event? Becomes pregnant? Dies? The events are assigned randomly, but the chance of having an event may be affected by the entity's characteristics. For example, the model will be specified so that an entity that is male cannot experience the event "Becomes pregnant." The computational program keeps a tally of numbers of events, time spent, and numbers of entities remaining alive. Programming discrete event models requires very large amounts of detailed clinical data and specially trained systems analysts for accurate results. After being programmed, discrete event models are amazingly versatile but also very complex to explain (Simpson et al., 2013). For these reasons, most published decision analysis models are either decision trees or Markov models. Decision trees and Markov models are discussed in detail below.

DECISION TREE EXAMPLE

Decision trees depict what may be expected to happen to a group of patients who receive different treatments. Each treatment choice is organized as one major branch originating from a central point, called a decision node. The population for each branch is then grouped into subgroups by:

1. The process of care common to patients, and
2. The intermediate and final outcomes experienced by patients over an episode of the illness

Figure 11-1 illustrates how a decision tree may be employed to use a combination of observational data from the evaluation of a guideline implementation with data from the published literature to compare current practice and use of a clinical practice guideline for the evaluation of pediatric appendicitis (Russel et al., 2013). Convention dictates that treatment choices are represented by square decision nodes and probability distributions are represented by round nodes or simple branches, with the proportion of patients who fall into a group indicated below each branch and the type of group written above the branch. For example, in **Figure 11-1**, the probability of having an ultrasound test is 55% for patients treated according to the guidelines. Of these patients, 88% may be expected to be true positive and 12% false negative. Five percent of the missed patients will get a computed tomography (CT) scan based on parent or physician preferences, and 95% of the missed patients on this branch are at risk of developing peritonitis because of the missed diagnosis. To calculate how many children may be expected to have the outcome specified by each branch, we "roll back" the tree. That is, we use the contingent probabilities organized by the decision tree format to estimate outcomes for a population of patients. In **Figure 11-1**, we used 1000 patients per branch to compare outcomes for patients treated by the guideline versus current practice. The numbers at the ends of the branches represent "rolling back" the decision tree. In this example, following the treatment guidelines dramatically reduced the number of CT studies from about two thirds of the patients to less

than 10%. This has the great advantage of reducing radiation exposure to young patients. The downside is that slightly more patients developed peritonitis, a complication of missing the diagnosis earlier because fewer CT studies were being performed.

We can also use the decision tree to calculate the differences in expected cost of care for the two treatment approaches. We simply multiply the number of patients on each branch of the tree by the mean expected treatment cost for their clinical path. In this example, the costs vary by ultrasonography ($257) and CT ($1418) as well as by the cost of a hospital admission for appendectomy ($9009) or admission with peritonitis ($12,703). We sum the cost for the branches above and below the square decision node. The summed costs will then represent best expected cost for treating 1000 children with each approach. In this case, it appears that using the guideline may both save money and reduce radiation risk but that it will slightly increase the number of missed cases with a higher incidence of peritonitis.

As illustrated in this example, a decision tree is a useful organizing framework for calculating the different types of outcomes that would be expected for acute events under different treatment assumptions and costing perspectives. Although decision trees can be used to inform many clinical and management decisions in health care, published papers using decision trees often focus on comparing emerging clinical or preventive health interventions at a time when the evidence for a new intervention is sparse. In such cases, a decision analysis can combine the limited new efficacy data available with disease history, epidemiologic data, and cost data to estimate differences in expected outcomes under a clearly articulated set of assumptions. Although the results of this type of analysis do not provide strong evidence either for or against the adoption of a new therapy, they often provide an invaluable framework for policy discussions and nearly always increase our understanding of the key factors that are associated with the desired outcomes from a particular therapy (Briggs, 1998).

MARKOV-TYPE DECISION MODELS

A Markov or state-transition decision analysis model structure is used to organize the data for conditions when a patient's health experience can be defined as a progression through different disease stages. Each stage in a Markov-type model is defined as a health state, and it may be possible to progress through stages of increasing severity, as well as from very severe stages to less severe stages or even to be cured. Markov models are especially useful for predicting long-term outcomes such as survival, for

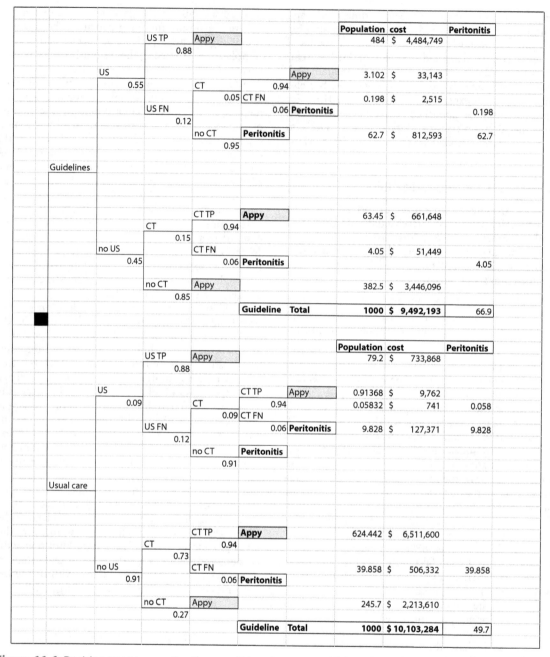

Figure 11-1. Decision tree representing the comparison between guideline use and usual care for pediatric appendicitis evaluation. CT, computed tomography; FN, False Negative; TP, True Positive.

clinical trials which are inclined to rely on less definitive intermediate health outcomes or surrogate markers such as CD4 cell counts to measure the clinical efficacy, effectiveness, and safety of treatments for complex chronic conditions such as HIV/AIDS (Sonnenberg and Beck, 1993). Markov-type structures often are used for modeling in cases when a decision tree would have a large number of subbranches that are nearly identical except for differences in their preceding probability nodes. Thus, a Markov-type structure may be used to simplify very dense, "bushy" decision trees.

The definition of the health states in a Markov model may change from very simple to more complex as the information about a condition improves. This relationship is readily observed in the AIDS models that have been published in the past 20+ years. The efficacy measures in the early trials of antiretroviral drugs were progression from asymptomatic HIV disease to AIDS or death, and early models used simple decision trees or state-transition models with few health states based on AIDS and death. As CD4 cell counts became a routinely reported measure of immune deficiency and RNA viral load began to be considered a strong indicator of the risk of disease progression, the health states used in the published decision models of treatments for HIV disease became defined by these markers. Furthermore, as our understanding of HIV disease progressed and our medical armamentarium increased, published HIV disease models progressed to using Markov-type structures with many health states, even linking sequential state-transition structures to capture the complexity of a condition which was transforming from a rapidly fatal disease to a severe chronic illness requiring lifelong monitoring and therapy. The AIDS modeling papers by Simpson et al. (1995, 2004, 2013), Chancellor et al. (1997), and Freedberg et al. (2001) illustrate this progression.

In a state-transition or Markov model, the disease process is carved into time periods of equal length defined by a set of health states. Each health state has a specific average quality of life, risk of progression or cure, and cost expected to be experienced with the defining clinical markers. The progression for a specific group of patients is then defined by the length of time they spend in each health state. Some health states are final or absorbing, meaning that when a patient reaches this state, no further progression or improvement will occur. Death is always an absorbing health state, but other states, such as cured or "surgical removal of . . ." may also be defined as absorbing states if they are assumed to happen no more than once to any one individual. Each health state lasts for a specific time period (e.g., 1 hour, day, week, month, or year); this is called the length of a cycle in the model. The choice of length for a cycle depends on the length of the illness episode modeled; the length of time included in the efficacy and epidemiologic data available; and the average time included in cost data, which usually are reported as aggregates, such as a hospital admission. The choice of a model cycle time is an optimization process. The objective is to find the longest time period that fits the majority of the patient's natural disease episodes, the efficacy data, and the cost reporting while making sure that the model does not inadvertently exclude differential outcomes for patients with very short episodes of care.

Estimates for patient groups with very long episodes of care can be accommodated by having patients occupy a health state for more than one cycle. Thus, the selection of cycle length often is more of an art than a science.

After a model's health states and cycle time has been defined, the available data can be analyzed to populate the model. Two types of data are needed: parameters and transition probabilities. Parameters are mean values for measures of interest that are specific to each health state. For example, an AIDS Markov model would use parameters that accounted for the mean risk of getting an AIDS event, the mean cost of treating an average AIDS event, and the mean quality of life weight (utility) that patients assign to living in that health state.

Transition probabilities are similar to the probability nodes in the decision tree. They function like gates between connected health states. Each transition probability defines the proportion of patients in a current health state who are allowed to move to another state after the cycle time has been completed. For example, the transition probability of moving from health state A to health state B is the percent of individuals who would progress from health state A to health state B during the time of one model cycle under the treatment conditions that are tested in the model. This seems simple, but getting these data can be complicated because the standard epidemiologic measures of risk, such as risk ratio or odds ratios account for the overall risk of disease progression across health states included in a model, not the contingent risk of progression from one health state to another, which is what we need to calculate transition probabilities. These transition probabilities are the critical variables that contain the differences in efficacy between the therapies compared in the model. They are the "engine" that drives the population through the model at different rates for different treatments. Correctly estimating the model transition probabilities, especially the differences in transition probabilities for the treatments compared in a Markov model, is the most critical aspect of designing a Markov model. The effects of even small variations in the transition probability differences often swamp the effects of relatively large differences in parameter values for cost, events, or quality of life in most models.

The probabilities of moving from health state A to health state B during a model cycle, as well as the probability of moving from state B to state A, are entered into a table called a transition matrix (**Figure 11-2**). This table has one row and one column for each health state. Thus, a transition matrix for a model with five health states will have five rows and five columns, with a total of 25 cells. In a Markov model in which

	Poststroke	MI Event	MI Death	Total
Poststroke	0.70	0.15	0.15	1.00
MI Event	0.50	0	0.50	1.00
MI Death	0	0	1.00	1.00

	Age-Specific Deaths	Poststroke	MI Event	MI Deaths	Age Deaths	Total Deaths	Check Sum
START		100	0	0	0		
Age 70	3.8%	67.3	14.4	14.4	3.8	18.23	100.0
71	4.1%	52.1	9.7	31.0	7.2	38.2	100.0
72	4.5%	39.5	7.5	43.1	9.9	53.1	100.0
73	4.9%	29.8	5.6	52.3	12.2	64.5	100.0
74	5.4%	22.4	4.2	59.2	14.1	73.4	100.0
75	5.9%	16.8	3.2	64.4	15.7	80.1	100.0
76	6.6%	12.4	2.3	68.2	17.0	85.2	100.0
77	7.2%	9.2	1.7	71.0	18.1	89.1	100.0
78	8.0%	6.7	1.3	73.1	19.0	92.0	100.0
79	8.8%	4.9	0.9	**74.6**	**19.7**	**94.2**	100.0
Total MI Events=		**51**					

Figure 11-2. Markov model for estimating the rate of myocardial infarctions (MIs) for 70-year-old stroke survivors: *Asterisk* indicates assumptions for the average cohort of 100 70-year-old stroke survivors.

patients can move from any one state to any other state at the end of each cycle, all 25 cells must contain an accurate contingent probability of a patient's move from one health state to the next. A Markov model with 10 health states, which allows movement between all health states, requires 10 × 10 = 100 contingent probability calculations. If at least 30 observations are needed for each calculation (a good rule of thumb for such calculations), then populating the transition matrix would require a minimum of 3000 patient observations in such a model. Given that the value of a decision modeling study is to inform discussions before sufficient efficacy data are available, it is easy to see the virtue of keeping the number of model health states low and making as many simplifying assumptions as possible to disallow movements between some model health states.

After the health states and cycle times have been specified and the transitions and parameters calculated, the model can be programmed.

Markov models can be solved as mathematical equations using matrix algebra, they can be programmed in spreadsheets using one column for each health state and one row for each cycle, or they can be programmed in special modeling software. **Figure 11-2** shows a simple Markov model for risk of a myocardial infarction (MI) in stroke survivors. Such a model might have just three health states: poststroke, MI, and death. Thus, if we have a cohort of 100 70-year-old male patients who are discharged alive from a hospital after a stroke, and we know that the annual risk of MIs is expected to be 30% and that 50% will die from their MIs, then we can calculate the number of expected MI deaths at 10 years. However, it would be too high unless our model also accounted for competing deaths from all other causes. To correct for competing deaths, we can use actuarial life table data on the probability of death by year of age and gender (Social Security Administration, 2011). For ease of calculation, we can use spreadsheet software.

For the purpose of this illustration, we will assume that (1) the MI and death rates are constant, (2) all events happen at the end of each year, and (3) the age-specific death rates do not have to be adjusted for this stroke population. (These assumptions would be too primitive for an actual model.) This simple Markov model is depicted in **Figure 11-2**. The "engine" of the model is in the top box, called the "transition matrix." In this matrix, we have translated the risks of having an MI and surviving and having an MI and dying into annual probabilities. All the row probabilities in the matrix add to 1, indicating that patients either change to a new column or stay where they are. This reflects the "mutually exclusive and jointly exhaustive" rule for Markov models. For ease of calculation, we apply the Centers for Disease Control and Prevention's death risk first to all live patients because this death risk is age specific and increases each year. After we have estimated who dies of "old age," then we apply the probabilities in the transition matrix to all patients on the next line of the model. Starting with 100 patients in the "poststroke" health state, at the end of the first year, we will have 14.4 patients with MIs who remain alive, 14.4 patient deaths from MI, and 3.8 deaths from old age. During the next year, we apply the same assumption to the remaining live population, and the model calculates the new numbers. In this simple example, one can see how MIs and MI deaths happen each year. You can also see how competing deaths from "old age" capture a larger and larger proportion of deaths as the population ages. If you look at the bottom of **Figure 11-2**, you can see that over the 10 years in the model, we had 51 MI events in which patients survived, 74.6 in which patients died, and 19.7 deaths from old age. Furthermore, the model indicates that 94.2 patients have died over the 10 years modeled. In real life, patients do not die in fractions. However, because a Markov model applies contingent probabilities repeatedly to the starting number of patients, one of its artificial features is that it will estimate fractions of people. We can circumvent this problem by calculating outcomes for large numbers of patients, or we can simply think of the Markov model results in terms of percentages of individual surviving.

SENSITIVITY ANALYSIS

Models are only as good as the assumptions and the data that are used for their construction. Decision makers, therefore, need some reassurance that predictions are not completely irrelevant to informing decisions. There are two ways to provide information about the validity of modeling results, model validation and model sensitivity analysis. Models must have **face validity**; that is, *they must seem reasonable to experienced clinicians*. If they do not, it is unlikely that they will inform any real-world clinical decisions. *Models should also, at a minimum, be able to predict the prevalence of key conditions and costs for populations other than those on which they were designed* (**predictive validity**). Unfortunately, because models are mainly needed to inform practice and policy for when strong evidence is not available, good data on outcomes for populations for the new therapies that are being modeled are often rare. If such data were readily available, then we might not need to construct a decision model in the first place. Thus, modelers must rely on *examining how their estimates change as model parameters are changed*. This is called **sensitivity analyses**. Sensitivity analyses test a model's response to variations in the levels of parameters variables included; they answer the "what if" questions. Although parameter values are usually entered into the model as discrete values, they may be drawn from a range of potential values (i.e., confidence intervals) based on random chance or the approach to measuring. Moreover, practitioners and researchers may want to adapt the model results to slightly different populations or scenarios than those used in a model.

To test the effect of these variations on the model results, the value of a single parameter may be replaced with ones that are less likely but still possible. For example, these could include values at the limits of the parameter's confidence interval or best or worst case scenario values. This is an example of one-way sensitivity analysis. A two-way sensitivity analysis changes the values of two parameters simultaneously. The stability of model predictions may also be tested by randomly varying many of the key parameter values within their confidence intervals. This type of testing may be done using a Monte Carlo approach.

If the model results do not change much when parameters are varied, the model is said to be **stable** *or* **robust**. Otherwise, the model is characterized as sensitive or volatile. One of the very important results from a modeling study is the information about which parameters most strongly affect the results. For sensitive models, we often calculate the value of the parameter at which the model yields a different conclusion; this is the model's "tipping point." In modeling language, this point is known as the threshold value.

SUMMARY

Comparative effectiveness research (CER) has been defined as "rigorous evaluation of the impact of different options that are available for treating a given medical condition" (CBO, 2007). Four types of research designs fall within the domain of CER: (1) systematic review or quantitative synthesis, (2) decision analysis, (3) OSs, and (4) large pragmatic clinical trials. In this chapter, we have explored how these various designs can contribute to informing treatment selection.

Large, pragmatic clinical trials offer the advantage of providing the highest quality of evidence because they randomize patients to treatment alternatives under consideration. Unfortunately, large RCTs are expensive to conduct, take comparatively long to complete, and often have restrictive inclusion criteria, making it difficult to extrapolate findings to other patient populations.

Meta-analysis or quantitative synthesis generally provides high-quality information, particularly when summarizing RCT data, but often is limited to the published literature, which may be biased toward studies with positive results. The ability to extrapolate data to populations similar to those encountered in "real–world" clinical practice also may be limited.

Models based on decision analysis are becoming more widely used because they can incorporate large and complex data that reflect routine clinical care situations. A variety of methods can be used for decision analysis purposes, ranging from relatively simple decision trees to complex Markov models. Fundamental to interpreting the results of a decision analysis is affirming both that (1) the structure of the model is valid and (2) that the data used in the model are free from bias or other errors.

Observational data may be limited by potential sources of bias related to the absence of randomization of treatment assignment. However, data from these studies may represent the typical clinical practice setting more appropriately than the constrained parameters of a clinical trial. Observational data also are available on a wide range of topics from routinely collected data and therefore may be much less expensive and time consuming for the investigator to amass.

Observational data sources include clinical record systems, as well as administrative data used for billing and regulatory purposes. These data sources often include very large patient populations that are followed over time. The lack of randomization, however, raises the question of whether the treatment groups being compared are balanced with respect to both known and unknown prognostic factors. A variety of methods have been developed to "pseudo-randomize" the study subjects, that is, to mathematically eliminate any potential bias in underlying differences between the groups being compared.

In this chapter, we have illustrated the use of a simple decision tree to evaluate a treatment guideline for managing appendicitis in children. The guideline attempts to reduce the number of children exposed to diagnostic radiation through the use of ultrasonography. The decision analysis affirmed that application of the treatment guideline dramatically lowers the use of ionizing radiation and cost. At the same time, the treatment guideline results in a slight increase in "missed diagnoses," with a greater number of resulting peritoneal infections.

We also applied a simple Markov model to gain insight into the risk of MI incidence and mortality after a stroke. The model helps to provide an appreciation of the relative contribution of cardiac disease to poststroke mortality over time, with more nonfatal MIs in the early years, more fatal MIs and other causes in the later years, and MIs accounting for more than three of four total deaths in this group.

Comparative effectiveness research is becoming an increasingly important approach for the evaluation of treatment options and making optimal care decisions. The ability to interpret the results of CER will emerge as a crucial skill for clinicians, regardless of care setting and focus of practice.

STUDY QUESTIONS

1. Which of the following is NOT an example of comparative effectiveness research?
   A. An observational study using propensity matching
   B. A meta-analysis
   C. An efficacy-based randomized control trial
   D. A decision tree–based analytical study

2. What is one of the weaknesses related to meta-analyses?
   A. They combine information from across multiple studies
   B. Most of the data available will be efficacy data, not data on effectiveness
   C. Similar endpoints from multiple studies are used to generate a combined effect size
   D. They are not well accepted

3. Which of these is NOT a strength of observational studies?
   A. Their longitudinal nature or ability for researchers to follow patients over very long periods of time that are most often contiguous
   B. Their ready availability at little expense
   C. Their ability to control for selection bias with randomization of subjects
   D. Their ability to answer research questions that cannot be answered with RCTs such as effects of changes in policy or clinical practice

4. A stochastic decision analysis model is
   A. A statistical approaches used to analyzed data to identify patterns of relationships between variables and to test hypotheses.
   B. Mathematical structures that are used to link evidence from multiple sources to predict outcomes such as effectiveness, costs, or cost effectiveness often over a long time period.
   C. A method used to control selection bias.
   D. A way to assess the efficacy of treatment effect in clinical trials.

5. Which of these is NOT a type of propensity score method?
   A. Matching
   B. Stratification
   C. Weighting
   D. Randomization

6. *What is selection bias?*

    A. A systematic error that can affect the integrity of a study (internal validity), causing some members of the population to be less likely to be included than others in the study sample

    B. A bias that makes the results of a study difficult to generalize to a broader population

    C. Error caused by study personnel being aware of the treatment allocation

    D. Problems that occur related to the inability of study participants to accurately remember personal details

7. *Which of these is NOT a type of data that can be used in observational studies?*

    A. Administrative billing data

    B. Abstracted medical records

    C. Survey data

    D. Clinical trial data

8. *The process of examining how decision analysis model estimates change as model parameters are changed is called*

    A. regression analysis.

    B. sensitivity analysis.

    C. guessing.

    D. survival analysis.

9. *What is NOT a benefit of large pragmatic clinical trials?*

    A. Maximize external validity

    B. Maximize internal validity

    C. Randomization controls for selection bias

    D. Less expensive

10. *Which of these is NOT a weakness of observational studies?*

    A. May lack representation of certain population groups

    B. Do not contain data on patient centered outcomes such as quality of life

    C. May take many years and be very expensive to obtain data

    D. Diagnosis codes may not differentiate things such comorbidity, complication, or clinical severity

FURTHER READING

Austin PC. The relative ability of different propensity score methods to balance measured covariates between treated and untreated subjects in observational studies. *Med Decis Making.* 2009;29(6):661-677.

Meyer AM, Wheeler SB, Weinberger M, Chen RC, Carpenter WR. An overview of methods for comparative effectiveness research. *Semin Radiat Oncol.* 2014;24:5-13.

Mitchell JB, Bubolz T, Paul JE, et al. Using Medicare claims for outcomes research. *Med Care.* 1994;32(7 suppl):JS38-JS51.

Sher DJ, Punglia RS. Decision analysis and cost effectiveness research—a primer. *Semin Radiat Oncol.* 2014;24:14-24.

REFERENCES

AHRQ Clinician Research Summaries. (2012, March). Non-pharmacologic interventions for treatment-resistant depression in adults. Pub.11(12)-EHC056-3.

Antman EM, Lau J, Kulpenick B, Mosteller F, Chalmers TC. A comparison of results of meta-analysis of randomized controlled trials and recommendations of clinical experts: treatments for myocardial infarction. *JAMA.* 1992;268:240-248.

Benson K, Hartz AJ. A comparison of observational studies and randomized, controlled trials. *N Engl J Med.* 2000; 342(25):1878-1886.

Berger ML, Dreyer N, Anderson F, Towse A, Sedrakyan A, Normand SL. Prospective observational studies to assess comparative effectiveness: the ISPOR good research practices task force report. *Value Health.* 2012;15(2):217-230.

Briggs A, Schulpher M. An introduction to Markov modelling for economic evaluation. *PharmEcon.* 1998;13(3):397-409.

Campbell MJ, Walters SJ. *How to Design, Analyze, and Report Cluster Randomized Trials.* Hoboken, NJ: Wiley; 2014.

Carpenter LL, Janicak PG, Aaronson ST, et al. Transcranial magnetic stimulation (TMS) for major depression: a multisite, naturalistic, observational study of acute treatment outcomes in clinical practice. *Depress Anxiety.* 2012;29(7):587-596.

Chalmers I, Hayes B. Systematic reviews: reporting, updating, and correcting systematic reviews of effects of health care. *BMJ.* 1994;309:862.

Chalmers I. The work of the National Perinatal Epidemiology Unit. One example of technology assessment in perinatal care. *Int J Technol Assess Health Care.* 1991;7(4):430-459.

Chancellor JV, Hill AM, Sabin CA et al. Modeling the cost effectiveness of lamivudine/zidovudine combination therapy in HIV infection. *PharmacoEconomics.* 1997;12(1):54-63.

Clark A, Jaurequi B, Griffith U, et al. TRIVAC decision-support model for evaluating the cost-effectiveness of *Haemophilus influenza* type b, pneumococcal and rotavirus vaccination. *Vaccine.* 2013;31(suppl 3):C19-C29.

Congressional Budget Office. Research on the comparative effectiveness of medical treatments. December, 2007. www.cbo.gov/publication/41655. Accessed on May 10, 2014.

Desch CE, Penberthy L, Newschaffer CJ, et al. Factors that determine the treatment for local and regional prostate cancer. *Med Care.* 1996;34(2):152-162.

Eddy DM, Hasselblad V, McGivney W, Hendee W. The value of mammography screening in women under age 50. *JAMA.* 1988;259:1512-1519.

Fava M, Rush AJ, Wisniewski SR, et al. A comparison of mirtazapine and nortriptyline following two consecutive failed medication treatments for depressed outpatients: a STAR*D report. *Am J Psychiatry.* 2006;163(7):1161-1172.

Freedberg KA, Losina E, Weinstein MC et al. The cost effectiveness of combination antiretroviral therapy for HICV disease. *N Eng J Med.* 2001;344(11):824-831.

Freedberg KA, Scharfstein JA, Seage GR et al. The cost-effectiveness of preventing AIDS-related opportunistic infection. *JAMA*. (1998;279(2):130-136.

Gold M, Siegel J, Russell L, et al., ed. *Cost-Effectiveness in Health and Medicine*. New York: Oxford University Press; 1996.

Greenfield S, Platt R. Can observational studies approximate RCTs? *Value Health*. 2012;15(2):215-216.

Gum PA, Thamilarasan M, Watanabe J, Blackstone EH, Lauer MS. Aspirin use and all-cause mortality among patients being evaluated for known or suspected coronary artery disease: a propensity analysis. *JAMA*. 2001;286(10):1187-1194.

Iezzoni LI, ed. *Risk Adjustment for Measuring Health Care Outcomes*. Ann Arbor, MI: Health Administration Press 1994.

Iezzoni LI. Assessing quality using administrative data. *Ann Interna Med*. 1997;127(8 Pt 2):666-674.

Institute of Medicine. Initial national priorities for comparative effectiveness research. Report Brief June, 2009. www.iom.edu/cerpriorities. Accessed on May 10, 2014.

Landrum MB, Ayanian JZ. Causal effect of ambulatory specialty care on mortality following myocardial infarction: a comparison of propensity score and instrumental variable analyses. *Health Serv Outcomes Res Methodol*. 2001;2(3-4):221-245.

Lohr K. IOM study urges a major shift in QA strategy. *QA Rev*. 1990;2(5):1, 7-8.

Lubitz JD, Gornick ME, Mentnech RM, Loop FD. Rehospitalizations after coronary revascularization among Medicare beneficiaries. *Am J Cardiol*. 1993;72(1):26-30.

McBean AM, Warren JL, Babish JD. Measuring the incidence of cancer in elderly Americans using Medicare claims data. *Cancer*. 1994;73(9):2417-2425.

Nahas Z, Short B, Burns C, et al. A feasibility study of a new method for electrically producing seizures in man: focal electrically administered seizure therapy [FEAST]. *Brain Stimul*. 2013;6(3):403-408.

Rosenbaum PR, Rubin DB. The central role of the propensity score in observational studies for causal effect. *Biometrika*. 1983;70(1):41-55.

Rosenbaum PR. *Design of Observational Studies*. New York: Springer; 2010.

Russell WS, Schuh AM, Hill JG et al. Clinical practice guidelines for pediatric appendicitis evaluation can decrease computer tomography utilization while maintaining diagnostic accuracy. *Ped Emerg Care*. 2013;29(5):568-573.

Shwartz M, Ash AS, Anderson J, Iezzoni LI, Payne SM, Restuccia JD. Small area variations in hospitalization rates: how much you see depends on how you look. *Med Care*. 1994;32(3):189-201.

Simpson AN, Bonilha HS, Kazley AS, Zoller JS, Ellis C. Marginal costing methods highlight the contributing cost of comorbid conditions in Medicare patients: a quasi-experimental case-control study of ischemic stroke costs. *Cost Eff Resour Alloc*. 2013;11(1):29.

Simpson KN. Economic modeling of HIV treatments. *Curr Opin HIV AIDS*. 2010;5(3):242-248.

Simpson KN. Modeling with clinical trial data: getting from the data researchers have to the data decision makers need. *Drug Info J*. 1995;29(4):1431-1440.

Social Security Administration. Actuarial life table: period life table, 2010. Published 2011. http://www.ssa.gov/oact/STATS/table4c6.html. Accessed December 27, 2014.

Sonnenberg FA, Beck JR. Markov models in medical decision making: a practical guide. *Med Decis Making*. 1993;13:322-338.

Stuart EA. Matching methods for causal inference: a review and a look forward. *Stat Sci*. 2010;25(1):1-21.

The Mount Hood Modeling Group. Computer Modeling of Diabetes and Its Complications: A report on the Fourth Mount Hood Challenge Meeting. *Diabetes care*. 2007;30(6): 1638-1646.

Wennberg JE, Freeman JL, Shelton RM, Bubolz TA. Hospital use and mortality among Medicare beneficiaries in Boston and New Haven. *N Engl J Med*. 1989;321(17):1168-1173.

Zhan C, Miller MR. Administrative data based patient safety research: a critical review. *Qual Saf Health Care*. 2003;12(suppl 2):ii58-ii63.

Planning a Systematic Review

Cathy L. Melvin and Carolyn Jenkins

HEALTH SCENARIO

Late on a Monday afternoon, a nurse researcher received a call from a community leader in a rural church in Bamberg County, South Carolina. Their annual community health fair was scheduled for the following month, and they were requesting "diabetes screening" using an analysis of glucose in the blood or the "finger stick screening for diabetes." According to the community leader, the church works with members of the congregation and surrounding community to bring free health services and linkages to health care providers to community members. Many people in this community may see their health care providers only when sick, may have inadequate health insurance coverage, or may be unable to afford to pay for preventive care and recommended screenings. The community leader knows that diabetes is a problem among members of the congregation and the broader community in Bamberg County.

The nurse researcher knows that epidemiologic data from the Behavioral Risk Factor Surveillance System (BRFSS) show that almost 15% of Bamberg County's 16,000 residents report a diagnosis of diabetes (South Carolina Department of Health and Environmental Control, 2013), a rate nearly twice the national average, and that three quarters of the county's residents report being overweight or obese. She also knows that about 60% of the county's population is African American (U.S. Census Bureau, 2014) and that according to national estimates, about 12.6% of non-Hispanic black adults have been diagnosed with diabetes (Centers for Disease Control and Prevention [CDC], 2014). Data and the personal experience of the nurse researcher suggest that Bamberg County's low median household incomes and rural location restrict residents' access to comprehensive medical care, opportunities for physical activity, and affordable healthy food options. Moreover, local and state news media recently covered the closure of the area hospital that provided basic resources for diabetes identification and education in the county. Now no diabetes prevention or diabetes self-management education programs are available in the area. Clearly, the church leader is responding to a pressing need in an underresourced community, which is, unfortunately, a typical situation faced by many rural communities across the United States.

The question is: How should the nurse researcher respond to the request from the church leader based on available evidence or recommendations about who to screen for diabetes, how to conduct screenings for diabetes, and whether a community-based event such as a health fair is the best approach?

SYSTEMATIC REVIEWS: UTILITY AND DEFINITION

Questions such as those facing the nurse researcher and church leader arise almost every day. Researchers and health care providers are always looking for ways to meet an expressed need, improve practice, stimulate behavior change among patients, or create or change a program or policy. Using the diabetes screening example, health care providers may wonder how to best screen for diabetes, asking whether it is better to use a survey based on risk factors as recommended by the American Diabetes Association (CDC, 2014) or an analysis of glucose in the blood as requested by the church leader. Payers may want to know if they should reimburse for one test versus another or either one under different conditions or for people at various levels of risk. Patients may wonder how often they should be screened or if they are at high risk for diabetes. And a church leader and nurse researcher may need to know if a community health fair is the best way to reach and identify individuals most in need of diabetes screening and follow-up care.

There are a variety of ways to find answers to such questions. Experts may be consulted, just as the church leader did when the call was made to the nurse researcher. Community members may ask their peers about how community health fairs worked for them or hear about successful health fairs via social or mass media. Health care providers and payers may attend conferences and hear about evidence-based options for improving diabetes screening, diagnosis, and management as well as changes colleagues made in their practices to accomplish these goals. Researchers and others may look at existing epidemiology data, health systems capacity, available peer-reviewed literature, and evidence-based guidelines on screening for diabetes such as those from the American Diabetes Association and the U.S. Preventive Services Task Force.

All of these perspectives are important in determining whether there is sufficient evidence to support the choice of community-based screening for diabetes via a community health fair with the expectation that the fair would improve the diagnosis and management of diabetes in Bamberg County. Ideally, we would like to find at least one credible source to answer such a question based on sound epidemiologic data, current health systems capacity, the costs of screening, the appropriateness of alternative tests, community priorities, and ethical and political considerations (World Health Organization [WHO], 2003).

One way to answer these questions is to find an existing source of evidence for each specific question posed by a stakeholder or stakeholder group. In our Health Scenario, we would like to know if a community health fair is the best way to reach and identify individuals most in need of diabetes screening and follow-up care. A quick search on the Internet may turn up a specific article in a peer-reviewed journal about community health fairs, a recommendation about the use of community health fairs to reach underserved individuals, or a case report of a particularly successful event. Although any one or a set of articles may appear helpful in answering our questions, closer examination reveals that the studies were conducted in locations very different from Bamberg County. In addition, they each used different tests to screen for diabetes, and community health fairs were attended by only a small number of people. Furthermore, some people attended in greater proportions than expected given the demographics of the area. Finally, some studies had different outcomes than the desired outcome for such an event in Bamberg County. Some studies may have reported outcomes such as the number of attendees at the event; others the proportion of attendees screened for diabetes or the proportion found to have diabetes or to be prediabetic. All of this "noise" across articles makes it difficult to translate findings from individual studies into best practice or, in this case, to determine if a community health fair is the best thing to do in Bamberg County.

A systematic review (SR) is one option for compiling existing research and other types of information to answer questions such as the ones faced by the church

leader and the nurse researcher. There are many definitions of SR in the literature and in use by various professional, research, and guideline development groups. We use the following definition adapted from one proposed by the Agency for Healthcare Research and Quality (AHRQ): *an SR is a critical assessment and evaluation of all research studies that address a particular issue* (http://effectivehealthcare.ahrq.gov/glossary-of-terms/?pageaction=showterm&termid=70) (AHRQ, n.d.b.).

Researchers and other persons developing SR (review developers) use an organized method of locating, assembling, and evaluating a body of literature on a particular topic using a set of specific criteria. An SR typically includes a description of the findings of the collection of research studies and may tailor presentation of findings for specific target audiences, including the general public (http://effectivehealthcare.ahrq.gov/glossary-of-terms/?pageaction=showterm&termid=70) (AHRQ, n.d.b.).

Research studies published in peer review sources usually are the foundational literature for an SR, but other types of literature may also be included such as "grey" or unpublished literature. Types of grey literature may include unpublished manuscripts, manuscripts in press, clinical trial registries, conference papers, conference posters, evaluation reports, and grant close-out reports. Searches may be conducted by reviewing grey-literature databases (i.e., the Grey Literature Report by The New York Academy of Medicine at http://www.greylit.org, Trip at http://www.tripdatabase.com, DocuTicker at http://www.docuticker.com, or U.S. Government Documents at http://guides.library.upenn.edu/usgovdocuments) or by contacting authors of published work on the topic or others known to have a special interest in the topic. SR developers include grey literature to help balance the publication bias for a review because reviews are often biased in favor of randomized controlled trials or positive research findings.

The literature found in an SR may be analyzed in different ways depending on the outcome of interest, the type of studies included in the review, and the presentation of results. Options range from a narrative qualitative summary of review findings to quantitative pooling of data using meta-analytic statistical techniques. A meta-analysis is a statistical process that combines the findings from individual studies. Not all reviews include studies suitable for a meta-analysis of findings (http://effectivehealthcare.ahrq.gov/glossary-of-terms/?pageaction=showterm&termid=39) (AHRQ, n.d.a.).

In sum, SRs are an important tool for health care decision makers and other stakeholders in the health care system. These reviews offer the best summary of existing evidence about a specific topic or set of interventions based on the available literature. SRs identify, select, assess, and synthesize the findings of similar but separate studies and can help clarify what is known and not known about the potential benefits and harms of drugs, devices, and other health care services as well as behavioral and policy-based approaches to improving health and health care. SRs can be helpful for clinicians who want to integrate research findings into their daily practices, for patients who want to make well-informed choices about their own care, for professional medical societies who are preparing guidance for their members, payers, and policymakers (Institute of Medicine [IOM], 2011).

PLANNING A REVIEW

Many organizations offer guidance on how to create a plan for the conduct of an SR. We present an adaptation of several of these approaches by starting with a statement of the intended outcomes of the planning process itself and the use of existing reviews in deciding whether to plan and conduct a review.

Outcomes of a Planning Process for a Systematic Review

The review planning process should result in at least the following three outcomes:

1. *A well-framed question or set of questions* specifying the types of **p**opulations or participants, **i**nterventions, **c**omparisons, and **o**utcomes (PICO) to be included in the review. The specification of these types of information to frame the review is often referred to as the PICO for the SR (Higgins and Green, 2011; IOM, 2011).

2. In our example, the church leader and nurse researcher agree that the **p**opulation they are trying to reach is African American adults older than age 18 years in Bamberg County, and they would like to know if their proposed **i**ntervention of a community health fair is more effective when **c**ompared with other diabetes screening options such as clinic-based or other interventions to affect their chosen **o**utcome of increasing the percentage of adults screened for diabetes in Bamberg County.

3. *A statement of what types of studies* are to be included in the review (e.g., clinical trials, observational studies)

4. A description (often a logic model or analytic framework) that describes the relationship of PICO elements to one another

Decisions about these outcomes of the planning process frame the review and become the prespecified eligibility criteria for including specific studies in the review.

Table 12-1. Selected organizations producing systematic reviews.

SR Developers	Website
International:	
The Cochrane Collaboration	http://www.cochrane.org/
Centre for Reviews & Dissemination (CRD)	http://www.york.ac.uk/inst/crd/
The Campbell Collaboration	http://www.campbellcollaboration.org/
National Institute for Health & Clinical Excellence (NICE)	http://www.nice.org.uk/
US Private:	
BCBS Association Technology Evaluation Center	http://www.ahrq.gov/research/findings/evidence-based-reports/centers/bcbsatec.html
ECRI Institute	https://www.ecri.org/Pages/default.aspx
Hayes International, Inc.	http://www.haynesintl.com/\
U.S. Government:	
AHRQ Effective Health Care Program via Evidence-based Practice Centers	http://www.ahrq.gov/research/findings/evidence-based-reports/overview/index.html
Centers for Disease Control and Prevention (CDC)	http://www.cdc.gov/
The Substance Abuse and Mental Health Services Administration (SAMHSA)	http://www.samhsa.gov/

Data from Institute of Medicine. (2011). *Finding What Works in Health Care: Standards for Systematic Reviews.* Washington, DC: The National Academies

Search for Existing Reviews

Many organizations conduct SRs on a wide range of health and health care topics (**Table 12-1**). Anyone considering the conduct of a review would be well advised to search these and other available sources to determine if a timely SR has been done on the topic or question of interest. An existing review would be most helpful if it was found to:

• Answer the same key question(s) of interest

• Provide appropriate and timely information

• Offer feasible and reasonable approaches to answering the key question(s), solving a similar problem, or meeting specific needs

• Represent findings from similar situations or settings or among similar populations

- Use best practices to conduct the review and report its findings
- Engage relevant stakeholders in the design, conduct, and interpretation of the review findings

If the search identifies a review that meets most of these criteria, its findings may be adequate to answer the question at hand, prompt the implementation of findings in a specific setting, "tee up" research based on research gaps identified in the review, or inform program or policy design.

If the identified reviews do not include recent literature on the key question(s), the review developer may choose to update the existing review. In this case, the review developer may have a significantly shortened planning process because it should be possible (and preferable) to replicate the prior review's SR protocol as closely as possible with at least one notable exception—the inclusion dates for the review. The new review should start where the prior review ended and continue to the most recent, reasonable date. After searches for the new review are complete, the analysis can be replicated by either combining all the data, as would be necessary for a meta-analysis, or by examining the new findings and then doing a cross-walk with the findings of the existing review, an approach more suited to a qualitative synthesis strategy of determining review findings.

If the search for reviews is unsuccessful, the review developer may elect to complete a planning process for a new SR, taking into account the resources necessary to conduct the review and the research developer's capacity to undertake the review. Reviews of complex questions can be quite expensive and time consuming, so a consideration of the costs and time constraints is very important in deciding to conduct a review. In the context of the Health Scenario, for example, the nurse researcher would likely need to engage the services of a reference librarian to identify the most efficient search strategy for the literature; find a colleague to be a second reviewer of abstracts and articles; and develop a process to involve community members in planning, conducting, and interpreting the SR findings. Each of these steps requires a consideration of how financial support will be obtained to cover the time individuals spend on the SR and other expenses associated with the review such as article retrieval.

Plan Development Steps

Methods and processes to create an SR plan are recommended by primary developers of SRs. We present our adaptation of the IOM Standards for Systematic Reviews published in 2011 as an orientation to the essential components of an SR plan. It is vitally important to document decisions made for each step so that the chosen approaches can be described in the presentation of SR findings. More details on how to approach each step can be found at http://www.iom.edu/Reports/2011/Finding-What-Works-in-Health-Care-Standards-for-Systematic-Reviews/Standards.aspx (IOM, 2011).

We offer approaches to each of seven steps necessary to plan a "new" review such as the one needed by the church leader and the nurse researcher to answer the following question: Is community-based screening for previously undiagnosed type 2 diabetes mellitus among African Americans as effective in identifying affected individuals as is clinic-based screening for type 2 diabetes mellitus?

Step 1

Establish a team with appropriate expertise and experience to conduct the SR. The team should include individuals with expertise in the pertinent content areas, SR methods, searching for relevant evidence, quantitative and qualitative methods, and other expertise as appropriate.

Approach: The nurse researcher will confer with academic colleagues to identify members of an SR team with experience in designing and conducting SR and in methods necessary to conduct the SR. Individuals may be invited to join the team based on their experience in relevant content areas such as diabetes screening and treatment; primary care, especially as delivered in rural areas; and ways to reach underserved individuals in rural areas. A research librarian with experience in conducting searches for SR or for complex topics would be recruited along with a researcher well versed in the use of qualitative methods. This SR is not likely to need an expert in quantitative methods such as meta-analysis given the type of literature on this topic.

Step 2

Manage bias and conflict of interest (COI) of the SR team conducting the SR. A process should be established to require each team member to disclose potential COI and professional or intellectual bias, exclude individuals with a clear financial conflict, and exclude individuals whose professional or intellectual bias would diminish the credibility of the review in the eyes of the intended users.

Approach: Most academic institutions have COI processes in place, and if all team members are part of that process, the team leader may proceed to document any reported COI or inquire about any further COI that may be present given the location, content area, or scope of the SR. For any members of the team whose organizations may not require a COI, the team leader should establish a process for identifying and documenting COI. In some cases, it may be necessary to reconsider membership by a specific team member based on his or her declared COI.

Step 3

Ensure user and stakeholder input as the review is designed and conducted. Although user and stakeholder input is vital to planning the review, a process should be in place to protect the independence of the review team to make the final decisions about the design, analysis, and reporting of the review.

Recent efforts by the Patient Centered Outcomes Research Institute (PCORI) and others seek to assure greater transparency of the SR processes and to engage patients and other stakeholders in the review process. Stakeholder groups are identified variously by SR developers but are generally assumed in the areas of health and health care to include patients and their caregivers; clinicians, including physicians, nurses, and other health care professionals; payers; and policymakers, including guideline developers and other SR sponsors.

Patient and stakeholder involvement in each step of the SR process is critical. Their perspectives inform the development of key questions, primary and secondary outcomes, analytic frameworks, strength of evidence, and interpretation of findings. Including these perspectives help to ensure that reviews address outcomes meaningful to patients and other stakeholders and provides actionable recommendations for all stakeholder groups and their members.

Stakeholder participation may be hampered by their awareness and understanding of methods used to conduct an SR; their bias for or against SR processes, findings, and applications; their interpretation of the implications of review findings for themselves and their organizations; and their understanding of their role in the SR process.

Principles of community engagement can be applied to increase the quality of stakeholder involvement in SR processes. Stakeholders can be offered orientation sessions describing their roles and responsibilities as stakeholder advisory panel members. They can also be offered training to increase their knowledge of the SR process and appreciate the strengths and limitations of an SR. Materials associated with planning the SR can be presented in "plain language," and ample time can be given for discussion or clarification.

Just as stakeholders may need to gain familiarity with the SR process, some review team members may need to learn more about the contextual and other factors affecting the topic of the review from the stakeholder perspective. This bidirectional learning is likely to enhance the relevance, credibility, and acceptance of review findings.

Approach: The church leader and nurse researcher spent time together to develop a list of potential stakeholders to advise their review team. Because individuals and groups in Bamberg County are the most likely short-term users of the SR findings, they decided to form a stakeholder advisory panel composed of county and state residents representing adults with and without diabetes (three members), clinicians and other health care professionals who regularly participate in screening events in the community and within the health care system (two members), a representative from the primary insurers of individuals in the county (Medicaid and Medicare program representatives) (one member), community leaders from the faith-based community (two members), a member of a local advocacy group for patients with diabetes (one member), and a policymaker such as a local member of the legislature (on member). They think that this group of 10 individuals represents most of the major stakeholder groups and that the number will be manageable from a logistical perspective. One of the review team members will be identified as the primary point of contact for the stakeholder advisory panel.

Step 4

Manage bias and COI for individuals providing input into the SR. Similar to the process for COI for review team members, individuals providing input to the review should be required, through a transparent, consistently used and applied process, to disclose potential COI and professional or intellectual bias. A process should include an approach to identifying and excluding from individuals whose COI or bias would diminish the credibility of the SR in the eyes of the intended users.

Approach: The review team's point of contact will develop, with stakeholder input, a process for assuring identification and disclosure of COI for members of the stakeholder advisory panel.

Step 5

Formulate the topic for the SR. In this step, the review team should confirm the need for a new review and develop an analytic framework that clearly lays out the chain of logic linking the health intervention to the outcomes of interest and defining the key questions to be addressed by the SR. A standard format to articulate each question of interest should be developed that states the rationale for each question. Key questions should be shared with intended users and stakeholders and refined, if necessary, based on their input. Types of questions may encompass clinical, behavioral, systems, or policy concerns in a particular field (IOM, 2011).

Approach: During the first combined meeting of the review team and the stakeholder advisory panel, a new key question is developed from the original PICO statement: for the population of African

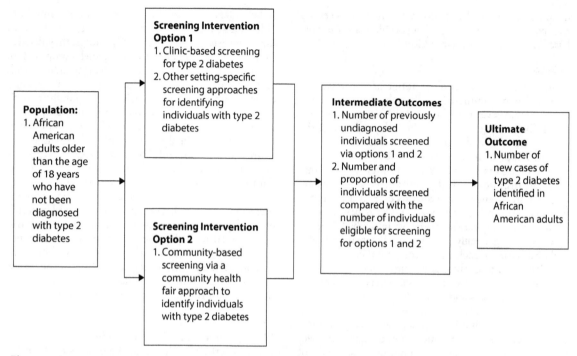

Figure 12-1. Analytic framework for a systematic review to compare community versus clinic-based screening options to increase the number of individuals screened for type 2 diabetes mellitus.

American adults older than age 18 years, is the proposed intervention of a community health fair more or less effective compared with other diabetes screening options such as clinic-based or other interventions to affect the outcome of increasing the percentage of adults screened for diabetes in a specific geographic area? During this meeting, the review team presents a preliminary analytic framework developed to link the PICO elements together and frame the review (**Figure 12-1**). The combined group agrees that this analytic framework is appropriate for taking the next two steps in the planning process.

Step 6

Develop an SR protocol describing the following elements of the SR process:

1. The context and rationale for the SR from both a decision-making and research perspective
2. The study screening and selection criteria (inclusion and exclusion criteria)
3. The precise outcome measures, time points, interventions, and comparison groups to be addressed
4. The search strategy for identifying relevant evidence
5. The procedures for study selection

6. The data extraction strategy
7. The process for identifying and resolving disagreement between researchers in study selection and data extraction decisions
8. The approach to critically appraising individual studies
9. The method for evaluating the body of evidence, including the quantitative and qualitative synthesis strategies
10. Any planned analyses of differential treatment effects according to patient subgroups, how an intervention is delivered, or how an outcome is measured
11. The proposed timetable for conducting the review
12. The conduct and timing of a public comment period for the protocol and publicly report on disposition of comments (IOM, 2011)

Approach: The review team develops a draft of the protocol in consultation with its expert members and with input from the stakeholder advisory panel as necessary. The iterative process is completed in about 6 months and defines the scope and conduct of the review to answer the key question.

Step 7

Submit the protocol for peer review.

Approach: The final protocol is made publicly available via email and an online posting to all members of the review team and the stakeholder advisory panel. Members share the protocol with their constituents along with a timeline for submitting comments on the protocol. Comments received during this time frame are compiled, and preliminary answers are prepared by the review team for joint discussion and consideration with the stakeholder advisory panel. Any necessary adjustments are made as amendments to the protocol and communicated to all relevant stakeholders.

SUMMARY

An SR is a critical assessment and evaluation of all research studies that address a particular issue. Typically, an SR relies principally on the results of investigations that are published in the peer-reviewed literature but may also include "grey" literature (e.g., unpublished manuscripts, conference papers and posters, grant close-out reports) The findings of an SR may be summarized in a variety of ways, ranging from a qualitative assessment to a formal statistical summary referred to as a meta-analysis.

Systematic reviews are useful to a range of stakeholders, from patients and patient advocates, to care providers, professional societies, payers for health care services, researchers, and policymakers. The conduct of an SR typically follows a standardized process. First, a question of primary interest is formulated around considerations of **p**opulations, **i**nterventions, **c**omparisons, and **o**utcomes (**PICO**). An SR also must specify the types of studies to be included, a time period for the literature to be reviewed, and any underlying assumptions about the relationships of the parameters that serve as a basis for the key elements of the PICO.

Systematic reviews are most useful if they are relevant to the population of interest, are timely, address the critical PICO elements, engage stakeholders in their design and conduct, and use best practices from initial development through final interpretation. If an SR has been conducted and published already, the need for a new review may be obviated. Often, however, there is no existing SR on the topic of interest, it may not apply to the population of interest, or it is out of date. Under these circumstances, one might entertain conducting a new SR.

Planning and conducting a formal SR should follow well-established guidelines, focusing on the topic of interest, assembling an interprofessional team to work together, identifying potential stakeholders from various interested parties and soliciting their input, identifying and managing any conflicts of interest, developing a protocol, and submitting the protocol for peer review. In the following chapters, the elements of performing an SR are presented in detail.

STUDY QUESTIONS

1. *A systematic review is*

    A. *a critical assessment and evaluation of all research studies that address a particular issue.*

    B. *a review of the literature for a topic relevant to health and health care.*

    C. *always a meta-analysis.*

    D. *a fair and balanced way to review available evidence.*

2. *PICO stands for*

    A. *patients, interventions, consultations, and outcomes.*

    B. *populations, inventions, comparisons, and observation.*

    C. *populations, interventions, comparisons, and outcomes.*

    D. *patients, inventions, comorbidities, and outcomes.*

3. *Which of the following is not true about systematic reviews?*

    A. *Researchers and other persons developing systematic reviews use an organized method of locating, assembling, and evaluating a body of literature on a particular topic using a set of specific criteria*

    B. *A systematic review typically includes a description of the findings of a collection of research studies*

    C. *A systematic review may tailor presentation of findings for specific target audiences, including the general public*

    D. *Systematic reviews present findings using only quantitative methods*

4. *Which item is not an expected outcome for a systematic review plan?*

    A. *A well-framed question or set of questions specifying the PICO*

    B. *A statement of what types of studies are to be included in the review (e.g., clinical trials, observational studies)*

C. A description of how stakeholders are to be involved in the review

D. A description (often a logic model or analytic framework) that describes the relationship of PICO elements to one another

5. An existing review would be most helpful if it addressed all but one of the following items:

A. provided appropriate and timely information.

B. offered feasible and reasonable approaches to answering the key question(s), solving a similar problem, or meeting specific needs.

C. used best practices to conduct the review and report its findings.

D. answered a slightly different but very similar key question.

6. Which of the following is not a type of grey literature?

A. Unpublished manuscripts

B. Conference papers and posters

C. Newspaper articles

D. Grant close-out reports

7. Which of the following groups would be likely stakeholders in a systematic review of community-based screening for diabetes?

A. Insurance payers

B. Health care providers

C. Community leaders

D. All of the above

8. A prior published systematic review may be deemed not useful for addressing a subsequent issue because of

A. the study populations included.

B. all relevant literature was not included.

C. the review and its source studies are not current.

D. all of the above.

9. Which of the following stakeholders has a potential conflict-of-interest in advising a systematic review on the topic of community-based screening for diabetes mellitus?

A. A diabetes expert who also serves as a paid consultant to a pharmaceutical company

B. A physician in a clinic that serves the community and moonlights in emergency departments

C. An administrator with the state Medicaid agency

D. A retired school teacher who lives in the community and volunteers with various not-for-profit organizations

10. Which of the following is **NOT** an essential of the protocol for developing a systematic review of the comparative effectiveness of community-based versus routine clinical screening for diabetes in an African American community?

A. Define the criteria for selecting individual studies for inclusion.

B. Identify the outcome measures, interventions, and comparison groups of interest.

C. Exclude all studies that have not been published in the peer-reviewed literature.

D. Extract the key data elements from the selected studies.

REFERENCES

Agency for Healthcare Research and Quality. Meta-analysis. In Glossary of Terms. http://effectivehealthcare.ahrq.gov/glossary-of-terms/?pageaction=showterm&termid=39. Published n.d.a. Accessed June 4, 2014.

Agency for Healthcare Research and Quality. Systematic review. In Glossary of Terms. http://effectivehealthcare.ahrq.gov/glossary-of-terms/?pageaction=showterm&termid=70. Published n.d.b. Accessed June 4, 2014.

Centers for Disease Control and Prevention. National Diabetes Fact Sheet: National Estimates and General Information on Diabetes and Prediabetes in the United States, 2011. Atlanta, GA: U.S. Department of Health and Human Services, Centers for Disease Control and Prevention. Published 2011. http://www.cdc.gov/diabetes/pubs/pdf/ndfs_2011.pdf. Accessed June 4, 2014.

Higgins JT, Green S, eds. *Cochrane Handbook for Systematic Reviews of Interventions* Version 5.1.0. Published March, 2011. http://www.cochrane-handbook.org. Accessed June 4, 2014.

Institute of Medicine. (2011). *Finding What Works in Health Care: Standards for systematic Reviews*. Washington, DC: National Academies Press. South Carolina Department of Health and Environmental Control, Bureau of Community Health and Chronic Disease Prevention. County Chronic Disease Fact Sheet. Published November, 2013. http://www.scdhec.gov/hs/epidata/county_reports.htm. Accessed June 4, 2014.

U.S. Census Bureau. State and County QuickFacts: Bamburg County, South Carolina. http://quickfacts.census.gov/qfd/states/45/45009.html. Published 2014. Accessed June 4, 2014.

World Health Organization. Screening for Type 2 Diabetes: Report of a World Health Organization and International Diabetes Federation meeting. Report no. WHO/NMH/MNC/03.1. Geneva: Department of Noncommunicable Disease Management, Author; 2003.

Assessing Evidence

Daniel T. Lackland

HEALTH SCENARIO

A 49-year-old African American man reports to the clinic after being told his blood pressure was "high" during a screening at a community health fair. His body mass index was calculated as 29. He has "pre-diabetes" from a previous examination with a current hemoglobin A1c of 6.4%. His total cholesterol is 150 mg/dL with a high-density lipoprotein cholesterol level of 30 mg/dL. His resting blood pressure was 168/96 mm Hg on the first assessment with 172/98 mm Hg 20 minutes later in the clinic. He has a family history of high blood pressure, with both parents and his sister and brother currently being treated for hypertension. He reports he tries to limit his salt intake and walks on his job as a sales associate at a hardware store. His blood pressure values are consistent with a diagnosis of high blood pressure with the questions:

- Should there be any intervention to reduce the blood pressure?
- How should the blood pressure be reduced and by what agent (s)?
- How low should the blood pressure be reduced?

For the caregivers at the clinic to determine the most appropriate treatment plan for this patient, it is essential to answer these clinical questions with the highest quality evidence available.

CLINICAL BACKGROUND

The three questions posed in the Health Scenario are fundamental to the optimal management of patients with high blood pressure. Hypertension typically is defined as a systolic blood pressure of 140 mm Hg or greater or a diastolic blood pressure of 90 mm Hg or greater.

Hypertension is one of the most common medical conditions among adults worldwide. For example, it is estimated that one in every four adults in the United States has high blood pressure. The prevalence of hypertension rises dramatically with age—among young adults age 35 to 44 years, only about one in seven persons has high blood pressure, but among adults age 65 years or older, more than half of all persons have this condition. Overall, men tend to have a slightly higher prevalence of high blood pressure than do women. African Americans have a higher risk of developing hypertension than do either non-Hispanic whites or Mexican Americans.

In addition to these demographic patterns, a number of risk factors have been identified for high blood pressure. Physical inactivity is one such predisposing factor, as are obesity, excessive alcohol consumption, and tobacco use. A diet too high in sodium content and too low in potassium content also is associated with risk of high blood pressure in some, if not all, populations. A positive family history also increases the risk of hypertension, although the extent to which this pattern reflects genetic predisposition, shared environmental exposures, or a mixture of both is unknown.

The most common form of high blood pressure, accounting for 90% or more of all occurrences, is so-called "essential hypertension." The mechanisms leading to essential hypertension are not known but likely involve elements of some of the following age-related phenomena: (1) increased peripheral vascular resistance, with thickening of the walls of small arteries; (2) altered regulation of adrenergic receptors, resulting in increased vascular tone; and (3) decreased sensitivity of pressure receptors (baroreceptors).

Most patients with essential hypertension are asymptomatic, and the condition typically comes to clinical attention because of a routine blood pressure measurement in a screening setting or a health care visit. The motivation for detecting and treating hypertension is that patients with this disorder are at increased risk for a variety of adverse health outcomes, including, but not limited to, coronary heart disease, stroke, and chronic kidney disease. The treatment of hypertension is motivated largely by the desire to reduce the risk of these multiple life-threatening consequences.

National survey data reveal an increase over time in the proportion of persons with hypertension who are aware that they have the condition (>80% in recent years); treated (nearly 75% in recent years); and achieving control, as defined by blood pressure levels of 140 mm Hg or less systolic and 90 mm Hg or less diastolic (nearly 70% in recent years). Nevertheless, there still is the recognition that many affected individuals remain unaware of their condition, and even if they are aware of it, they are not receiving treatment or achieving control. As attempts are made to address these gaps, we are drawn back to the central questions raised in the Health Scenario—to better define the true value of reducing blood pressure and to what levels it must be reduced and by what means to achieve these benefits.

Example 1: A Systematic Review

The Joint National Committee (JNC) on Prevention, Detection, Evaluation, and Treatment of High Blood Pressure was created to review the scientific literature and develop guidelines for the management of hypertension. The first such report was issued in 1976, and there have been regular, periodic updates since then. The eighth such report (JNC 8) was organized in 2008 with the appointment of a large, multidisciplinary team of experts in relevant areas of research and patient care. Five years later, the panel presented the results of its extensive review of the medical literature appearing between 1966 and 2009. Studies with sample sizes of less than 100 subjects or with observation periods less than 1 year were excluded because too few outcomes would occur in order to yield valid assessments of treatment effects. Only studies that evaluated overall mortality or morbidity or mortality from cardiovascular (CVD) or renal disease were considered. Moreover, the panel excluded observational studies (e.g., cohort and case-control studies) on the basis that these studies were prone to bias, and the strongest type of evidence about benefits of treatment would derive from randomized controlled trials (RCTs). Finally, the panel excluded prior quantitative or nonquantitative syntheses of the literature and confined the review to the source studies.

An external team performed the literature review and prepared summary tables based on data extracted from the studies that were included. These summaries then were used by the panel to construct evidence statements. For each of these statements that the panel approved, a rating was provided by the panel on the quality of the evidence. The resulting quality-scored evidence statements were used by the panel to prepare patient care recommendations, which were graded according to the strength of the evidence. An attempt was made to reach consensus on evidence

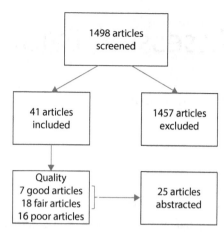

Figure 13-1. Flow diagram of article screening process for Joint National Committee 8 review of pharmacologic therapy of hypertension at specific blood pressure levels to improve outcomes. (Data from James PA, Oparil S, Carter BL, et al. 2014 evidence-based guideline for the management of high blood pressure in adults: report from the panel members appointed to the Eighth Joint National Committee (JNC 8). *JAMA*. 2014;311:507-520.)

statements and recommendations, but if a unanimous opinion was not possible, a two thirds majority was considered sufficient agreement to render an opinion.

In **Figure 13-1**, the screening process is illustrated for addressing one of the fundamental questions: "In adults with hypertension, does initiating antihypertensive pharmacologic therapy at specific blood pressure thresholds improve health outcomes?" In brief, a total of almost 1500 separate articles were identified as being potentially relevant to answering this question. Of these screened articles, 1457 (97%) were eliminated from further consideration because they failed to meet the prespecified inclusion criteria for the review. For each of the remaining 41 articles that were included, a rating of quality was provided. Seven studies (17%) were considered to be of good quality, and 18 studies (44%) were rated as being of fair quality. The remaining 16 studies (39%) were judged to be of poor quality, and therefore, were not considered further. The 25 studies that were determined to be of either good or fair quality were abstracted, and the data from these investigations served as the evidence base for formulating answers to the question.

The panel concluded on the basis of its review of the evidence that:

- In persons age 60 years or older, a strong recommendation was made for pharmacologic therapy of people with a systolic blood pressure of 150 mm Hg or higher or a diastolic blood pressure of 90 mm Hg or higher, with a goal of lowering their respective blood pressures below the specified levels.

- In persons between 30 and 59 years of age, a strong recommendation was made for pharmacologic therapy of people with a diastolic blood pressure of 90 mm Hg or higher, with a goal of lowering blood pressure below that level.
- For persons younger than the age of 60 years, there was insufficient evidence for a systolic blood pressure goal.
- For persons younger than the age of 30 years, there was insufficient evidence to establish a diastolic blood pressure goal.

When applied to the Health Scenario, the patient in question is age 49 years old, and his diastolic blood pressure exceeded the goal level of 90 mm Hg. Accordingly, he would fit the second recommendation for treating his high blood pressure with pharmacologic therapy to a target goal diastolic blood pressure of 90 mm Hg or lower. In terms of selecting the preferred pharmacologic agent for treating this patient, the recommendations went on to examine the data by agent and patient demographics. It was concluded that for African American patients, such as the individual in the Health Scenario, a moderate recommendation can be made to initiate antihypertensive treatment with a thiazide-type diuretic or calcium channel blocker. Of course, individual treatment needs to be customized to the particular situation for each patient, but these guidelines can help the caregiver focus on the treatment choices that are most likely to benefit this patient based on the best evidence that is available.

As illustrated in the review conducted by the JNC 8, the volume of medical literature on a particular topic can be very extensive. The number of RCTs and studies conducted has increased dramatically over the past few decades. For example, the number of RCTs published in MEDLINE increased five fold from 1978 to 1985 to 1994 to 2001. At the same time, not all of these studies produced results that are internally and externally valid. If results are biased or confounded or limited to selective subsets of patients, the evidence may have reduced value in guiding clinical practice. Routinely, clinicians are confronted with a vast volume of evidence of uncertain and unclear value. Thus, critically appraised and synthesized scientific evidence has become fundamental to clinical practice. Likewise, the "art of medicine" involves the incorporation of the best evidence in the integration of clinician skills and expertise with patient values and preferences.

Clinical practice guidelines and recommendations incorporate the interrelationships among these critical contributors to clinical decision making. Such guidelines should enhance clinical decision making by clearly describing and appraising the scientific evidence behind clinical recommendations. Some common limitations in developing high-quality and trustworthy clinical practices and guidelines include:

- Variable quality of individual scientific studies
- Limitations in systematic reviews
- Inadequate consideration of evidence quality in appraisals
- Failure to include multidisciplinary groups
- Failure to adequately include conflicting studies
- Failure to use rigorous methodologies in the considered studies

The Institute of Medicine (IOM) issued two reports that established new "best practice" standards for generating systematic evidence reviews and developing clinical guidelines for evidence-based clinical practices. Similarly, the National Heart, Lung, and Blood Institute (NHLBI) has implemented evidence-based practice development for the prevention, detection, and treatment of cardiovascular, lung, and blood diseases. To continually improve the quality and impact of the evidence reviews, the evidence review process should ensure rigor and minimize bias. The process based on the IOM recommendation should:

- Be based on a systematic review of the existing evidence.
- Consider important patient subgroups and patient preferences.
- Be based on an explicit process that minimizes distortion, biases, and conflicts of interest.
- Provide a clear explanation of logical relationships between alternative care options and health outcomes.
- Provide ratings of both the quality of evidence and the strength of the recommendations.

This type of a review should be implemented in a systematic manner. As illustrated in the JNC 8 review of hypertension research, there are several components of the review process:

1. **Construction of the clinical questions most relevant to clinical practice.** In general, these questions follow "PICOTSS" (population, intervention or exposure, comparison group, outcome, time, setting, and study design) format.

2. **Identification (a priori) of inclusion/exclusion (I/E) criteria for each clinical question.** This process includes the development of a search strategy based on I/E criteria. The more restrictive the I/E criteria, the greater the limits on extrapolating the results to other groups.

3. **Implement a systematic electronic search of the published literature from relevant bibliographic databases for each clinical question.**

The first activity is the screening process to identify relevant original articles, systematic reviews, or meta-analyses. Rigorous validation procedures should be applied to ensure that the selected articles meet the preestablished detailed I/E criteria before being included in the final review.

4. **Assessment of quality (good, fair, or poor) of each included study.** This is typically accomplished with study-rating instruments.

5. **Abstraction of relevant information from the included studies into an electronic database.** These data elements can be completed by constructing templates with lists of data elements that were pertinent to I/E criteria.

6. **Construction of detailed evidence tables from the abstraction database.** Included in the evidence tables are summary tables displaying the evidence in a manageable format to answer specific parts of each clinical question.

7. **Evaluate summary tables to develop evidence statements for each clinical question.** The quality of evidence for each evidence statement can be graded as high, moderate, or low. The grade is based on scientific methodology, scientific strength, and consistency of results.

SYSTEM FOR GRADING THE BODY OF EVIDENCE

The assessment system is used to grade the body of the evidence and the strength of the clinical intervention. The evidence statements typically are graded as high, moderate, or low quality. **Table 13-1** presents an example of an evidence quality grading system. Studies with results considered with high confidence to reflect the true effect, and further research is unlikely to change the high confidence are considered to be of *high* quality. Studies with moderate confidence that the evidence reflects the true effect, and further research may change the moderate confidence in the estimate of effect and may change the estimate are considered to be of *moderate* quality. Studies with low confidence that the evidence reflects the true effect, and further research is likely to change the low confidence in the estimate of effect and is likely to change the estimate are considered to be of *low* quality.

Example 2: When Experimental and Observational Studies Differ

The strength of the body of evidence represents the degree of certainty, based on the overall body of evidence, that an effect or association is correct. Different types of studies often agree about the general direction

Table 13-1. Evidence quality grading system including types of evidence and strength of evidence grade.

Well-designed, well-executed RCTs that adequately represent populations to which the results are applied and directly assess effects on health outcomes	High
Meta-analyses of such studies	High
RCTs with minor limitations that affect confidence in or applicability of the results, including minor flaws in design or execution.	Moderate
Well-designed, well-executed nonrandomized controlled studies and well-designed, well-executed observational studies	Moderate
Meta-analyses of such studies	Moderate
RCTs with major limitations	Low
Nonrandomized intervention studies and observational studies with major limitations affecting confidence in or applicability of the results	Low
Uncontrolled clinical observations without an appropriate comparison group (e.g., case series, case reports)	Low
Physiological studies in humans	Low
Meta-analyses of such studies	Low

RCT, randomized controlled trial.

of the evidence but vary concerning the strength. However, there are scenarios in which evidence from observational studies varies significantly from RCTs. A classic example of the limitations of observational studies compared with RCTs is the hormone replacement therapy (HRT) experience. Early on, the clinical enthusiasm for the use of HRT was based in part on the perception that it could lower women's risk for heart disease, with some estimations as much as 50%. This attitude was encouraged by the consistent finding from observational studies that postmenopausal women users of HRT had substantially lower rates of cardiovascular events than nonusers. In addition, in vitro investigations and animal study results indicated favorable effects of HRT on cardiovascular risk factors, further supporting the observational study results. These findings and perceptions made HRT one of the most frequently prescribed medications in the United States despite the absence of any large RCTs.

The Heart and Estrogen/progestin Replacement Study (HERS) was the first major RCT of HRT for secondary prevention of heart disease. This study found an increased risk of heart disease rather than an overall benefit of hormone treatment. Further RCTs confirmed the conclusions of no benefit of HRT on atherosclerosis in women with established CVD, with a consistent suggestion that HRT might increase cardiovascular risk.

The discrepancy in the results of the observational studies and RCTs might be explained in part by healthy user bias in the observational studies because HRT users typically are healthier and have higher socioeconomic status than nonusers. Although most of the observational studies of HRT included adjustment for potential confounders, many failed to delete or adjust the apparent benefit in the analyses. Another explanation for the discordance between observational studies and clinical trials relates to differing ages and exposure durations to HRT. In many of the observational studies, HRT users included longer term users compared with subjects exposed experimentally in RCTs, and users in the general population tend to also use better tolerated HRTs, leading to increased exposure times. By ignoring timing persistence and tolerance of exposure to HRTs, different results and conclusions about potential risks and benefits for observational and RCT studies could be seen.

The HRT and heart disease scenario leads to two major considerations when judging evidence from observational studies:

• Observational data, clinical studies of intermediate endpoints, and in vitro and animal model research are useful for hypothesis generation, but they should not be considered adequate on their own to justify a broad-based pattern of clinical practice.
• The cardiovascular effects of estrogen are complex, with impacts on lipids, endothelial function, and other aspects of vascular biology producing a net increase in clinical cardiovascular events.

In the following sections, we will consider separately the assessment of quality of evidence from both experimental (RCT) and observational studies. In some settings, such as the JNC 8 review of hypertension, there may be substantial evidence from RCTs, so it is not necessary to include observational studies in the review. For other clinical questions, there may so few RCTs conducted that it is necessary to rely primarily on the results of observational studies. In between these two extremes is the relatively common situation in which there may be some RCTs but not enough to justify ignoring the results of observational studies. In this setting, even bearing in mind the potential for differing conclusions from RCTs and observational studies, there may be value to maximizing the use of all available information by including both types of research in the systematic review.

Regardless of the types of studies included, a fundamental task in a systematic review is to judge the quality of the evidence in the studies included. In essence, for each of the studies involved, one is trying to address two fundamental questions:

1. To what extent are the results of the study attributable to the intervention rather than to flaws in the design and conduct of the study (**internal validity**)?
2. To what extent can the results of the study be extrapolated to populations other than the one included (**external validity**)?

The answer to the first question relates primarily to judging the likelihood that the results could be attributable, in part or in whole, to distortions because of bias in the selection of subjects, the collection of information, or the mixture of the effect of interest with other determinants of the outcome (**confounding**). If a judgment is made that there is a high likelihood for bias, as occurred presumably in the observational studies on HRT use and risk of heart disease, the quality of evidence would be rated as poor. If the likelihood of bias is low, as in the HERS RCT of HRT, then the corresponding quality of evidence would be rated as high.

The answer to the second question concerning external validity relates to the extent to which the study population is likely to be broadly representative or not. The types of constraints that often are placed on a study population include considerations such as willingness to participate, age, gender, health status, treatment facility, region, and time period, among many other possible attributes. These constraints might be incorporated for purely logistical reasons for ease of accessing and following the subjects. Alternatively, the sample might be narrowed with the goal of reducing the potential influence of other prognostic factors. Regardless of the reason for restricting the characteristics of participants, narrow I/E criteria limit the ability to extrapolate the results to other populations.

In the following sections, we provide a framework for evaluating the quality of individual studies to be included in a systematic review. This framework is organized by the design of the research study involved because the type of issues that one must consider varies somewhat for RCTs, cohort studies, and case-control studies.

Quality Assessment of Controlled Intervention Studies

The guidance document below is organized from the tool for quality assessment of controlled intervention studies.

1. Described as randomized

   A study does not satisfy quality criteria as randomized simply because the authors call it **randomized**. Nonetheless, the study is reviewed initially if randomization is indicated.

2. Treatment allocation adequacy

   The randomization is adequate if it occurred according to the play of chance (e.g., computer-generated sequence in more recent studies or random number table in older studies). Randomization is inadequate if there is a preset plan (e.g., alternation in which every other subject is assigned to treatment arm or another method of allocation is used, such as time or day of hospital admission or clinic visit, ZIP code, or phone number). This type of allocation is not true randomization. The assessment of randomization requires careful reading and consideration for the role of chance in assignment. For example, in group randomization, sites are randomized to receive treatment or not. All individuals at the site thereby are assigned to the same treatment group. Another approach is allocation concealment in which one does not know in advance, or one cannot guess accurately, to what group the next person eligible for randomization will be assigned. Methods include sequentially numbered, opaque, sealed envelopes; numbered or coded containers; central randomization by a coordinating center; and computer-generated randomization that is not revealed ahead of time.

3. Blinding

   Blinding, or masking, means that one does not know to which group—intervention or control—the participant is assigned. It is important to consider who is blinded to knowledge of treatment assignment, which may include one or more of the following groups:

   A. The person assessing the primary outcome(s) for the study (e.g., taking the measurements, examining medical records to determine type of event as in an adjudication committee)

   B. The person receiving the intervention (e.g., the patient or volunteer participant)

   C. The person providing the intervention (e.g., the physician, nurse, or behavioral interventionist)

   Generally placebo-controlled medication studies are blinded to patient, provider, and outcome assessors; behavioral or lifestyle studies may often be blinded only to the outcome assessors. Sometimes the person providing the intervention is the same person doing the outcome assessment.

4. Similar characteristics of study groups at baseline

   This assessment considers if the intervention and control groups have similar characteristics on average. A primary purpose of a randomization is to create similar groups to enable valid comparisons of intervention effects between or among groups. If there is a significant imbalance in prognostic factors between or among the groups, it may be detected during the review of baseline characteristics. Baseline characteristics for intervention groups usually are presented in a table in the article, typically the first table. It is possible for study groups to differ at baseline without adversely affecting the results if the differences are not of prognostic importance (i.e., would not be expected to have any bearing on the interventions and outcomes).

5. Dropout

   Dropout refers to *participants for whom there are no endpoint measurements*. The most common reason for dropping out of the study is being lost to follow-up. Typically, an acceptable overall dropout rate is considered 20% or less of participants who were randomized or allocated into each group, and an acceptable differential dropout is considered an absolute difference between groups of no more than 15% (calculated by subtracting the dropout rate of one group minus the dropout rate of the other group). These are, however, general considerations and not absolute rules. Higher overall dropout rates might be acceptable in a longer term study or one that is particularly complicated. Likewise, a simple short-term trial might be expected to have a lower dropout rate. Regardless of overall dropout rates, if a differential of more than 15% exists between groups, there is a serious potential for bias.

6. Adherence

   Adherence refers to *whether the participants in each treatment group comply with the protocols for assigned interventions*. For example, one might ascertain the percentage of patients who took the intervention (and comparison) drugs as prescribed.

7. Competing interventions

   Changes that occur in the study outcomes being assessed should be attributable to the interventions being compared in the study. Distortion could occur if participants in any of the study groups receive other interventions that are not part of the study protocol but could affect the outcomes being assessed. If the use of other interventions is balanced between comparison groups, the expected effect is to reduce the apparent effect of the intervention. If the use of other interventions is unbalanced, however, the impact could be either to increase or decrease the observed effect.

8. Outcome measures assessment

The methods that were used to measure outcomes in the study should be assessed for validity, accuracy, reliability, and objectivity. This assessment is important because it indicates the confidence in the reported outcomes. Even more important is whether the outcomes were assessed in the same manner within groups and between groups.

9. Power calculation

In general, the current standard is to have at least 80% statistical power to detect a clinically relevant difference in an outcome using a two-sided type I error rate of 0.05. Negative results in small, underpowered studies do not provide compelling evidence of no effect.

10. Prespecified outcomes

Outcomes reported in the study must have been prespecified and define the whole purpose of doing an RCT. If outcomes are not prespecified, then the study may be reporting ad hoc analyses—simply looking for differences that support the findings they wanted. In addition to outcomes, the subgroups being examined should be prespecified. Multiple subgroup analyses can lead to spurious findings if statistical significance levels are not adjusted accordingly. Bearing this caveat in mind, it also is true that most RCTs conduct numerous post hoc analyses as a way of exploring findings and generating additional hypotheses. This may be justified given the time and expense of collecting these intervention data. Nevertheless, such findings must be considered exploratory and subject to confirmation in other studies.

11. Intent-to-treat (ITT) analysis

Intent to treat is an analysis approach that means participants who were randomized are analyzed according to the original group to which they are assigned even if they do not receive the treatment completely. This is an important concept because ITT analysis preserves the intended benefits of randomization. When the ITT analysis philosophy is not followed, it is not certain that the groups being compared are balanced in other important attributes. Some studies use a completer's analysis (which analyzes only the participants that completed the intervention and the study), which introduces significant potential for bias because characteristics of participants who do not complete the study are unlikely to be comparable to those who do. The likely impact of participants who withdraw from the study treatment must be considered carefully.

12. General guidance for determining the overall quality rating

In addition to the considerations of quality identified above, some additional study attributes should be included in the overall assessment.

If a study has a *fatal flaw*, then the risk of bias is significant, and the study is of poor quality. Examples of fatal flaws in RCTs include high dropout rates, high differential dropout, no ITT analysis, or unsuitable statistical analysis (e.g., completers-only analysis). Typically in published studies, fatal flaws are not evident, but indicators of the risk of bias are found. By focusing on the concepts of quality, studies can be appraised uniformly and critically. It is important to think about the assessment categories and potential for bias within any study.

Quality Assessment of Cohort and Cross-Sectional Studies

The quality assessment for cohort and cross-sectional studies includes the clarity of the research question or research objective; the definition, selection, composition, and participation of the study population; the definition and assessment of exposure and outcome variables; the measurement of exposures before outcome assessment; the study timeframe and follow-up; study analysis and power; and other factors.

1. Research question

The study goal and research question should be clearly defined and appropriate to the research design. The research question should be obvious in the early assessment of the study.

2. Study population

This is the study participants who were selected or recruited, with regard to demographics, location, and time period. In cohort studies, it is crucial that the population at baseline is free of the outcome of interest. Also, if fewer than 50% of eligible persons participated in the study, then there is concern that the study population does not adequately represent the target population.

3. Groups recruited from the same population and uniform eligibility criteria

The I/E criteria developed before recruitment or selection of the study population should be clearly defined, as well as the underlying criteria used for all of the subjects involved. Most cohort studies begin with the selection of the source population(s); participants in this cohort are then measured or evaluated to determine their exposure status. However, some cohort studies may recruit or select exposed participants in a different time or place than unexposed participants. This approach typically is seen in retrospective cohort studies, which is when data are obtained from the past (retrospectively), but the analysis still examines exposures before outcomes.

4. Sample size justification

A discussion of statistical power may be found in the Discussion section of the paper (e.g., the study had 85% power to detect a 20% increase in the rate of an outcome of interest, with a two-sided alpha of 0.05). Observational cohort studies, however, often do not report anything about statistical power or sample size because the analyses are exploratory in nature. This is not necessarily a "fatal" flaw but rather indicates that the study was exploratory or hypothesis generating.

5. Exposure assessed before outcome measurement

Temporality is important because to determine whether an exposure causes an outcome, the exposure must occur before the outcome. For some prospective cohort studies, the investigator enrolls the cohort and then determines the exposure status of various members of the cohort. Elsewhere, the cohort is selected based on its exposure status. An example of the latter is a cohort identified by its exposure to fluoridated drinking water and then compared with a cohort living in an area without fluoridated water. Another example is a cohort of military personnel exposed to combat compared with a cohort of military personnel not deployed in a combat zone. With either of these types of cohort studies, the cohort is followed forward in time to assess the outcomes that occur subsequently among the exposed compared with the nonexposed.

For retrospective cohort studies, the same principle applies. The difference is that rather than identifying a cohort in the present and following them forward in time, the investigators go back in time (i.e., retrospectively) and select a cohort based on their exposure status in the past and then follow them forward to assess the subsequent outcomes that occurred in the exposed and nonexposed cohort members. In retrospective cohort studies, the exposure and outcomes both may have occurred already, so it is important to make sure that the exposure preceded the outcome.

Sometimes cross-sectional studies are conducted (or cross-sectional analyses of cohort study data) in which the exposures and outcomes are measured during the same timeframe. As a result, cross-sectional analyses provide weaker evidence than cohort studies regarding a potential causal relationship between exposures and outcomes because the sequence of occurrence (temporality) of exposure and outcome are obscured.

6. Sufficient timeframe for an effect

The issue of timeframe is important to enable meaningful analysis of the relationships between exposures and outcomes to be conducted. This depends on the research question and outcomes being examined. When looking at chronic health outcomes, it often requires at least several years.

Cross-sectional analyses allow no time to see an effect because the exposures and outcomes are assessed at the same time.

7. Different levels of the exposure of interest

If the exposure can be defined in graded levels (e.g., drug dosage, amount of physical activity, amount of sodium consumed), were multiple categories of that exposure assessed (e.g., for medications: no use, low dose, medium dose, high dose; for dietary sodium intake: higher than average U.S. consumption, average consumption, and lower than average consumption)? Sometimes discrete categories of exposure are not used, but instead exposures are measured as continuous variables (e.g., milligrams per day [mg/day] of dietary sodium or millimeters of mercury [mm Hg] for blood pressure values).

In any case, studying different levels of exposure (when possible) enables investigators to assess trends or dose-response relationships between exposures and outcomes. The presence of trends or dose-response relationships lends credibility to the hypothesis of causality between exposure and outcome.

For some exposures, however, this question may not be applicable; for example, the exposure may be a dichotomous variable (e.g., living in a rural setting vs. an urban setting or vaccinated vs. not vaccinated).

8. Exposure measures and assessment

When exposures are measured with less accuracy or validity, it is harder to see an association between exposure and outcome even if one exists. Also important is whether the exposures were assessed in the same manner within groups and between groups; if not, bias may result.

For example, retrospective self-report of dietary salt intake is not as valid and reliable as prospectively using a standardized dietary log plus testing participants' urine for excreted sodium. Another example is measurement of blood pressure; there may be quite a difference between usual care (e.g., routine measurements in physician's practices) or use of trained blood pressure assessors using standardized equipment and a standardized protocol.

If individuals with hypertension (exposed cohort) are seen by their providers more frequently than normotensives (nonexposed group), it also increases the chances of detecting and documenting changes in health outcomes, including CVD-related events. Therefore, it may produces the conclusion that hypertension produces more CVD events when it is just a product of greater surveillance. Thus, it could bias the results and lead to an erroneous conclusion.

9. Repeated exposure assessment

Multiple measurements with the same result increase confidence that the exposure status was classified correctly. Multiple measurements also enable investigators to look at changes in exposure over time (e.g., individuals who ate high dietary sodium throughout the follow-up period compared with those who started out high and then reduced their intake compared with those who ate low sodium throughout). Again, this may not be applicable in all cases. In many older studies, exposure was measured only at baseline. Multiple exposure measurements provide stronger evidence for exposure–outcome associations.

10. Outcome measures

The study outcomes should be defined in detail. The tools and methods for measuring outcomes should be accurate and reliable with clear quality indicators. Also important is whether the outcomes were assessed in the same manner within groups and between groups.

An example of an outcome measure that is objective, accurate, and reliable is death—the outcome measured with more accuracy than any other. But even with a measure as objective as death, there can be differences in the accuracy and reliability of how death was assessed by the investigators. For example, was the cause of death assigned from an autopsy report, death certificate, death registry, or report from a family member? Sometimes the outcome is based on a biomarker. For example, in a study of whether dietary fat intake is related to blood cholesterol level, the cholesterol level is measured from fasting blood samples that are all sent to the same laboratory. Similar to the example cited earlier, results may be biased if one group (e.g., hypertensive individuals) is seen more frequently than another group (e.g., normotensive individuals) because more frequent encounters with the health care system increases the chances of outcomes being detected and documented.

11. Blinding of outcome assessors

Blinding in this case means that outcome assessors did not know whether individual participants were exposed or unexposed. It is also sometimes called "masking." The objective is to look for evidence in the article that the person(s) assessing the outcome(s) for the study (e.g., examining medical records to determine the outcomes that occurred in the exposed and comparison groups) is masked to the exposure status of the participant. Sometimes the person measuring the exposure is the same person who conducts the outcome assessment. In this case, the outcome assessor would most likely not be blinded to exposure, although in very large cohorts, recall of individual subjects may be limited. It is important to consider whether it is likely that the person(s) doing the outcome assessment would know (or be able to figure out) the exposure status of the study participants. If the answer is "no," then blinding is adequate. One approach to blinding of the outcome assessors is to create a separate committee, whose members were not involved in the care of the patient and had no information about the study participants' exposure status. The committee would then be provided with copies of participants' medical records, which would be stripped of any potential exposure information or personally identifiable information. The committee would then review the records for prespecified outcomes according to the study protocol. In some situations, blinding is not possible, and the potential for bias must be weighed.

12. Follow-up rate

Higher overall follow-up rates always are better than lower follow-up rates, even though higher rates are expected in shorter studies, and lower overall follow-up rates often are seen in studies of longer duration. For example, a 6-month cohort study examining the relationship between dietary sodium intake and blood pressure level may have a more than 90% follow-up rate, but a 20-year cohort study examining effects of sodium intake on stroke may have only a 65% follow-up rate. As a guideline, an acceptable overall follow-up rate is considered 80% or more of participants whose exposures were measured at baseline. The greater loss-to-follow-up is a potential concern if subjects who are lost differ from those followed.

13. Statistical analyses

Statistical analyses need to control for potential confounders, in contrast to an RCT in which randomization tends to limit the potential of confounders. All key factors that may be associated both with the exposure of interest and the outcome—that are not intermediaries in the association of interest—should be controlled for in the analyses.

For example, in a study of the relationship between cardiorespiratory fitness and heart attacks and strokes, the study should control for age, blood pressure, blood cholesterol, and body weight because all of these factors are associated both with low fitness and with heart attacks and stroke.

14. General guidance for determining the overall quality rating

Internal validity for cohort studies *is the extent to which the results reported in the study can truly be attributed to the exposure being evaluated and not to flaws in the design or conduct of the study.* In other words, can one draw associative conclusions about the effects of the exposures being studied on outcomes?

Critical appraisal involves considering the risk for potential for selection bias, information bias, measurement bias, or confounding (the mixture of exposures that one cannot tease out from each other). Examples of confounding include co-interventions or differences at baseline in patient characteristics. A high risk of bias in a study requires that it be rated as being of "poor" quality. A low risk of bias in a study allows it to be rated of good quality. In addition, the more attention in the study design to issues that can help determine whether there is a causal relationship between the exposure and outcome, the higher the quality of the study. These attributes include exposures occurring before outcomes, evaluation of a dose-response gradient, accuracy of measurement of both exposure and outcome, sufficient timeframe to see an effect, and appropriate control for confounding.

Quality Assessment of Case-Control Studies

The quality assessment tool for case-control studies includes clarity of the research objective or research question; definition, selection, composition, and participation of the study population; definition and assessment of case or control status; exposure and outcome variables; use of concurrent controls; confirmation that the exposure occurred before the outcome; statistical power; and other factors.

1. Research question

Was the study designed to answer a clear predetermined question, or was it exploratory in nature?

2. Study population

Case-control study populations are determined by the location, time period, and inclusion criteria for cases (individuals with the disease or health problem) and controls (individuals without the disease or health problem). Selection criteria should address how the disease was diagnosed, whether cases were limited to those newly diagnosed, when and where cases were sampled, and any other selection factors. The choice of controls is even more challenging in order to assemble an unbiased comparison group, and the source and approach to sampling should be appropriate to the study question.

Other studies may use disease registries or data from cohort studies to identify cases, in which case the populations are individuals in the area covered by the disease registry or included in a cohort study (i.e., nested case control or case cohort). For example, a study of the relationship between vitamin D intake and myocardial infarction (MI) might use patients identified via a database of heart attack patients.

3. Target population and case representation

For a study to truly address the research question, the target population, the population from which the study population is drawn and to which study results are believed to apply, should be defined carefully. Some authors may compare characteristics of the study cases with characteristics of cases in the target population. When study cases are shown to be representative of cases in the appropriate target population, it increases the likelihood that the study was well designed for the research question.

Because these statistics frequently are difficult or impossible to measure, however, publications should not be penalized unduly if case representativeness is not documented.

4. Sample size justification

Generally, the sample size needed to detect differences in exposures should be discussed or a presentation should be made about the statistical power to detect an association of the magnitude anticipated.

5. Groups recruited from the same population

To determine whether cases and controls were recruited from the same source population, it is important to consider if a control was to develop the outcome of interest (the condition that was used to select cases), would she or he have been eligible to become a case? For example, cases and controls may be recruited from hospitals in a given region. It may be reasonable to assume that controls in the catchment area for the hospitals, or those already in the hospitals for a different reason, would attend those hospitals if they became a case; therefore, the controls are drawn from the same population as the cases.

In a prospective case-control study, participants are enrolled as cases at the time they are found to have the outcome of interest; the number of cases increases as time progresses. In this type of study, controls may be recruited or selected from the population without the outcome of interest at the time the case is diagnosed. Cases may be identified or recruited through a surveillance system, with controls selected from the population covered by that surveillance system; this is an example of population-based controls. If cases are selected from a cohort study population, then controls may be sampled from the cohort study population as well. This is known as a nested case-control study.

6. I/E criteria prespecified and applied uniformly

The same selection criteria should be used for cases and controls except, of course, for whether or not they had the disease or condition of interest. Typical criteria include age (or age range), gender, race, and so on. If the inclusion criteria are highly selective, the ability to extrapolate results beyond the study population may be limited.

7. Case and control definitions

A specific description of "case" and "control" should be defined, with a discussion of the validity of the case and control definitions and the processes or tools used to identify study participants. The more definitive the diagnostic process, the better for the purposes of validity. All cases should be identified using the same methods. Study results cannot be used to draw valid conclusions unless the distinction between cases and controls is accurate and reliable.

8. Random selection of study participants

If a case-control study did not use 100% of eligible cases and controls (e.g., not all disease-free participants were included as controls), did the authors indicate that random sampling was used to select controls? When it is possible to identify the source population fairly explicitly (e.g., in a nested case-control study or in a registry-based study), then random sampling of controls is preferred. If consecutive sampling was used, as frequently occurs for cases in prospective studies, then study participants were not randomly selected, but unless there is some inherent lack of independence between cases, this is not necessarily an issue of great concern.

9. Concurrent controls

A concurrent control is selected at the same time as a case. This means that one or more controls are recruited or selected from the population without the outcome of interest at the time a case is diagnosed. Concurrent controls tend to reduce the potential for bias if exposure patterns vary over time. This can be done in both prospective case-control studies and retrospective case-control studies. It also can be done in hospital-based

samples, population-based samples, and case-control studies nested within a cohort.

The use of concurrent controls can be done in the presence or absence of matching and vice versa. Just because a study incorporates matching does not necessarily mean that concurrent controls were used.

10. Exposure assessed before outcome measurement

Because the case or control status is determined first (based on the presence or absence of outcome of interest) and then the exposure history of the case or control is assessed, it is important to make sure that the exposure actually occurred before the outcome. For example, if tissue samples were used to determine exposure, were the tissue samples collected from patients before their diagnosis? If hospital records were used, did investigators verify that the date that a patient was exposed (e.g., received medication for hypertension) occurred before the date that a person became a case (e.g., was diagnosed with MI)? For an association between an exposure and an outcome to be considered causal, the exposure must occur before the outcome.

11. Exposure measures and assessment

Are measures of exposure accurate and reproducible? Equally important is whether the exposures were assessed in the same manner within groups and between groups. In a case-control study, one often has to rely on historical information about exposure. Personal recall is a relatively weak method of exposure classification, but it may be all that is available to the investigator. If disease status could affect recall, a potential bias ("recall bias") may occur.

12. Blinding of exposure assessors

Blinding in this case means that persons assessing the exposure status of study participants did not know whether the participant was a case or a control. The objective is to look for evidence in the article that the person assessing the exposure(s) (e.g., examining medical records to determine the exposures that occurred in the cases and controls) is masked to the case or control status of the participant. Sometimes it is not possible to blind the disease status because it is so obvious (e.g., many serious illnesses). If interviews are conducted with the cases and controls, it would be important to ensure that the interviewers are blinded to the research question of interest.

If the investigators used medical records to assess exposure, the following attributes favor blinding:

- Assessors not directly involved in the care of the study subjects because they would probably have knowledge of the conditions of their patients.

- If the medical record contained information on the patient's condition that identified him or her as a case (which is likely), that information would have to be removed before the exposure assessors reviewed the records.
- At a minimum, the record abstractors should be blinded to the research question of interest.

13. Statistical analysis

Logistic regression or other multiple regression methods often are used to adjust for the influence of variables other than the exposure of interest. This is a key issue in case-control studies, in contrast to an RCT in which the randomization process tends to control for potential confounders. All key factors that may be associated both with the exposure of interest and the outcome should be controlled for in the analyses. Most well-designed case-control studies control for multiple potential confounders.

Matching *is a technique used in an effort to improve study efficiency and control for known confounders.* For example, in a study of smoking and CVD events, one might identify cases who had a heart attack or stroke and then select controls of similar age, gender, and body weight to the cases. For case-control studies, it is important that if matching was performed during the selection or recruitment process, it should be considered in the analysis.

14. General guidance for determining the overall quality rating

Internal validity for case-control studies *is the extent to which the associations between disease and exposure reported in the study can truly be attributed to the exposure being evaluated and not to flaws in the design or conduct of the study.* In other words, what is the ability of the study to draw associative conclusions about the effects of the exposures being studied on outcomes? Any such study limitations and weaknesses can increase the risk of bias. Critical appraisal involves considering the risk for potential for selection bias, information bias, measurement bias, or confounding (the mixture of exposures that one cannot tease out from each other). Examples of confounding include co-interventions, differences at baseline in patient characteristics, and other issues throughout the questions above. The greater the risk of bias, the lower the quality rating of the study.

a. Risk of bias

Risk of bias refers to *the likelihood that the body of included studies for a given question or outcome is distorted because of flaws in the results of design or conduct of the studies.* Risk of bias and internal validity are similar concepts that are inversely correlated. A study with a low risk of bias has high internal validity and is more likely to provide correct results than one with high risk of bias and low internal validity. At the individual study level, risk of bias is determined by rating the quality of each individual study using standard rating instruments. Overall risk of bias for the body of evidence regarding a particular question, summary table, or outcome is then assessed by the aggregate quality of studies available for that particular question or outcome. If the risk of bias is low, then it increases the rating for the strength of the overall body of evidence. If the risk of bias is high, then it decreases the strength of evidence rating.

b. Consistency

Consistency *is the degree to which reported effect sizes are similar across the included studies for a particular question or outcome.* Consistency, when present, enhances the overall strength of evidence and is assessed through effect sizes being in the same direction (i.e., multiple studies demonstrate an improvement in a particular outcome) and the range of effect sizes across studies being narrow. Inconsistent evidence is reflected in:

- Effect sizes that are in different directions
- A broad range of effect sizes
- Non-overlapping confidence intervals
- Unexplained clinical or statistical heterogeneity

Studies included for a particular question or outcome can have effect sizes that are consistent, inconsistent, or unknown (or not applicable). The latter occurs when only a single study is available.

c. Directness

Directness has two aspects: *the direct line of causality and the degree to which findings can be extended from a specific population to a more general population.* The first defines directness as whether the evidence being assessed reflects a single direct link between the intervention (or service, approach, or exposure) of interest and the ultimate health outcome under consideration. Indirect evidence relies on intermediate or surrogate outcomes that serve as links along a causal pathway. Evidence that an intervention results in changes in important health outcomes (e.g., mortality, morbidity) increases the strength of the evidence. Evidence that an intervention results in changes limited to intermediate or surrogate outcomes (e.g., a blood measurement) decreases the strength of the evidence. However, the importance of each link in the chain should be considered, including existing evidence that a change in an intermediate outcome affects important health outcomes.

Another example of directness involves whether the bodies of evidence used to compare interventions are the same. For example, if drug A is compared with placebo in one study and drug B is compared with placebo in another study, using those two studies to compare drug A with drug B yields indirect evidence and provides a lower strength of the evidence than direct head-to-head comparisons of drug A versus drug B.

The second aspect of directness refers to the degree to which participants or interventions in the study are different from those to whom the study results are being applied. This concept is referred to as *applicability* or *generalizability*. If the population or interventions are similar, then the evidence is direct and strengthened. If they are different, then the evidence is indirect and weakened.

d. Precision

Precision is *the degree of statistical certainty about an estimate of effect for a specific outcome of interest*. Indicators of precision are statistical significance and confidence intervals. Precise estimates enable conclusions to be drawn about an intervention's effect relative to another intervention or control. An imprecise estimate is one in which the confidence interval is so large that the superiority or inferiority of an intervention cannot be defined with relevant specificity. Precision is related to the statistical power of the study. An outcome that was not the primary outcome or not prespecified generally will be less precise than the primary outcome of a study. In a meta-analysis, precision is reflected by the confidence interval around the summary effect size. For systematic reviews, which include multiple studies but no quantitative summary estimate, the quantitative information from each study should be considered in determining the overall precision of the body of included studies because some studies may be more precise than others. Determining precision across many studies without conducting a formal meta-analysis is challenging and requires judgment. Whereas a more precise estimate increases the strength of evidence, less precision reduces the strength of a body of evidence.

Quality Assessment of Systematic Reviews and Meta-Analyses

The quality assessment for systematic reviews and meta-analyses includes elements of prespecified eligibility criteria, use of a comprehensive and systematic literature search process, dual review for abstracts and full-text articles, quality assessment of individual studies, assessment of publication bias, and other factors. Some specific factors to consider are detailed next.

1. Focused question

    The review should be based on a question that is clearly stated and well formulated. An example would be a question that uses the PICO (population, intervention, comparator, outcome) format, with all of the components clearly described.

2. Eligibility criteria

    The eligibility criteria used to determine whether studies were included or excluded from the review should be clearly specified and predefined.

3. Literature search

    The search strategy should employ a comprehensive, systematic approach to capture all of the evidence possible that pertains to the question of interest. At a minimum, a comprehensive review should have the following attributes:

- Electronic searches were conducted using multiple scientific literature databases such as MEDLINE, EMBASE, Cochrane Central Register of Controlled Trials, PsychLit, and others as appropriate for the subject matter.

- Manual searches of references found in articles and textbooks should supplement the electronic searches.

    Additional search strategies that may be used to improve the yield of potential studies include the following:

- Studies published in a range of countries and different populations

- Studies published in languages other than English

- Use of content area experts to identify studies and articles that may have been missed

- Search of the grey (non–peer-reviewed) literature, which includes technical reports and other papers from government agencies or scientific groups or committees, presentations and posters from scientific meetings, conference proceedings, unpublished manuscripts, and so on. A search of the grey literature is important (whenever feasible) because sometimes only positive studies with significant findings are published in the peer-reviewed literature, which can bias the results of a review.

The literature search strategy should be described clearly in the review and be reproducible by others.

4. Dual review for determining which studies to include and exclude

Titles, abstracts, and full-text articles (when indicated) should be reviewed by two independent reviewers to determine which studies to include or exclude from the review. Disagreements between the reviewers should be resolved by discussion and consensus or with third-party involvement. The process for review, including methods for adjudicating disagreements, should be stated clearly.

5. Quality appraisal for internal validity

Each included study should be appraised for internal validity (study quality assessment) using a standardized approach for rating the quality of the individual studies. Ideally, this should be done by at least two independent reviewers. However, because there is not one commonly accepted, standardized tool for rating the quality of studies, at a minimum, the goal should be to show that individual study quality was assessed and adequately described by the authors.

6. List and describe included studies

All of the included studies should be listed in the review along with descriptions of their key characteristics. This can be presented in narrative or tabular format.

7. Publication bias

Publication bias is *when studies with positive results have a higher likelihood of being published, being published rapidly, being published in higher impact journals, being published in English, being published more than once, or being cited by others.* Publication bias can be linked to favorable or unfavorable treatment of research findings by any of the following: the investigators, editors, industry sponsors, or peer reviewers. A strategy that can minimize the potential for publication bias is to conduct a very comprehensive literature search. A funnel plot is a commonly used graphical method for detecting publication bias. The funnel plot is a scatter plot of component studies in a meta-analysis. The graph looks like a symmetrical inverted funnel if there is no significant publication bias.

8. Heterogeneity

Heterogeneity is *used to describe important differences in the included studies of a meta-analysis that may make it inappropriate to combine the results of studies.* Heterogeneity can be clinical (e.g.,

important differences between study participants, baseline disease severity, interventions), methodologic (e.g., important differences in the design and conduct of the study), or statistical (e.g., important differences in the quantitative results or reported effects). *Clinical or methodologic heterogeneity* usually is assessed qualitatively by determining whether it makes sense to combine studies. An example of *clinical heterogeneity* is whether a study that involves elderly male smokers with hypertension could be combined with a study that involves healthy, nonsmoking adults ages 18 to 40 years. *Methodologic heterogeneity* is illustrated by the question of whether studies that use an RCT design could be combined with studies that use observational study designs.

Statistical heterogeneity describes the degree of variation in the effect estimates from a set of studies and is assessed quantitatively. The two most common methods used to assess statistical heterogeneity are the Q test (also known as the χ^2 or chi-square test) or I2 test.

An assessment for heterogeneity should be conducted and clearly described. If the studies are found to be heterogeneous, the investigators should explore and explain the causes of the heterogeneity, and they should determine what influence, if any, the study differences had on the overall study results.

SUMMARY

In this chapter, we have introduced the process involved in the assessment of medical literature using as an illustrative model the work of the JNC 8 review of the treatment of hypertension. A systematic review conducted for the purpose of developing treatment guidelines should have a number of key elements, including (1) framing of a question(s) that is (are) relevant to clinical practice, (2) choosing I/E criteria appropriate to the questions of interest, (3) conducting a thorough screening process for literature relevant to the question of interest, (4) assessing the quality of each study included in the review, (5) abstracting essential information from each included study into a database, (6) constructing evidence tables that summarize the abstracted data from the database, and (7) evaluating the summary tables in order to derive evidence statements about the questions of interest.

One of the most fundamental and challenging tasks in this process is the fourth item above—judging the quality of each included study. A framework for doing so is included in this chapter, recognizing that such an assessment must be adapted to the types of studies being reviewed. In general, the strongest evidence comes from RCTs. In situations, such as the literature reviewed by the JNC 8, when many RCTs have been performed, a judgment may be made to exclude from consideration evidence derived from observational studies. In many other situations, however, there may be too few RCTs available, or those that are available have such major design limitations that the evidence base needs to be augmented by the inclusion of observational studies.

Assessment of the quality of studies is motivated by the desire to determine the level of confidence that can be placed in the accuracy (**validity**) of their conclusions. It is useful to dissect out two different aspects of validity. The first domain is the extent to which the study provides a correct answer for the population that was studied (**internal validity**). Limitations in internal validity relate to aspects of the design or execution of the study that may have led to a distorted result. We refer to such a distortion as a **bias** and conventionally group these distortions into broad categories related to the **selection** of study subjects, the **information** collected on the study participants, and the mixing (or **confounding**) of the effect of interest with other factors that may influence the outcome. A second broad category of validity is so-called **external validity**, which relates to the ability to extend the findings from the study population to other groups who were not studied. In general, the more restrictive the inclusion criteria for the study sample, the more one is concerned about the ability to extrapolate the findings to other people who were not studied.

For RCTs, the typical elements of quality assessment include whether randomization was performed correctly and achieved the intended results, whether the observers were adequately blinded, whether the sample size was sufficient, whether dropout rates were acceptably low, whether the subjects adhered to their assigned treatment regimens, and whether the appropriate analysis was performed. For cohort studies, the principal elements of quality assessment include whether the study groups were chosen appropriately, whether the exposure was measured adequately and assessed before outcome determination, whether the sample size was sufficient to observe an effect, whether sufficient time was allowed to observe an effect and the dropout rate was acceptable, whether the outcome was measured adequately, whether a gradient of effect was assessed, and whether the appropriate analysis was performed. For case-control studies, the key elements of quality assessment include whether the definition of cases was sufficient, whether controls came from the same time period and source population that gave rise to the cases, whether exposure occurred before outcome development and was measured appropriately, whether the sample size was sufficient to observe an effect, and whether the appropriate analysis was performed.

The JNC 8 review of RCTs led to some clear recommendations for pharmacologic treatment of high blood pressure. Specifically, for all persons 60 years of age or older, patients with blood pressures above 150 mm Hg systolic or 90 mm Hg diastolic should receive pharmacologic therapy with a goal of reaching those specified blood pressure targets. For persons 30 to 59 years of age, the same diastolic blood pressure target was established, but a systolic blood pressure target could not be established for persons younger than age 60 years. These and other findings can help guide appropriate evidence-based care for patients with high blood pressure.

STUDY QUESTIONS

1. All of the following would be considered providing low quality of evidence EXCEPT

    A. RCTs with major limitations.

    B. case reports of clinical observations.

    C. physiological measurement studies.

    D. well-designed, well-executed observational studies.

    E. none of the above.

2. Which of the following types of studies typically is considered to provide the strongest quality of evidence?

    A. Well-designed, well-executed nonrandomized intervention studies

    B. Well-designed, well-executed randomized intervention studies

    C. Well-designed, well-executed observational studies

    D. Well-designed, well-executed case series

    E. Well-designed, well-executed physiological measurement studies

3. Which of the following associations is an example in which the results of observational studies and RCTs reached differing conclusions?

    A. Cholesterol reduction and lowered risk of recurrent MIs

    B. Hypertension control and reduced risk of stroke

    C. Hormone replacement therapy and reduced risk of cardiovascular disease

    D. Aspirin use and reduced risk of cardiovascular disease

    E. Blood glucose control and reduced risk of complications of diabetes mellitus

4. The IOM's "best practice" standards for developing evidence-based clinical guidelines include all of the following EXCEPT
   A. use of a systematic review.
   B. consideration of patient subgroups and preferences.
   C. a process to minimize biases.
   D. ratings of the quality of the evidence.
   E. none of the above.

5. A study with highly restrictive inclusion criteria is likely to be limited with respect to
   A. internal validity.
   B. face validity.
   C. ecologic validity.
   D. external validity.
   E. construct validity.

6. Which of the following study designs is LEAST susceptible to the potential distortion from confounding?
   A. An RCT
   B. A correlation (ecologic) study
   C. A cross-sectional study
   D. A case-control study
   E. A cohort study

7. Which of the following is NOT a potential fatal flaw for an RCT?
   A. High dropout rates
   B. Too short a follow-up period for the outcome of interest
   C. Restrictive inclusion criteria
   D. No intention-to-treat analysis
   E. None of the above

8. A study with too few subjects to detect an effect of moderate magnitude is said to be limited with respect to statistical
   A. significance.
   B. power.
   C. sampling.
   D. control.
   E. dispersion.

9. Which of the following study designs has the greatest potential for recall bias?
   A. A crossover RCT
   B. A prospective cohort study of hospital records of elderly subjects
   C. An RCT conducted many years ago

D. A prospective cohort study using administrative data
   E. A case-control study with exposures classified from subject interviews

10. In an evaluation of a systematic review, which of the following is a strategy to maximize the yield of studies reviewed?
   A. Include research from a broad range of countries
   B. Include studies published in a wide variety of languages
   C. Include research not published in the peer-reviewed literature
   D. Include content area experts to identify any missing studies
   E. All of the above

FURTHER READING

Eccles MP, Grimshaw JM, Shekelle P, Schünemann HJ, Woolf S. Developing clinical practice guidelines: target audiences, identifying topics for guidelines, guideline group composition and functioning and conflicts of interest. *Implement Sci.* 2012;7:60.

Guyatt GH, Oxman AD, Kunz R, Vist GE, Falck-Ytter Y, Schünemann HJ, GRADE Working Group. What is "quality of evidence" and why is it important to clinicians? *BMJ.* 2008;336:995-998.

Shekelle P, Woolf S, Grimshaw JM, Schünemann HJ, Eccles MP. Developing clinical practice guidelines: reviewing, reporting, and publishing guidelines; updating guidelines; and the emerging issues of enhancing guideline implementability and accounting for comorbid conditions in guideline development. *Implement Sci.* 2012;7:62.

Woolf S, Schünemann HJ, Eccles MP, Grimshaw JM, Shekelle P. Developing clinical practice guidelines: types of evidence and outcomes; values and economics, synthesis, grading, and presentation and deriving recommendations. *Implement Sci.* 2012;7:61.

REFERENCES

Clinical Background

Egan BM, Zhao Y, Axon RN. US trends in prevalence, awareness, treatment, and control of hypertension, 1988-2000. *JAMA.* 2010;303:2043-2050.

James PA, Oparil S, Carter BL, et al. 2014 evidence-based guideline for the management of high blood pressure in adults: report from the panel members appointed to the Eighth Joint National Committee (JNC 8). *JAMA.* 2014;311:507-520.

Example 1: A Systematic Review

Goff DC Jr, Lloyd-Jones DM, Bennett G, et al. American College of Cardiology/American Heart Association Task Force on Practice Guidelines. 2013 ACC/AHA guideline on the assessment of cardiovascular risk: a report of the American College of Cardiology/American Heart Association Task Force on Practice. *Circulation.* 2014;29(suppl):S49-S73.

Herrington DM. Hormone replacement therapy and heart disease: replacing dogma with data. *Circulation.* 2003;107:2-4.

Institute of Medicine. *Clinical Practice Guidelines We Can Trust.* Washington, DC: National Academies Press; 2011.

Wright JT Jr, Fine LJ, Lackland DT, Ogedegbe G, Dennison Himmelfarb CR. Evidence supporting a systolic blood pressure goal of <150 mm Hg in patients >60 year: the minority view. *Ann Intern Med.* 2014;160:499-503.

System for Grading the Body of Evidence

Balshem H, Helfand M, Schünemann HJ, et al. GRADE guidelines: 3. Rating the quality of evidence. *J Clin Epidemiol.* 2011;64:401-406.

Guyatt GH, Oxman AD, Kunz R, Falck-Ytter Y, Vist GE, Liberati A, Schünemann HJ, GRADE Working Group. Going from evidence to recommendations. *BMJ.* 2008;336:1049-1051.

Example 2. When Experimental and Observational Studies Differ

Harman SM. Menopausal hormone treatment cardiovascular disease: another look at an unresolved conundrum. *Fertil Steril.* 2014;101:887-897.

Quality Assessment of Controlled Intervention Studies

Manchikanti L, Benyamin RM, Helm S, Hirsch JA. Evidence-based medicine, systematic reviews, and guidelines in interventional pain management: Part 3: systematic reviews and meta-analyses of randomized trials. *Pain Phys.* 2009;12:35-72.

Manchikanti L, Hirsch JA, Smith HS. Evidence-based medicines, systematic reviews, and guidelines in interventional pain management: Part 2: randomized controlled trials. *Pain Phys.* 2008;11:717-773.

Quality Assessment of Cohort and Cross-Sectional Studies

Sanderson S, Tatt ID, Higgins JPT. Tools for assessing quality and susceptibility to bias in observational studies in epidemiology: a systematic review and annotated bibliography. *Int J Epidemiol.* 2007;36:666-676.

von Elm E, Altman DG, Egger M, Pocock SJ, Gøtzsche PC, Vandenbroucke JP, STROBE Initiative. The strengthening of reporting of observational studies in epidemiology (STROBE) statement: guidelines for reporting observational studies. *J Clin Epidemiol.* 2008;61:344-349.

Quality Assessment of Case-Control Studies

Manchikanti L, Datta S, Smith HS, Hirsch JA. Evidence-based medicine, systematic reviews, and guidelines in interventional pain management: Part 6. Systematic reviews and meta-analyses of observational studies. *Pain Phys.* 2009;12:819-850.

Manchikanti L, Singh V, Smith HS, Hirsch JA. Evidence-based medicine, systematic reviews, and guidelines in interventional pain management: Part 4: observational studies. *Pain Phys.* 2009;12:73-108.

Quality Assessment of Systematic Reviews and Meta-Analyses

Sinha MK, Montori VM. Reporting bias and other biases affecting systematic reviews and meta-analyses: a methodological commentary. *Expert Rev Pharmacoecon Outcome Res.* 2006;6:603-611.

Quantitative Systematic Review

14

Giovanni Filardo, Briget da Graca, and David J. Ballard

HEALTH SCENARIO

Mr. P. is a 67-year-old, retired engineer who has had Canadian Cardiovascular Society class III angina for the past 3 months and symptomatic intermittent claudication for the past 12 months. His medical history shows no previous cardiovascular interventions, but he does have a number of vascular risk factors, including smoking, hypertension, and diabetes. Coronary angiography showed blockages in three vessels, with involvement of the left anterior descending coronary artery; his ejection fraction is 45%, and chest radiography showed a possible calcified ascending aorta. Mr. P. was referred to Dr. S. for consideration of coronary artery bypass graft surgery (CABG). After discussion of Mr. P.'s health goals and priorities and of the risks and benefits associated with CABG, Dr. S. and Mr. P. agree that surgery is the best treatment option for Mr. P. Mr. P., however, has an additional question: He has looked up some information on CABG procedures, as well as questioning friends and family members who have undergone revascularization procedures themselves or who work in medicine and has learned that CABG can be performed in more than one way, specifically, on pump (which uses cardiopulmonary bypass to enable surgeons to work on a still heart that has been arrested temporarily) versus off pump (which is performed on a beating heart). He wants to know if he is a candidate for both types of surgery, and, if so, what the risks and benefits of each type are and which is likely to offer him the best outcome. Dr. S. only performs on-pump CABG, and although he knows some of his colleagues strongly believe in the superiority of the off-pump procedure, he is not familiar enough with it to provide Mr. P. with the answers he is looking for. Because Mr. P.'s surgery is not immediately urgent, Dr. S. suggests that they schedule another appointment in a few days, giving him the opportunity to review the relevant literature regarding the two techniques.

CLINICAL BACKGROUND

More than 1 million patients worldwide undergo isolated CABG each year. In Asia, the majority (>60%) of these procedures are performed off pump (i.e., beating-heart surgery), but in the Western world, more than 80% of CABG procedures are performed on pump (i.e., with cardiopulmonary bypass). Off-pump CABG is relatively cheaper and is thought to reduce the risk of some adverse complications (i.e., postoperative atrial fibrillation, pulmonary complications, infection, and stroke) associated with conventional on-pump CABG. Drawbacks associated with this technique are the reduced graft patency and completeness of revascularization. To date, more than 200 studies have investigated the efficacy (randomized controlled trials [RCTs]) and effectiveness (observational studies) of off-pump CABG compared with on-pump CABG in terms of short- and long-term mortality. Study results are inconsistent and conflicting and leave the question regarding the best treatment option unanswered. In such situations, reviewing the primary research literature is unlikely to be of great help to physicians who find themselves in similar positions to Dr. S. Even if Dr. S. had time to read the large volume of articles available, the inconsistency of the results would likely prevent him from drawing any meaningful conclusions. A systematic review of the available evidence, however, can be extremely valuable. The results of such reviews not only form the basis for the development or revision of clinical guidelines but can also be used by clinicians and patients to accurately assess the risks and benefits of the available options during the shared decision-making process, better enabling the patient's priorities to drive the decision.

In this chapter, we will use the example of comparing off-pump and on-pump CABG to provide an overview of the process and methods involved in executing a rigorous quantitative systematic review.

SYSTEMATIC REVIEW DEFINITION

A **systematic review** *is a critical assessment and evaluation of all research studies that address a particular issue* (from Agency for Healthcare Research and Quality, as noted in Chapter 12). Systematic reviews summarize the empirical evidence found in the literature that meets prespecified eligibility criteria associated with a specific research question. Integrating individual clinical expertise with the best available external clinical evidence from systematic research is the basis for evidence-based health care (use of current best evidence in making decisions about the care of individual patients or the delivery of health services) and clinical practice (see Table 12-1). Therefore, systematic reviews play a central role in modern health care delivery. In particular, quantitative systematic reviews (also known as meta-analyses), which combine multiple studies with similar characteristics to achieve vastly greater statistical power and precision than can be obtained in any one study, can settle controversies from conflicting studies and inform clinical guidelines and health care decisions.

Methods to conduct systematic reviews include both quantitative and qualitative approaches. Both approaches offer advantages and disadvantages, and their use often is predicated upon the types of studies available to answer a specific question. This chapter focuses on the use of meta-analysis, a quantitative method for synthesizing and summarizing data from empirical studies. Whether the approach to a review is qualitative or quantitative, each review should be planned so that the standards for conducting a systematic review as described in Chapter 12 are met. Specific standards recommended by the Institute of Medicine include:

STANDARD 2.1: Establish a team with appropriate expertise and experience to conduct the systematic review.

STANDARD 2.2: Manage bias and conflict of interest of the team conducting the systematic review.

STANDARD 2.3: Ensure user and stakeholder input as the review is designed and conducted.

STANDARD 2.4: Manage bias and conflict of interest for individuals providing input into the systematic review.

STANDARD 2.5: Formulate the topic for the systematic review, confirm the need for a new review, and develop an analytic framework that clearly lays out the chain of logic that links the health intervention to the outcomes of interest and defines the key clinical questions to be addressed in the systematic review.

STANDARD 2.6: Develop a systematic review protocol.

STANDARD 2.7: Submit the protocol for peer review.

STANDARD 2.8: Make the final protocol available publicly and add any amendments to the protocol in a timely fashion.

PERFORMING A QUANTITATIVE SYSTEMATIC REVIEW: META-ANALYSIS

When the study designs, populations, treatments or interventions, exposures, and outcomes (including how and when these were assessed) of the studies included in the systematic review are similar, it is possible to summarize the published evidence quantitatively (using statistical methods) by performing a meta-analysis. Key components of a meta-analysis are:

- A clearly stated set of objectives with predefined eligibility criteria for studies
- An explicit, reproducible methodology
- A systematic search that attempts to capture all studies that would meet the eligibility criteria
- An assessment of the validity of the findings of the included studies (e.g., through the assessment of risk of bias)
- A systematic presentation and synthesis of the characteristics and findings of the included studies

In the case of the off-pump versus on-pump CABG example, our research question might be: "Does the recent evidence show that off-pump or on-pump CABG offers patients undergoing elective CABG a lower risk of operative mortality or a better probability of 1-year survival?" The meta-analysis to answer this question would then include all published studies that compared the efficacy and effectiveness of off-pump and on-pump CABG, in terms of operative or in-hospital or 1-year mortality, in the general CABG population (i.e., not limited to specific subgroups, such as "patients with diabetes") and enrolled study subjects no earlier than January 1, 2000. Such a meta-analysis should be executed, step-by-step, using the following framework and steps:

1. **Search strategy:** The search strategy should be based on the main concepts being examined. The terms to be used to conduct the literature search should be determined by the study hypothesis, the research questions, and the database in which the search is to be conducted. Moreover, the search should be reproducible. An experienced medical librarian can be invaluable in designing and executing a comprehensive search. The specification of search terms should be vetted thoroughly with the review team to ensure

that appropriate studies are identified and that systematic bias related to the search criteria is avoided.

The best place to start is PubMed (http://www.ncbi.nlm.nih.gov/pubmed), a free search engine developed and maintained by the National Library of Medicine, which provides access to MEDLINE, PreMEDLINE, HealthSTAR, the Cochrane Database of Systematic Reviews, publisher-supplied citations, and other related databases. Other search engines that one may have access to (depending on personal or institutional subscriptions) include OVID and Embase. Because these databases do not overlap entirely, it may be worth searching all of those one has access to, to ensure comprehensive coverage. Although the specific methods of searching within each of them are different, the basic principles outlined here apply across the board. For simplicity here, we will focus on PubMed.

The first important search tool to be aware of in PubMed is the Medical Subject Heading (MeSH) browser (http://www.nlm.nih.gov/mesh/meshhome.html). MeSH terms are a detailed taxonomy of keywords developed by the National Library of Medicine to cover all the topics in biomedicine. They automatically "explode out" to search for alternate or related terms and spellings so that one does not have to identify and search for each of these separately. Depending on the particular MeSH term searched, this can cast a very wide net. However, at this point in the search, one wants to be more inclusive than exclusive; it is much easier to discard nonrelevant papers as the review process continues than to identify studies missed by too narrow a search. The MeSH browser should be used to identify the relevant MeSH terms for the research question.

MeSH terms do, however, have one important limitation to keep in mind. Because the process of indexing articles and assigning the relevant MeSH terms and characteristics (e.g., language, study type) that can be used to filter search results takes time, recently published articles listed in PubMed may not be captured by a search that relies entirely on MeSH terms. If one is researching a topic that has been receiving substantial recent attention, one might need to include free-text terms as well as MeSH terms so as to not miss the most recent evidence.

After search terms are chosen, PubMed allows one to combine them using Boolean connectors (AND, OR, NOT). For more information about searching in PubMed, see the tutorial available online (http://www.nlm.nih.gov/bsd/disted/pubmedtutorial/cover.html).

In the example of the on-pump versus off-pump CABG meta-analysis, a search such as the following might be used: **"Coronary Artery Bypass"[Mesh] AND ("Coronary Artery Bypass, Off-Pump"[Mesh] OR off-pump) AND on-pump AND mortality**.

This search returns far more than the articles that will help answer our research question; for example, it will capture editorials that do not report any original research results. PubMed provides filtering options that can help reduce the number of unwanted articles one has to sift through. For example, here the search results might be limited to (1) Article types: randomized controlled trial, comparative study, meta-analysis, review, and systematic review; (2) species: humans, (3) language: English; and (4) publication dates: after January 1, 2000, which reduced the number of articles returned by the search from 474 to 291. The meta-analysis, review, and systematic review articles were included in the search not because they will provide results to be included in our meta-analysis but rather because checking their bibliographies for additional articles our search may have missed is another important step in conducting a systematic search. This method identified 12 additional articles to be considered for the on-pump versus off-pump CABG meta-analysis.

2. **Inclusion/exclusion (I/E) criteria:** A key feature of a systematic review is the prespecification of criteria for including and excluding studies in the review (eligibility criteria). As for the search strategy, the I/E criteria should be based on the study hypothesis and research questions. Features of the target population to whom the results of the systematic review are intended to apply should also be considered in determining the study I/E criteria so that findings can be generalized (external validity) accordingly. For example, if the systematic review is intended to inform the development of clinical guidelines for the treatment of coronary artery disease in elderly adults, a study in which enrollment was limited to patients younger than age 50 years should not be included because its results are not relevant to the systematic review's purpose. The I/E criteria also impact the systematic review's internal validity; for example, including non-RCT studies that do not rigorously account for confounding factors or excluding RCT studies that have a high cross-over rate (even if the analysis was correctly executed using an *intention-to-treat* approach) might significantly bias the meta-analysis findings.

Inclusion of non-RCT studies in a meta-analysis: By definition, a meta-analysis is a summary of

all empirical evidence associated with the specific research question. Therefore, it is critical to consider **all** rigorous and well-executed studies, including non-RCTs, regarding the topic of interest. Rigorously adjusted (by recognized and other possible confounders of the association of interest) non-RCTs provide critical evidence on the impact of the intervention or exposure on the outcome being evaluated in a real-world setting. Although RCTs continue to be considered the gold standard in empirical research, they suffer from one very important weakness: **limited external validity** (generalizability) because of narrow inclusion criteria and the difficulty this creates in translating study findings beyond the experimental cohort being evaluated. Including non-RCTs in the meta-analysis helps address this lack of external validity. Accordingly, both RCTs and non-RCTs should be considered in a meta-analysis, and findings should be presented by study type and overall.

In our example, all studies (RCTs and non-RCTs) comparing patient outcomes following isolated on-pump versus off-pump CABG; and included all-cause mortality (in-hospital, 30-day, or 1-year mortality) among the outcomes reported were considered. Upon reviewing the titles and abstracts of the 291 articles identified through the PubMed search plus the 12 articles identified from the bibliographies of past reviews, the review team narrowed down the candidates for inclusion to 217 articles.

Next, the review team examined the full text of each of the 217 articles to apply the following exclusions: (1) enrolled patients before January 1, 2000; (2) were restricted to patients with a specific demographic characteristic (i.e., male), cardiac condition (i.e., ST-elevation myocardial infarction), comorbidity (i.e., diabetes), or undergoing a specific type of CABG procedure (i.e., urgent or emergent procedures, redo procedures, minimally invasive or robotic-assisted procedures, or CABG with a simultaneous or synchronous additional procedure); (3) RCT but did not randomize patients between on-pump versus off-pump CABG; (4) observational study that did not report risk-adjusted mortality or survival for on-pump versus off-pump CABG; or (5) the mortality results reported duplicated those reported in another included article.

After applying these exclusion criteria, 27 articles remained (**Figure 14-1**).

3. **Data abstraction:** The processes used to abstract the data from the articles considered in the meta-analysis are critical and should be designed to warrant the highest validity and reliability of the

information collected. A standardized data collection tool that clearly specifies exactly what information needs to be collected from each article should be created and used by the research team abstracting data.

Continuing with the off-pump versus on-pump CABG meta-analysis, two members of the research team independently abstracted the necessary data from each article. This duplication of data collection increases the reliability of the process because any discrepancies between the abstractors' data sets are investigated and resolved. For our meta-analysis, we collected data from each article regarding the participants (cohort size and number of subjects in each study group), the interventions (off-pump or on-pump CABG), type of study (RCT or observational study), and the number of all-cause deaths (or adjusted estimated all-cause deaths for observational studies) at each time point reported in the article. These data are entered into RevMan 5.2 (meta-analysis software). **Table 14-1** shows the characteristics of the included studies.

4. **Assessment of risk of bias:** The internal validity of the meta-analysis depends on whether the data and results from the included studies are valid (i.e., the studies were conducted rigorously) and generalizable. Accordingly, a meta-analysis of poor-quality studies will have low internal validity and is likely to produce biased results. The evaluation of the risk of bias of the included studies is critical because it influences interpretation and the conclusions of the review.

The specifics of how to collect and report the risk of bias data depend very much on the tool chosen to assess it. A good option, particularly when all or most of the included studies are RCTs, is the Cochrane Collaboration's RCT Bias Assessment Tool (see http://handbook.cochrane.org/chapter_8/table_8_5_a_the_cochrane_collaborations_tool_for_assessing.htm), in which the risk of bias in a specified set of categories is judged to be at low, high, or unclear risk. Other tools may be more appropriate when focusing on observational studies, and including both RCTs and observational studies in the same systematic review may require some adaptation to enable one tool to be applied consistently across all studies.

For the on-pump versus off-pump CABG meta-analysis, which includes both RCTs and risk-adjusted observational studies, we used an adaptation of the Cochrane Collaboration tool, assessing each article for the following domains:

- Random sequence generation (applicable to RCTs only): Were patients properly randomized?

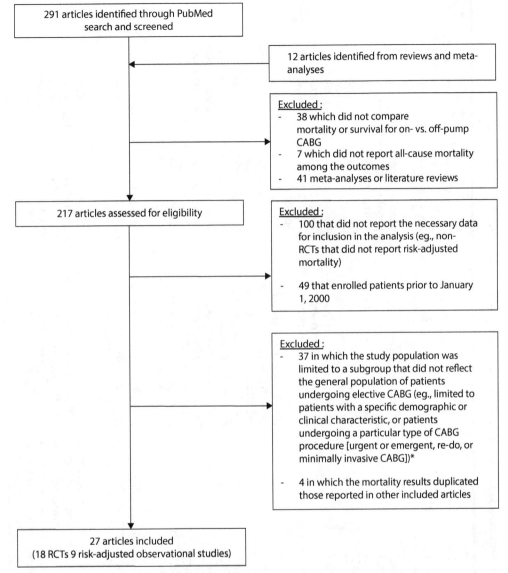

Figure 14-1. Flow chart showing inclusion/exclusion of studies in the off-pump versus on-pump coronary artery bypass graft surgery (CABG) meta-analysis.
*Sensitivity analyses that included the studies excluded because they were limited to subgroups based on particular demographic or clinical characteristics (e.g., patients age ≥75 years, or patients with diabetes) or because they used risk adjustment strategies that did not account for the relevant risk factors for mortality recognized by the Society of Thoracic Surgeons were conducted to ensure these exclusions did not bias our results. The sensitivity analyses extended to these excluded studies confirmed the study results.

- Selection bias
  - For RCTs, (1) were the intervention groups balanced (e.g., gender)? (2) Was intention-to-treat analysis used (i.e., patients randomized to off-pump CABG who underwent on-pump CABG were analyzed as patients belonging to the off-pump group)?

- For observational studies, (1) were the same I/E criteria applied to the on-pump and off-pump CABG groups? (2) Did the reported characteristics of the two groups show imbalance? c) Were the appropriate risk adjustment methods applied?

- Detection bias: Were different methods used to assess mortality or survival between the on-pump versus off-pump CABG groups?

Table 14-1. Characteristics of the studies included in the on-pump vs. off-pump CABG meta-analysis.

	Study Type	Cohort Size	Period During Which Surgeries Were Performed	Time Points at Which Mortality Results Were Reported or Included in the Meta-Analysis
Randomized Controlled Trials(RCTs)				
Muneretto et al. (2003)	RCT	88 off pump, 88 on-pump	1/2000 to 1/2002	Operative 1 year
Carrier et al. (2003)	RCT	28 off pump, 37 on-pump	10/2001 to 9/2002	Operative
Chen et al. (2004)	RCT	150 off pump, 150 on-pump	6/2001 to 4/2003	Operative
Straka et al. (2004)	RCT	204 off pump, 184 on pump	5/2000 to 6/2002	Operative
Hernandez et al. (2007)	RCT	99 off pump, 102 on pump	1/2001 to 1/2004	Operative
Motallebzadeh et al. (2007)	RCT	108 off pump, 104 on pump	8/2002 to 3/2004	Operative
Bednar et al. (2008)	RCT	40 off pump, 40 on pump	5/2005 to 12/2006	Operative
Medved et al. (2008)	RCT	30 off pump, 30 on pump	1/15/2006 to 6/30/2007	Operative
Nogueira et al. (2008)	RCT	105 off pump, 97 on pump	1/2002 to 12/2006	Operative
Shroyer et al. (2009)	RCT	1104 off pump, 1099 on pump	2/2002 to 5/2008	Operative 1 year
Hueb et al. (2010)	RCT	155 off pump, 153 on pump	3/2001 to 3/2006	Operative
Møller et al. (2010)	RCT	176 off pump, 163 on pump	4/2002 to 3/2006	Operative
Serrano et al. (2010)	RCT	40 off pump, 41 on pump	3/2001 to 3/2006	Operative 1 year
Sousa Uva et al. (2010)	RCT	75 off pump, 75 on pump	4/2005 to 7/2007	Operative 1 year
Puskas et al. (2011)	RCT	98 off pump, 99 on pump	3/2000 to 8/2001	Operative 1 year
Lamy et al. (2012)	RCT	2375 off pump, 2377 on pump	11/2006 to 10/2011	Operative
Lemma et al. (2012)	RCT	208 off pump, 203 on pump	12/2006 to 4/2010	Operative
Lamy et al. (2013)	RCT	2375 off pump, 2377 on pump	11/2006 to 10/2011	1 year
Risk-Adjusted Observational Studies				
Lamy et al. (2005)	Retrospective cohort study	1233 off pump, 1233 on pump	3/2001 to 12/2002	Operative 1 year
Roscitano et al. (2005)	Retrospective cohort study	87 off pump, 87 on pump	5/2000 to 5/2002	Operative
Stamou et al. (2005)	Retrospective cohort study	315 off pump, 198 on pump	1/1/2000 to 12/31/2000	Operative
Hannan et al. (2007)	Retrospective cohort study	13889 off pump, 35941 on pump	2001 to 2004	Operative
Konety et al. (2009)	Retrospective cohort study	26011 off pump, 99344 on pump	2000 to 2004	Operative
Abdulrahman et al. (2010)	Retrospective cohort study	416 off pump, 578 on pump	2006 to 2009	Operative
Chawla et al. (2012)	Retrospective cohort study	158561 off pump, 584348 on pump	1/2004 to 12/2009	Operative
Marui et al. (Sept. 2012)	Retrospective cohort study	1091 off pump, 1377 on pump	1/2000 to 12/2002	Operative
Polomsky et al. (2013)	Retrospective cohort study	186138 off pump, 689943 on pump	1/2005 to 12/2010	Operative

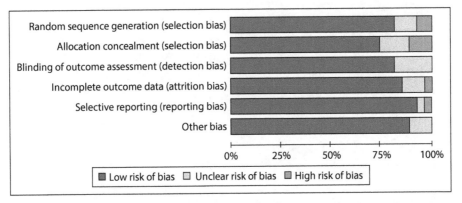

Figure 14-2. Results of risk of bias assessment of studies included in the off-pump versus on-pump coronary artery bypass graft surgery meta-analysis using an adapted version of the Cochrane Collaboration's RCT Bias Assessment Tool.

- Attrition bias: Was there a high rate (>20%) of loss to follow-up?
- Reporting bias: Were some prespecified outcomes not reported?
- Other sources of bias: Were patients converted from off-pump to on-pump CABG during surgery analyzed as part of the off-pump group or on-pump group, or were they excluded?

As for the data collection, we had two members of the research team independently review each article and enter the risk of bias data into RevMan 5.2. **Figure 14-2** summarizes the results of the risk of bias assessment, showing an overall fairly low risk of bias.

5. **Publication bias:** In some instances, studies' publication is affected by the study findings; most commonly, this takes the form of studies showing nonsignificant associations between the intervention and the outcome of interest not reaching publication. Publication bias is an important issue to consider when conducting a systematic review because the internal validity of the systematic review heavily depends on the evidence included in (or omitted from) the review. Because the researcher conducting a systematic review seldom has any practical means of determining which studies have remained unpublished, let alone of obtaining their results, reporting bias frequently has to be assessed solely based on the published studies. This can be done via a scatter plot (funnel plot) that depicts the intervention effect estimates from individual studies against some measure of each study's size or precision. An asymmetrical plot suggests publication bias may be present (i.e., some studies showing non-statistically significant effects are not published).

Figure 14-3 shows a funnel plot for the studies included in the off-pump versus on-pump CABG meta-analysis, produced using RevMan 5.2 and plotting the intervention effect (odds ratios for operative mortality) on a logarithmic scale. This plot does not show asymmetry (skewing of results to either the right or left), indicating that there is little risk of publication bias.

6. **Measures of association (statistical analysis and data synthesis):** The estimation of the measure of the association depends on the type of outcome: binary, continuous, categorical (more than two level outcome) or ordinal, counts or rates, or time to event. **Table 14-2** summarizes the measures of association for each type of outcome.

In the on-pump versus off-pump CABG meta-analysis example, we estimated an odds ratio (operative mortality), risk ratio (1-year mortality rate), and 95% confidence intervals (95% CI) based on Mantel-Haenszel chi-squares to compare mortality after off-pump versus on-pump CABG.

7. **Heterogeneity:** The intervention effects of the studies included in a meta-analysis might vary because of random error alone or due to differences in studies' methodologies (e.g., outcome assessment procedures, study population, study design). This variation is commonly known as heterogeneity. When intervention effects show **different directions** and magnitudes between studies, the heterogeneity is more likely to be attributable to methodologic differences between studies, and a meta-analysis **cannot** be performed. In this case, a qualitative review of the evidence may be presented instead. In contrast, when the intervention effects have the **same direction** but different magnitudes between studies, the heterogeneity is more likely to be attributable to chance, and it is appropriate to conduct a meta-analysis to summarize the available evidence. In this case, a random-effect model

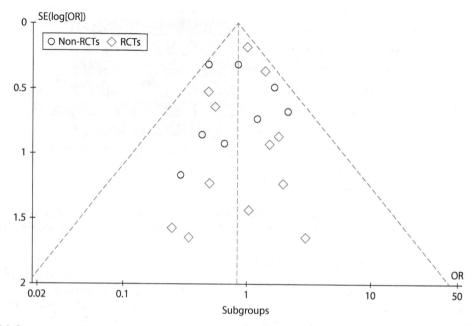

Figure 14-3. Funnel plot to assess reporting bias in the off-pump versus on-pump coronary artery bypass graft surgery meta-analysis. OR, odds ratio; RCT, randomized controlled trial; SE, standard error.

Table 14-2. Systematic review measures of association by outcome.

Type of Outcome	Measure of Association
Binary	Risk ratio
	Odds ratio
	Risk difference
Continuous	Mean difference
	Standardized mean difference
Ordinal	Proportional odds ratio
Counts or rate	Rate ratio
Time to event	Hazard ratio

(which assumes that the effects being estimated in the different studies are not identical but that the studies methods are similar) should be used. A fixed-effect meta-analysis should be used when there is no heterogeneity, as this model assumes that the true effect of the intervention is similar (in both magnitude and direction) across studies. It is important to specify a priori whether a random- or fixed-effect model will be used.

Reviewing the articles included in our on-pump versus off-pump CABG example, the methods are sufficiently similar for a meta-analysis to be appropriate, and a random-effect model is clearly called for, given the conflicting results

between studies and the possible variation associated with the intervention effects' differences. Using RevMan 5.2 to assess the heterogeneity that existed among the included studies, we see in **Figure 14-4** that although all studies' intervention effects had the same direction, their magnitudes greatly and significantly varied. This confirms that the choice of a random-effect model to summarize the available evidence was appropriate.

8. **Sensitivity analysis:** Performing a meta-analysis involves a series of decisions, specifically, choosing a search strategy, the study I/E criteria, and the measures of association that are of interest; assessing the sources of heterogeneity (and deciding whether a meta-analysis is appropriate); and choosing the types of sensitivity analysis that need to be performed. In some situations, decisions might be arbitrary, making the meta-analysis findings susceptible to bias. To assess whether the meta-analysis results are independent from the investigator's decisions, a sensitivity analysis should be performed by repeating the primary analysis, substituting alternative decisions that were arbitrary or unclear (e.g., include the excluded studies in the analysis).

In our on-pump versus off-pump CABG meta-analysis example, we needed to assess whether our findings were biased by our study exclusion criteria. Accordingly, we repeated our primary analysis and included the studies we excluded

Study or Subgroup	Off-Pump Events	Total	On-Pump Events	Total	Weight	Odds Ratio M-H, Random, 95% CI	Odds Ratio M-H, Random, 95% CI
Non-RCTs							
Abdulrahman et al. (2010)	1	416	13	578	0.3%	0.10 [0.01, 0.80]	
Chawla et al. (2012)	1892	158561	7849	584348	20.9%	0.89 [0.84, 0.93]	
Hannan et al. (2007)	926	13889	3013	35941	19.7%	0.78 [0.72, 0.84]	
Konety et al. (2009)	564	26011	3279	99344	18.9%	0.65 [0.59, 0.71]	
Lamy et al. (2005)	18	1233	21	1233	2.5%	0.86 [0.45, 1.61]	
Marui et al. (Sept 2012)	9	1091	30	1377	1.8%	0.37 [0.18, 0.79]	
Polomsky et al. (2013)	2793	186138	11630	689943	21.2%	0.89 [0.85, 0.93]	
Roscitano et al. (2005)	2	87	3	87	0.3%	0.66 [0.11, 4.04]	
Stamou et al. (2005)	19	315	23	198	2.5%	0.49 [0.26, 0.92]	
Subtotal (95% CI)		387741		1413049	88.2%	0.77 [0.68, 0.87]	
Total events	6224		25861				

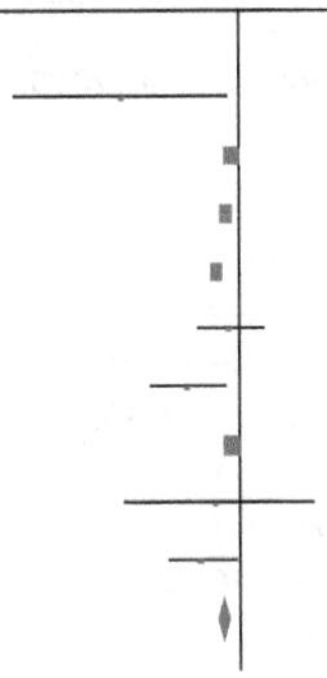

Heterogeneity: $Tau^2 = 0.02$; $Chi^2 = 57.44$, df = 8 (p < 0.00001); $I^2 = 86\%$
Test for overall effect Z = 4.32 (p < 0.0001)

Figure 14-4. Heterogeneity test results for the non–randomized controlled trials included in the off-pump versus on-pump coronary artery bypass graft surgery meta-analysis. CI, confidence interval; M-H, Mantel-Haenszel.

because the study population was limited to patients with a particular demographic or clinical characteristic, and we compared the results with the results from the primary analysis. The results (not shown here) were very similar; therefore, the sensitivity analysis supported our study findings.

9. **Presentation of results:** A very intuitive and clear way of presenting findings from a meta-analysis is with a Forest plot. The Forest plot shows not only the overall effect (and associated 95% CI) estimated from the meta-analysis, but for each included study, it shows the raw summary data, including the total number of patients by intervention or control group, the total number of events (mean and standard deviation are used for continuous outcomes) by intervention or control group, the percent weight (the "weight" the individual study contributes to the overall effect), and the weighted (depending on the cohort size) point estimate (i.e., intervention effect). Revman 5.2 further automatically includes the results of a heterogeneity test, a chi-squared statistic, and a test for differences across subgroups in the Forest plot, which aid in interpretation.

Figures 14-5 and **14-6** show the Forest plots, respectively, for short-term and 1-year mortality rates from the on-pump versus off-pump CABG meta-analysis produced using RevMan 5.2. For short-term mortality, the results when all studies were included favored off-pump CABG (odds ratio [95% CI] = 0.80 [0.72, 0.88]), although no significant difference was observed in the subgroup of RCTs (odds ratio [95% CI] = 1.00 [0.76, 1.32]). At 1 year, there was no significant difference in mortality regardless of whether all studies were considered (risk ratio [95% CI] = 1.03 [0.86, 1.25]) or only the subgroup of either RCTs (risk ratio [95% CI] = 1.08 [0.87, 1.33]) or observational studies (risk ratio [95% CI] = 0.90 [0.60, 1.34]).

Finally, when writing up the systematic review for publication, the standards laid out in the Preferred Reporting Items for Systematic Reviews and Meta-Analyses (PRISMA) Statement should be followed. Most peer-reviewed journal articles require this (including submission of the PRISMA checklist) for publication. Details on the PRISMA statement, including the PRISMA checklist and a template for creating the flow diagram for studies included and excluded in the systematic review, are available at http://www.prisma-statement.org.

It is a good idea to consult the PRISMA checklist at the start of the systematic review process to ensure one records all of the information necessary to comply with the PRISMA standards (e.g., reasons why studies were excluded) along the way.

HEALTH SCENARIO CONCLUSION

When Dr. S. and Mr. P. from the opening Health Scenario meet again as scheduled, Dr. S. explains the findings from this quantitative systematic review of the evidence to Mr. P. Given that there is little evidence of even a short-term benefit with off-pump CABG and none that lasts through the first year after surgery, Dr. S. recommends that Mr. P. also take into account the fact that although some local surgeons do perform off-pump CABG, the surgical teams are generally, like himself, more experienced with the on-pump technique. Mr. P. considers all the information

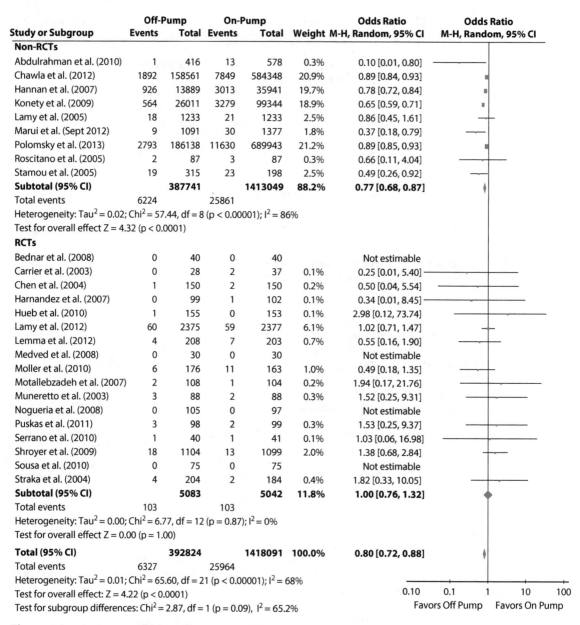

Figure 14-5. Systematic review example: Forest plot summarizing meta-analysis results for short-term mortality (operative or in-hospital). CI, confidence interval; M-H, Mantel-Haenszel; RCT, randomized controlled trial.

provided to him and decides that, in light of the evidence and the local practice experience, on-pump CABG is the best option for him.

SUMMARY

In this chapter, we looked at the process and methods involved in conducting a quantitative systematic review of the published literature using the example of comparing mortality rates after off-pump versus on-pump CABG.

Before starting a quantitative systematic review, it is critical to develop a meta-analysis protocol, specifying the systematic search that will be conducted, the I/E criteria that will be applied, how the data will be abstracted from included studies, how the risk of bias will be assessed, and how the data will be analyzed (fixed-effect vs. random-effect model) and presented.

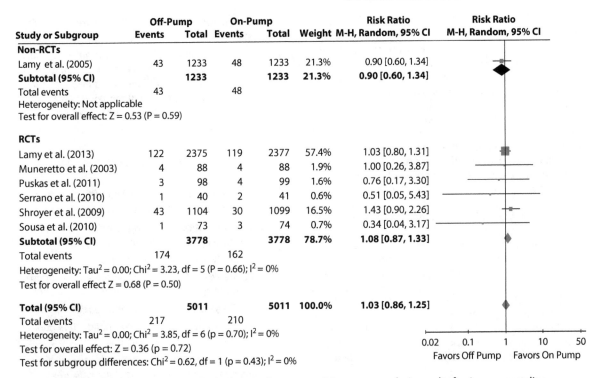

Study or Subgroup	Off-Pump Events	Total	On-Pump Events	Total	Weight	Risk Ratio M-H, Random, 95% CI	Risk Ratio M-H, Random, 95% CI
Non-RCTs							
Lamy et al. (2005)	43	1233	48	1233	21.3%	0.90 [0.60, 1.34]	
Subtotal (95% CI)		**1233**		**1233**	**21.3%**	**0.90 [0.60, 1.34]**	
Total events	43		48				
Heterogeneity: Not applicable							
Test for overall effect: Z = 0.53 (P = 0.59)							
RCTs							
Lamy et al. (2013)	122	2375	119	2377	57.4%	1.03 [0.80, 1.31]	
Muneretto et al. (2003)	4	88	4	88	1.9%	1.00 [0.26, 3.87]	
Puskas et al. (2011)	3	98	4	99	1.6%	0.76 [0.17, 3.30]	
Serrano et al. (2010)	1	40	2	41	0.6%	0.51 [0.05, 5.43]	
Shroyer et al. (2009)	43	1104	30	1099	16.5%	1.43 [0.90, 2.26]	
Sousa et al. (2010)	1	73	3	74	0.7%	0.34 [0.04, 3.17]	
Subtotal (95% CI)		**3778**		**3778**	**78.7%**	**1.08 [0.87, 1.33]**	
Total events	174		162				
Heterogeneity: Tau² = 0.00; Chi² = 3.23, df = 5 (P = 0.66); I² = 0%							
Test for overall effect Z = 0.68 (P = 0.50)							
Total (95% CI)		**5011**		**5011**	**100.0%**	**1.03 [0.86, 1.25]**	
Total events	217		210				
Heterogeneity: Tau² = 0.00; Chi² = 3.85, df = 6 (p = 0.70); I² = 0%							
Test for overall effect: Z = 0.36 (p = 0.72)							
Test for subgroup differences: Chi² = 0.62, df = 1 (p = 0.43); I² = 0%							

Figure 14-6. Systematic review example: Forest plot summarizing meta-analysis results for 1-year mortality. CI, confidence interval; RCT, randomized controlled trial.

The systematic search must identify the relevant studies to include. PubMed is an excellent—and free—tool for such work, and it is worth taking the time to learn how to effectively use MeSH terms to search efficiently. It is also worth seeking the help of a medical librarian in designing the search! A step that should not be skipped in any systematic review is reviewing the reference lists of previous reviews and recent large studies addressing the topic to be sure there are no additional relevant articles that the search missed.

The second vital step in a rigorous systematic review is the prespecification of clearly defined I/E criteria for the articles that will be considered for inclusion. If possible, at least two people should independently review the candidate articles for I/E, their results compared, and discrepancies resolved to ensure that these criteria are applied accurately and consistently.

After the final set of included articles has been determined, abstraction of the study data and assessment of the risks of bias can begin. A standardized data collection form should be developed and used, and, again, two people should independently abstract and review each article to increase reliability through the identification and resolution of discrepancies. After resolution, the data can be entered into

meta-analysis software such as RevMan 5.2 for easy data management and analysis.

The assessment of bias is essential because the internal validity of a meta-analysis depends on the validity of its included studies. In addition to biases the included studies may carry, the possibility of publication bias—in which studies reporting nonsignificant results are less likely to be published—needs to be considered and assessed via a funnel plot. Whereas a symmetrical funnel indicates low risk of publication bias, an asymmetrical funnel suggests it may be present.

Heterogeneity of the results between included studies needs to be considered as it determines, first, whether a meta-analysis (summarizing results into a single point estimate) is appropriate, and, second, if it is, the type of statistical model needed to summarize the results. When the magnitude **and** direction of the effect size vary between studies **and** the heterogeneity test is significant, a meta-analysis **should not** be performed, and the summary of the evidence should be qualitative. When the intervention effects have the **same direction** but their magnitudes vary between studies and the heterogeneity test is significant, a random-effect model is needed. When no significant heterogeneity is present, a fixed-effect model should be used. Because rigorous methodology requires the type of model to be specified **before** any analysis is done, formal tests for heterogeneity are typically done after the analysis is complete to confirm that the right model was chosen.

Results from the chosen model are typically best presented in a Forest plot, which combines a graphic and tabular display of the individual included studies' intervention effect sizes, as well as the summary result and information about heterogeneity and differences between any subgroups that were broken out.

Quantitative systematic reviews of the evidence are immensely valuable to the practice of evidence-based medicine. When a large volume of published studies with contradictory or inconsistent results has developed for a particular topic, quantitative systematic reviews can distil those findings down to a meaningful, synthesized result. Such summaries of the evidence can support the development (or updating) of evidence-based clinical practice guidelines or be applied directly by clinicians to treatment recommendations and by both clinicians and patients during shared decision making. Systematic reviews are also valuable in demonstrating when evidence—or, at least, good-quality evidence—is lacking and further research is needed before any conclusions about a "best practice" can be drawn.

 STUDY QUESTIONS

1. Is it appropriate to summarize available evidence when study designs, populations, treatments or interventions, exposures, and outcomes of the studies included in the systematic review are not similar?
   A. No
   B. Yes, if the heterogeneity test is not significant
   C. Yes, independently of the heterogeneity test is not significant
   D. It depends on the number of studies considered in the meta-analysis

2. What should be considered in determining the search strategy for a meta-analysis?
   A. The time that it will take to read the manuscripts identified from the search
   B. The study hypothesis and number of possible studies that the search will return
   C. The study hypothesis, research questions, and the database in which the search is to be conducted
   D. The research questions and the number of possible studies that the search will return

3. Can a meta-analysis be limited to non-RCTs studies only?
   A. Yes, if published non-RCTs have similar methods, sound findings and report adjusted results, and all published RCTs evidence suffer from evident methodologic problems or their study designs and method vary significantly
   B. No
   C. It depends on the number of studies included in the meta-analysis
   D. Yes, independently of the non-RCTs' methods and whether RCT evidence is available

4. Why it is critical to assess the risk of bias of the evidence considered in a meta-analysis?
   A. Study analysis will be easier
   B. Studies suffering from bias are difficult to understand
   C. The sensitivity analysis will be easier
   D. To ensure that the meta-analysis has good internal and external validity

5. Dr. F. is executing a meta-analysis, and he is uncertain on whether he can use a fixed-effect model to estimate the overall effect. In which of the following scenarios is it appropriate to use a fixed-effect model?
   A. The intervention effect is similar (in both magnitude and direction) across studies, but the study designs and methods are very different
   B. The intervention effect is similar (in both magnitude and direction) across studies, and the study designs and methods are very similar
   C. The heterogeneity test result is significant
   D. All estimates from the studies included in the meta-analysis were computed using fixed-effect models

6. Dr. B. is executing a sensitivity analysis to confirm her meta-analysis findings. Which of the following scenarios is appropriate?
   A. Remove all the studies with significant estimates and rerun the primary analysis
   B. Remove all the studies with nonsignificant estimates and rerun the primary analysis
   C. Add all the studies removed due to differences in how they assessed the study outcome and rerun the primary analysis
   D. Add all the studies removed because they focused on particular patient populations and rerun the primary analysis

7. Dr. B. has been asked to comment on the outcome he investigated in his meta-analysis; the overall effect odds ratio (95% CI) was 0.80 (0.72, 0.88). Which type of outcome did Dr. B. consider in his analysis?

A. Ordinal

B. Rate

C. Continuous

D. Binary

FURTHER READING

Higgins JPT, Green S, eds. *Cochrane Handbook for Systematic Reviews of Interventions* Version 5.1.0 [updated March 2011]. The Cochrane Collaboration. Published 2011. http://www.cochrane-handbook.org.

Ioannidis JP, Patsopoulos, Evangelou E. Uncertainty in heterogeneity estimates in meta-analyses. *BMJ.* 2007;335:914-916.

Moher D, Liberati A, Tetzlaff J, Altman DG; The PRISMA Group. Preferred reporting items for systematic reviews and meta-analyses: the PRISMA statement. *Ann Intern Med.* 2009;151(4):264-269.

Moher D, Liberati A, Tetzlaff J, Altman DG; The PRISMA Group. Preferred reporting items for systematic reviews and meta-analyses: the PRISMA statement. *PLoS Med.* 2009;6(6):e1000097.

Thompson SG, Higgins JP. How should meta-regression analyses be undertaken and interpreted? *Stat Med.* 2002;21:1559-1573.

REFERENCES

Clinical Background

Afilalo J, Rasti M, Ohayon SM, Shimony A, Eisenberg MJ. Off-pump vs. on-pump coronary artery bypass surgery: an updated meta-analysis and meta-regression of randomized trials. *Eur Heart J.* 2012;33(10):1257-1267.

Athanasiou T, Saso S, Rao C, et al. Radial artery versus saphenous vein conduits for coronary artery bypass surgery: forty years of competition—which conduit offers better patency? A systematic review and meta-analysis. *Eur J Cardiothorac Surg.* 2011;40(1):208-220.

Hattler B, Messenger JC, Shroyer AL, et al. Off-pump coronary artery bypass surgery is associated with worse arterial and saphenous vein graft patency and less effective revascularization: results from the Veterans Affairs Randomized On/Off Bypass (ROOBY) trial. *Circulation.* 2012;125(23):2827-2835.

Hijazi EM. Is it time to adopt beating-heart coronary artery bypass grafting? A review of literature. *Rev Bras Cir Cardiovasc.* 2010;25(3):393-402.

Huffmyer J, Raphael J. The current status of off-pump coronary bypass surgery. *Curr Opin Anaesthesiol.* 2011;24(1):64-69.

Patel NN, Angelini GD. Off-pump coronary artery bypass grafting: for the many or the few? *J Thorac Cardiovasc Surg.* 2010;140(5):951-953.

Polomsky M, He X, O'Brien SM, Puskas JD. Outcomes of off-pump versus on-pump coronary artery bypass grafting:

impact of preoperative risk. *J Thorac Cardiovasc Surg.* 2013; 145(5):1193-1198.

Society of Thoracic Surgeons. Adult Cardiac Surgery Database: Executive Summary 10 Years (STS Period Ending December 31, 2012). Published 2013. http://www.sts.org/sites/default/files/documents/1stHarvestExecutiveSummary.pdf. Accessed October 3, 2013.

Taggart DP, Altman DG. Off-pump vs. on-pump CABG: are we any closer to a resolution? *Eur Heart J.* 2012;33(10):1181-1183.

Definition of a Systematic Review

Cochrane AL. Archie Cochrane in his own words. Selections arranged from his 1972 introduction to "Effectiveness and Efficiency: Random Reflections on the Health Services" 1972. *Control Clin Trials.* 1989;10(4):428-433.

Performing a Quantitative Systematic Review: Meta-Analysis

Harrell FE Jr. *Regression Modeling Strategies: With Application to Linear Models, Logistic Regression, and Survival Analysis.* New York: Springer-Verlag; 2001.

Higgins JP, Altman DG, Gotzsche PC, et al. The Cochrane Collaboration's tool for assessing risk of bias in randomised trials. *BMJ.* 2011;343:d5928.

Higgins JPT, Green S, eds. *Cochrane Handbook for Systematic Reviews of Interventions* Version 5.1.0 [updated March 2011]. The Cochrane Collaboration. Published 2011. http://www.cochrane-handbook.org.

Review Manager (RevMan) [Computer program]. *Version 5.3.* Copenhagen: The Nordic Cochrane Centre, The Cochrane Collaboration; 2012.

U.S. National Library of Medicine. PubMed.gov. http://www.ncbi.nlm.nih.gov/pubmed. Accessed August 1, 2014.

Studies Included in the Example Off-Pump vs On-Pump CABG Meta-Analysis

Abdulrahman RI, Parvizi R. Outcome of coronary artery bypass grafts: comparison between on pump and off pump. *Acta Med Iran.* 2010;48(3):158-163.

Bednar F, Osmancik P, Vanek T, et al. Platelet activity and aspirin efficacy after off-pump compared with on-pump coronary artery bypass surgery: results from the prospective randomized trial PRAGUE 11-Coronary Artery Bypass and REactivity of Thrombocytes (CABARET). *J Thorac Cardiovasc Surg.* 2008;136(4):1054-1060.

Carrier M, Perrault LP, Jeanmart H, Martineau R, Cartier R, Page P. Randomized trial comparing off-pump to on-pump coronary artery bypass grafting in high-risk patients. *Heart Surg Forum.* 2003;6(6):E89-E92.

Chawla LS, Zhao Y, Lough FC, Schroeder E, Seneff MG, Brennan JM. Off-pump versus on-pump coronary artery bypass grafting outcomes stratified by preoperative renal function. *J Am Soc Nephrol.* 2012;23(8):1389-1397.

Chen X, Xu M, Shi HW, Mu XW, Chen ZQ, Qiu ZB. Comparative study of on-pump and off-pump coronary bypass surgery in patients with triple-vessel coronary artery disease. *Chin Med J (Engl).* 2004;117(3):342-346.

Hannan EL, Wu C, Smith CR, et al. Off-pump versus on-pump coronary artery bypass graft surgery: differences in short-term outcomes and in long-term mortality and need for subsequent revascularization. *Circulation.* 2007;116(10):1145-1152.

Hernandez F Jr, Brown JR, Likosky DS, et al. Neurocognitive outcomes of off-pump versus on-pump coronary artery bypass: a prospective randomized controlled trial. *Ann Thorac Surg.* 2007;84(6):1897-1903.

Hueb W, Lopes NH, Pereira AC, et al. Five-year follow-up of a randomized comparison between off-pump and on-pump stable multivessel coronary artery bypass grafting. *Circulation.* 2010;122(11 Suppl):S48-52.

Konety SH, Rosenthal GE, Vaughan-Sarrazin MS. Surgical volume and outcomes of off-pump coronary artery bypass graft surgery: does it matter? *J Thorac Cardiovasc Surg.* 2009;137(5):1116-1123 e1111.

Lamy A, Devereaux PJ, Prabhakaran D, et al. Effects of off-pump and on-pump coronary-artery bypass grafting at 1 year. *N Engl J Med.* 2013;368(13):1179-1188.

Lamy A, Devereaux PJ, Prabhakaran D, et al. Off-pump or on-pump coronary-artery bypass grafting at 30 days. *N Engl J Med.* 2012;366(16):1489-1497.

Lamy A, Farrokhyar F, Kent R, et al. The Canadian off-pump coronary artery bypass graft registry: a one-year prospective comparison with on-pump coronary artery bypass grafting. *Can J Cardiol.* 2005;21(13):1175-1181.

Lemma MG, Coscioni E, Tritto FP, et al. On-pump versus off-pump coronary artery bypass surgery in high-risk patients: operative results of a prospective randomized trial (on-off study). *J Thorac Cardiovasc Surg.* 2012;143(3):625-631.

Marui A, Okabayashi H, Komiya T, et al. Benefits of off-pump coronary artery bypass grafting in high-risk patients. *Circulation.* 2012;126(11 suppl 1):S151-S157.

Medved I, Anic D, Zrnic B, Ostric M, Saftic I. Off-pump versus on-pump—intermittent aortic cross clamping—myocardial revascularisation: single center experience. *Coll Antropol.* 2008;32(2):381-384.

Møller CH, Perko MJ, Lund JT, et al. No major differences in 30-day outcomes in high-risk patients randomized to off-pump versus on-pump coronary bypass surgery: the best bypass surgery trial. *Circulation.* 2010;121(4):498-504.

Motallebzadeh R, Bland JM, Markus HS, Kaski JC, Jahangiri M. Neurocognitive function and cerebral emboli: randomized study

of on-pump versus off-pump coronary artery bypass surgery. *Ann Thorac Surg.* 2007;83(2):475-482.

Muneretto C, Bisleri G, Negri A, et al. Off-pump coronary artery bypass surgery technique for total arterial myocardial revascularization: a prospective randomized study. *Ann Thorac Surg.* 2003;76(3):778-782.

Nogueira CR, Hueb W, Takiuti ME, et al. Quality of life after on-pump and off-pump coronary artery bypass grafting surgery. *Arq Bras Cardiol.* 2008;91(4):217-222, 238-244.

Polomsky M, He X, O'Brien SM, Puskas JD. Outcomes of off-pump versus on-pump coronary artery bypass grafting: impact of preoperative risk. *J Thorac Cardiovasc Surg.* 2013;145(5):1193-1198.

Puskas JD, Williams WH, O'Donnell R, et al. Off-pump and on-pump coronary artery bypass grafting are associated with similar graft patency, myocardial ischemia, and freedom from reintervention: long-term follow-up of a randomized trial. *Ann Thorac Surg.* 2011;91(6):1836-1842; discussion 1842-1833.

Roscitano A, Benedetto U, Capuano F, et al. Off-pump versus on-pump coronary artery bypass: does number of grafts performed represent a selection bias in comparative studies? Results from a matched cohort comparison. *Ital Heart J.* 2005;6(9):740-744.

Serrano CV Jr, Souza JA, Lopes NH, et al. Reduced expression of systemic proinflammatory and myocardial biomarkers after off-pump versus on-pump coronary artery bypass surgery: a prospective randomized study. *J Crit Care.* 2010;25(2):305-312.

Shroyer AL, Grover FL, Hattler B, et al. On-pump versus off-pump coronary-artery bypass surgery. *N Engl J Med.* 2009;361(19):1827-1837.

Sousa Uva M, Cavaco S, Oliveira AG, et al. Early graft patency after off-pump and on-pump coronary bypass surgery: a prospective randomized study. *Eur Heart J.* 2010;31(20):2492-2499.

Stamou SC, Jablonski KA, Hill PC, Bafi AS, Boyce SW, Corso PJ. Coronary revascularization without cardiopulmonary bypass versus the conventional approach in high-risk patients. *Ann Thorac Surg.* 2005;79(2):552-557.

Straka Z, Widimsky P, Jirasek K, et al. Off-pump versus on-pump coronary surgery: final results from a prospective randomized study PRAGUE-4. *Ann Thorac Surg.* 2004;77(3):789-793.

SECTION IV

Translating Evidence into Medical Practice

Quality of Care

David J. Ballard, Briget da Graca, and David Nicewander

HEALTH SCENARIO

Mrs. E., a 69-year-old, Spanish-only-speaking Hispanic woman with a history of congestive heart failure (CHF), is admitted to Hospital A complaining of shortness of breath and difficulty breathing when lying down. During her stay, she is not evaluated for left ventricular systolic dysfunction (LVSD); as a result, she does not receive a prescription for an angiotensin-converting enzyme inhibitor (ACEI) or angiotensin receptor blocker (ARB) for LVSD despite having no contraindications. She receives postdischarge instructions verbally and in writing but only in English because Hospital A does not have onsite translators or a translation service. Two days after discharge, she is readmitted through the emergency department (ED) with an ejection fraction of 15% and severe pulmonary edema. Despite treatment, she dies.

Hospital A starts looking closely at its delivery of heart failure care when it receives the maximum 1% reimbursement penalty under the Medicare Readmissions Reduction program based on higher-than-expected 30-day readmission rates in the Medicare patients it treats for heart failure, pneumonia, and acute myocardial infarction (AMI) and a 1.1% penalty under Medicare's Hospital Value-Based Purchasing Program based on its below average compliance with publicly reported, evidence-based practices in heart failure, pneumonia, AMI, and surgical care and on patients' experience of care in fiscal year 2013. Hospital A finds that there are significant

opportunities for improvement, and it seeks to address these issues to improve its patients' experience and outcomes, and to avoid further financial penalties.

CLINICAL BACKGROUND

More than 5 million adults in the United States have heart failure, and more than 500,000 new cases are diagnosed each year. Approximately 275,000 deaths and more than 1 million hospitalizations are attributable to heart failure annually in the United States; it is the most common discharge diagnosis in persons older than 65 years, and nearly 25% of patients require rehospitalization within 30 days. The total cost of care for heart failure in 2013 was estimated at $32 billion; this number is expected to rise to $72 billion by 2020.

Clinical practice guidelines strongly recommend the evidence-based practices of left ventricular function assessment, ACEI and ARB prescription for left ventricular systolic dysfunction, smoking cessation counseling, and discharge instructions as part of standard care for heart failure, yet they remain underutilized: fewer than 60% of heart failure patients receive all recommended evidence-based diagnostic and therapeutic measures for which they are eligible.

The high prevalence and incidence of heart failure, together with its high burdens of mortality and morbidity and the availability of easily measurable, evidence-based treatments that reduce these burdens, makes it a high-priority target for quality improvement. It is one of the four conditions and categories for which Medicare has required hospitals to publicly report compliance with certain evidence-based recommendations since 2005 and performance on 30-day readmission and mortality rates since 2009. Most recently, Medicare has linked hospital reimbursement to these performance measures through its Readmissions Reduction Program and its Hospital Value-Based Purchasing (VBP) Program. Heart failure care also is a focus of the National Quality Strategy, falling within the priority of "promoting the most effective prevention and treatment practices for the leading causes of mortality, starting with cardiovascular disease."

EPIDEMIOLOGY AND QUALITY OF CARE

Although the public tends to associate "epidemiology" with investigations of dramatic outbreaks of contagious diseases, its principles have many more applications vital to day-to-day health care delivery. Prime among these are the measurement and improvement of health care quality. In such applications of epidemiology, we adjust the classic study of disease etiology (examining the possible relationship between a suspected cause and an adverse health effect) to focus on the provision of care as the independent or exposure variable and the reduction in adverse health effects as the dependent or outcome variable, taking into account environmental and other factors that may influence that relationship (**Table 15-1**).

WHAT IS "QUALITY OF CARE?"

"Quality of care" is a phrase that has become ubiquitous in the United States' health care system in the time that has passed since the landmark year of 1998, when reports detailing serious quality-of-care concerns were released by the Institute of Medicine (IOM), the Advisory Commission on Consumer Protection and Quality in the Health Care Industry, and the RAND Corporation. The revelations these reports contained about the harms suffered through overutilization of some health care services, the underutilization of others, errors of commission and omission, and inequitable access to needed health care resources placed a national spotlight on "quality of care." But what is "quality of care?" And how do we know when high-quality care has been provided? How can we tell which hospitals or physicians are the "best?" There are no easy answers to these questions, and "quality" will always remain somewhat subjective. However, significant strides have been made toward consensus on what "quality of care" should encompass and on essential attributes of measures used to document and compare it.

In the words of Robert Pirsig in *Zen and the Art of Motorcycle Maintenance*, "...even though Quality cannot be defined, *you know what Quality is!*" and it has been demonstrated and accepted that many aspects of quality of care are subject to measurement. Such measurement depends, however, on the perspective from which quality is examined and on the nature and extent of the care being examined.

Table 15-1. Objectives of epidemiology as applied to classic studies and to the measurement and improvement of quality of care.

	Classic Epidemiologic Study	Application of Epidemiologic Principles to Quality of Care
Objectives of Epidemiology	1. Identify the etiology or cause of a disease and the factors that increase a person's risks for the disease.	1. Identify the causes of poor quality care and the factors that increase a patient's risk for experiencing poor quality or a provider's risk of providing poor quality.
	2. Determine the extent of disease found in the community.	2. Determine the extent of poor quality care within an organization or community.
	3. Study the natural history and prognosis of disease.	3. Study the short- and long-term consequences of poor quality care for the patient and the community.
	4. Evaluate existing and new preventive and therapeutic measures and modes of health care delivery.	4. Evaluate existing and new strategies to improve quality of care and modes of health care delivery.
	5. Provide the foundation for developing public policy and regulatory decisions relating to environmental problems	5. Provide the foundation for developing public policy and regulatory decisions relating to quality of care standards

For example, patients choosing a health care provider or plan tend to view quality in terms of access, cost, choice of providers, the time the physician spends with them, and the physician's qualifications. In contrast, physicians are likely to view quality of care in terms of the specific services they provide to the patients they treat—the benefits gained and the harms caused. Most definitions of quality of care do, however, agree on two essential components:

1. *High technical quality of care*, meaning, broadly, the provision of care for which the benefits outweigh the risks by a sufficient margin to make the risks worthwhile; and

2. *Art of care*, which refers to patients' perception that they were treated in a humane and culturally appropriate manner and were invited to participate fully in their health decisions

Probably the most widely accepted definition of quality in the United States is the framework outlined in the IOM's 2001 report *Crossing the Quality Chasm*, which states that "[h]ealth care should be:

- Safe: Avoiding injuries to patients from the care that is intended to help them
- Effective: Providing services based on scientific knowledge to all who could benefit and refraining from providing services to those not likely to benefit (avoiding underuse and overuse, respectively)
- Patient centered: Providing care that is respectful and responsive to individual patient preferences, needs, and values and ensuring that patient values guide all clinical decisions
- Timely: Reducing waits and sometimes harmful delays for both those who receive and those who give care
- Efficient: Avoiding waste, including waste of time, money, equipment, supplies, ideas, and energy
- Equitable: Providing care that does not vary in quality because of personal characteristics such as gender, race, ethnicity, geographic location, and socioeconomic status"

Internationally, the World Health Organization uses a definition based on six similar dimensions but with language that more explicitly invokes both population health and individual patient care. This "population health" aspect has been added to the United States' definition through the Triple Aim for health care improvement, which has been adopted by the Department of Health and Human Services (DHHS) in the National Quality Strategy to achieve:

1. Better care: improve the overall quality by making health care more patient-centered, reliable, accessible, and safe.

2. Healthy people and healthy communities: Improve the health of the U.S. population by supporting proven interventions to address behavioral, social, and environmental determinants of health in addition to delivering higher quality care.

3. Affordable care: Reduce the cost of quality health care for individuals, families, employers, and government.

MEASURING HEALTH CARE QUALITY

Background

For most of the 20th century, there was a widespread belief that the individual training and skills of physicians were the most important determinants of health care quality.[18] As a result, policies related to ensuring high-quality care tended to focus on standards for medical education and continuing education for practicing physicians. Routine measurement and reporting of quality indicators started gaining prominence toward the end of the 20th century as competition in the health care marketplace increased (particularly in the form of managed care structures that use financial incentives to influence physician and patient behavior); geographic variation in use of medical services was documented, raising questions regarding appropriate use; clinical and administrative databases were developed; and computing capability increased.

Public reporting of quality measures in the United States began "accidentally" in 1987 when the predecessor of today's Centers for Medicare and Medicaid Services (CMS) produced a report of hospital-level mortality statistics. This report, which used only crude risk adjustment, was intended for internal use only but was obtained by members of the press under the Freedom of Information Act and widely released. Although this undoubtedly caused short-term furor, long-term benefits were realized in the form of demand for more fairly adjusted, quantitative quality reports in both the public and private sectors, which led to a proliferation of quality report cards for hospitals and health plans at national, state, and local levels. But even while applauding this increased transparency regarding quality of care, one must keep in mind not only the weaknesses of quality report cards in general (e.g., that they can capture only a few aspects of care and are hard to adjust for underlying differences in patient populations) but also that they are not all created equal. It is important to look closely at the kinds of measures used, the data sources from which these measures were collected, and the extent to which relevant differences in patient populations have been accounted for.

Structure, Process, and Outcome Measures

The dominant framework for quality of care evaluations is the "structure, process, and outcome" model developed by Avedis Donabedian in the 1960s. This model recognizes the fundamental interrelationships among these aspects of care: the necessary structures must be in place to facilitate delivery of the appropriate processes of care, which in turn achieve or increase the probability of the desired outcomes.

Donabedian defines *structure* as the relatively stable characteristics of providers of care, the tools and resources at their disposal, and the physical and organizational settings in which care is provided. As such, it encompasses factors such as the number, distribution, and qualifications of professionals; the number, size, equipment, and geographic distribution of hospitals and other care facilities; staff organization; internal structures for the review of clinical work; and the reimbursement strategies through which providers are paid. Structure measures are typically the easiest to collect data on—personnel and equipment, for example, can be counted in a straightforward manner—making it unsurprising that these are the initial foci of many quality evaluation programs. However, structure measures can indicate only general tendencies toward good- or poor-quality care. Meaningful evaluations of quality need to include measures more directly related to the care actually provided—in other words process or outcomes of care.

A *process* is an activity occurring within or between practitioners and patients, as determined through either direct observation or review of recorded data. The basis for using process measures to evaluate the quality of care provided is the scientific evidence of the relationship between the process and the consequences to the health or welfare of individuals or the community, taking into account the value placed on health or wellness by the individual or community in question. To use the terminology that has entered the health care lexicon in recent decades, process measures look at the practice of evidence-based medicine, or "the integration of best research evidence with clinical expertise and patient values." The strengths of process measures include the ability to specify criteria for and standards of good-quality care to establish the range of acceptable practice, the incentive they provide to document the care delivered, and the ability to attribute discrete clinical decisions to the relevant providers. They also are easy to interpret and sensitive to variations in care and provide a clear indication of what remedial action is needed in the case of poor performance. Weaknesses include the fact that they do not consider how well a process was carried out, only if it was performed or not, and may even give credit for wrongly delivered

processes, such as the wrong dosage of a recommended drug or use in patients at high risk for adverse reactions. Furthermore, their emphasis on technical interventions may encourage high cost care, and the priority they place on a narrow aspect of care may lead to loss of quality in other areas.

Outcome measures reflect changes in the patient's current or future health status (including psychosocial functioning and patient attitudes and behavior) that can be attributed to the antecedent care provided. In many ways, outcome measures provide the best evaluation of the quality of care as they capture the goals of the care being provided, and they reflect all aspects of the care provided. This may be particularly important when multiple providers and their teamwork, culture, and leadership, as well the patients themselves contribute to the care. However, the duration, timing, or extent of measurement of outcomes that indicate good-quality care can be hard to specify, and data can be difficult and expensive to obtain. Furthermore, outcomes can be substantially affected by factors outside the control of the provider who is being evaluated (e.g., patient characteristics), so that careful risk adjustment—typically requiring detailed clinical data and development of risk models by statisticians and epidemiologists—is required to avoid penalizing providers who treat higher risk patients. Currently, there is no standardized approach for risk adjusting outcome measures, and varying approaches may result in substantial differences in the measured performance. Furthermore, even after risk adjustment, outcome measures may be unstable over time and unable to provide reliable comparisons for small-volume providers or where the outcome of interest is a rare event. For example, in the 1990s, the Veterans Affairs (VA) cardiac surgery program implemented semiannual internal reports to identify hospitals with high or low risk-adjusted operative mortality rates among patients undergoing coronary artery bypass grafting (CABG); however, to detect a risk-adjusted mortality rate twice the VA average with 80% statistical power and at a significance level of 5%, a minimum 6-month hospital volume of 185 CABG surgeries was required—a volume reached by only one VA hospital, once, in 5.5 years.

As should be clear from these relative strengths and weaknesses of structure, process, and outcomes measures, they have varying degrees of usefulness according to the purpose of the quality evaluation. This question must be answered before any attempt at evaluation is initiated to ensure the correct sort of measure or mix thereof—is selected. Generally, the broader the perspective of the evaluation, the more relevant outcome measures are, since they reflect the inter-play of a wide variety of influential factors. For narrower perspectives—for example, care provided by an individual physician—process measures may prove more useful because they are less subject to causes of variation outside the provider's control. Structure measures can be very useful when one of the goals of the evaluation is to elucidate possible reasons for variations in quality between countries, regions, or providers because they provide insight into the resources available to providers and patients and the incentives to give and seek out certain kinds of care.

ATTRIBUTES OF QUALITY MEASURES

Measure Development

There is no formal consensus on how health care quality measures should be developed, although there are general consistencies among the methods applied. The first step in measure development is evaluating the need for quality indicators or measures based on the perspectives of all relevant stakeholders (e.g., patients, physicians, hospital leaders, payers, and policymakers). After this, the need for measure development should be prioritized according to (1) the incidence or prevalence of the condition and the health burden on the individual; (2) evidence, in the form of variable or substandard care, of an opportunity for quality improvement; (3) evidence that quality improvement will improve patient outcomes or population health; and (4) evidence that relevant quality measures do not already exist or are inadequate. Other relevant factors include the significance of resources consumed by and the cost effectiveness of treatments and procedures, variations in use, and controversies around use.

After an area has been identified as a measure development priority, key steps include:

1. Specifying a clear goal for the measurement
2. Using methodologies to incorporate research evidence, clinical expertise, and patient perspectives
3. Considering the contextual factors and logistics of implementing measurement

Included within these steps might be such requirements as that the quality measure be based on established clinical practice guidelines or that it undergo pilot testing to ensure that data collection and analysis are feasible and that the reporting meets the needs of the specified goal.

Broadly speaking, there are two approaches through which these steps are applied to the development of measures: the deductive approach (going from concept to data) and the inductive approach (going from data to concept). The former is more frequently used, with quality indicators or measures being based on recognized quality of care concepts and derived directly from existing scientific evidence or expert opinion. Although this deductive approach can help identify gaps in existing measurement systems, it can be limited by the lack of existing data sources through which the measure can be implemented and may focus efforts on quality of care issues that, although conceptually important, are not the ones most in need of improvement.

The less commonly used inductive approach starts with identifying existing data sources, evaluating their data elements, and then querying the data to identify variations from which quality indicators and measures can be developed. Strengths of this approach include the use of existing data and the ability to look at local variation to identify priorities and feasibilities, which may make providers more willing to accept measures to explore and track that variation. A third option is to combine the deductive and inductive approaches, as advocated by the Agency for Healthcare Research and Quality (AHRQ); this enables both the current scientific evidence and the availability and variability of existing data to be taken into account during the development process, supported by the engagement of relevant stakeholders and end users to ensure the measures developed are both relevant and meaningful.

In the United States, measures developed by the National Quality Forum (NQF) are considered the gold standard for health care quality measurement, based on the rigorous, consensus-based process through which they are developed. The NQF is a nonprofit organization with members drawn from patients, health plans, health professionals, health care provider organizations, public health agencies, medical suppliers/industry, purchasers, and those involved in quality measurement, research, and improvement, focused on the evaluation and endorsement of standardized performance measurement. The measure development process is designed to obtain input from and to consider the interests of all these stakeholders, as well as the scientific evidence supporting the rationale for the proposed quality measure.

Evaluation of Quality Measures

Essential Attributes of Quality Measures

At the most basic level, quality measures need to be:

- Important—the target audience(s) will find the information useful
- Scientifically sound—the measure will produce consistent and credible results
- Feasible—the measure can be implemented in the relevant health care context
- Usable—the target audience(s) can understand the results and apply them to decision-making processes

Whether one is involved in the measure development process, seeking relevant measures for quality reporting and improvement purposes, or interpreting reported performance on a quality measure, it is important to assess the essential attributes of the measure. These should be familiar from those discussed for variables used in the classical disease etiology applications of epidemiologic methods:

- *Reliability:* In the context of quality measurement, reliability can refer either to consistency of performance scores in repeated measurements or stability of performance scores over time. Reliability can be assessed in multiple ways: providers (whether they are individual physicians, or hospitals) can be classified according to their performance on the measure (or measure set) and the distribution of providers compared across measurement periods. Or, taking the providers individually, the correlation between successive measurement periods on a particular measure and the overall proportion of measures satisfied can be examined. Reliability can be affected by both variation in the provider's characteristics over time (e.g., seasonal variation in volume of patients admitted for a particular condition) and interobserver variation, whereby individuals collecting data relevant to the measure interpret identical data differently. These sources of variation need to be considered and accounted for in defining the measure and the data collection and reporting processes used to implement it.

- *Validity:* Three types of validity can be defined. First, *criterion validity* refers to how well the quality measure agrees with a reference standard measurement. When reference standard data can reasonably be obtained, this can be assessed by examining the agreement between the quality measure data and the reference standard data in terms of sensitivity and specificity and by calculating receiver operating characteristic (ROC) curves. For example, for quality measures based on hospital administrative data, patient charts could be reviewed for a subset of patients to obtain "reference standard" data for comparison. Another aspect of validity that is important for quality measures is *construct validity*, which refers to how well the measure represents the aspect of quality it is intended to target and relates to the strength of the evidence linking the two. For example, a hospital's incidence rate of central line–associated infections has good construct validity as a measure of patient safety because there is strong evidence showing that the majority of these infections can be avoided if preventive actions are consistently applied in a timely manner. Finally, a quality measure needs *face validity*, which refers to the extent to which it is perceived to address the concept it purports to measure. This is important in quality measurement in getting the relevant providers to "buy

in" to the importance of improving performance on the measure to improve the care provided to their patients. Although face validity does, to a large degree, overlap with construct validity, it is not necessarily implied by it. Steps may have to be taken to educate providers on the evidence demonstrating construct validity to establish face validity or to show that the evidence applies in the local context within which they provide care.

- *Bias:* Bias is a systematic error in the design, conduct, or analysis of a study that leads to a mistaken estimate of an exposure's effect on the outcome of interest. There are multiple types and sources of bias that are relevant to quality measures that should be considered in developing, choosing, and interpreting performance measures:

  o *Selection bias* occurs when the cases with the condition or procedure of interest that can be identified from the data source do not represent the entire population of patients with that condition or procedure. As a result, the measured performance will not reflect the true rate at which the quality measure occurs in the relevant population. For example, if one were examining the quality of care provided to patients undergoing cholecystectomy and considered only inpatient data sources, the results would likely be subject to selection bias because hospitals admit all patients requiring open cholecystectomy but only some of those undergoing laparoscopic cholecystectomy (the less complex, lower risk cases are treated in outpatient settings). Quality measures may also be subject to selection bias when there is inadequate or variable coding of key diagnoses, interfering with consistent identification of relevant cases.

  o *Information bias* occurs when the means of obtaining information about the subjects is inadequate, causing some of the information gathered to be incorrect. Sources of information bias relevant to quality measure data collection include the way in which data are abstracted from medical records or in how interviewers or surveys pose questions; *surveillance bias* (in which providers actively looking for particular events, e.g., venous thromboembolism, have better detection procedures in place and thus appear to have higher rates than providers investing less effort in or with fewer resources available for detection programs); and, particularly relevant to survey-based measures, *recall bias* (in which, for example, an individual who has an adverse outcome is more likely to recall a potentially relevant exposure than an individual who did not have such an outcome) and *reporting bias* (in which an individual is reluctant to report an exposure or an outcome because of his or her beliefs, attitudes, or perceptions). Hospital quality measures that rely on hospital discharge data sets may suffer from information bias through their lack of data on postdischarge outcomes. For example, when looking at conditions in which the 30-day mortality rate (determined from death certificates) substantially exceeds the in-hospital mortality rate, hospitals with shorter lengths of stay may appear to perform better if only in-hospital mortality data are considered because the period of observation is shorter for them. Information bias also encompasses *misclassification bias*, through which individuals who are not members of the target population (e.g., because of a contraindication to the recommended process of care) are included in the measurement or, conversely, individuals who should be included in the measurement are classified as falling outside the target population.

o *Confounding bias* occurs when patient characteristics, such as disease severity, comorbidities, functional status, or access to care, substantially affect performance on a measure and vary systematically across providers or areas. For example, hospitals treating patients across large geographic areas (national referral centers) may show artificially low risk-adjusted mortality rates because of the confounding effect of illness severity factors associated with referral selection and mortality. This produces lower-than-expected mortality rates in the subgroup of patients referred to the hospital over a distance that biases the hospital's overall rate downward if the risk-adjustment model does not adequately capture this patient characteristic. To the extent that confounders can be identified from the data sources available, risk adjustment can improve performance of the quality measure.

• *Case-mix and risk adjustment:* Differences in case mix make direct performance comparisons among providers or over time challenging. Case-mix adjustment can be controversial and is complicated in terms of both the analysis and the implementation of data collection and reporting. However, when using outcome measures, risk adjustment for patient and environmental factors outside the provider's control (e.g., severity of illness or comorbidities, patient access to resources) are essential to fair performance comparisons. Furthermore, building clinically appropriate exceptions into specifications for both outcome and process measures (e.g., excluding patients admitted for comfort care only from an in-hospital mortality measure) is necessary both for the validity of the measures and for clinician acceptance of the measures.

• *Currency:* Health care delivery is dynamic, and measures of quality need to be relevant to the contemporary context. As such, measures cannot simply be developed and evaluated once and then implemented in perpetuity. Studies show that more than half of clinical practice guidelines are outdated within 6 years of adoption and that systematic reviews of clinical effectiveness evidence can require updating as frequently as every 2 years. Quality measures require updates to remain current with advances in medical technology and clinical practice and to replace measures that have "topped out" (i.e., almost all providers routinely achieve near optimal performance) with measures reflecting new priorities.

Finally, an attribute of any quality measure that must be considered is its potential for manipulation and the perverse incentives its use may inadvertently create to improve measured performance without improving the quality of care actually provided. This might include "cherry picking" easy cases, encompassing both the refusal to treat complex, high-risk patients who might nonetheless benefit and treating less severe patients with dubious indications to inflate volumes and improve apparent performance; "teaching to the test," whereby the narrow focus on the particular area of care being measured leads to the neglect of the broader aspects of quality; and "upcoding" of severity or comorbidities used in risk adjustment to create an overadjustment and favorably influence the findings.

Data Sources

The purpose underlying a specific instance of quality measurement and the approach adopted to achieve it frequently dictate the type of data that needs to be collected. Conversely, given the limited resources typically available for quality measurement and improvement, the data that can be obtained at a feasible cost and within a reasonable timeframe need to be considered. The potential information sources run a broad gamut of data collection methods, but certain common sources and methods recur frequently in quality measurement.

Clinical records: Patient medical records are the source of information for most studies of medical care processes, for disease- or procedure-specific registries, and for quality improvement or monitoring initiatives in both ambulatory and inpatient settings. In the sense that they should contain detailed information about the patient's clinical condition as well as about the clinical actions taken, they are an excellent source of data for assessing the quality of care provided. However, they also have several practical drawbacks. First, the time and effort required to perform chart abstraction of traditional paper records make this an expensive form of data collection, severely limiting the size of the sample of providers or patients whose care is evaluated and making real-time performance measurement unfeasible. Second, it assumes complete and accurate documentation of the patient's condition and the actions taken, an assumption that the research literature does not bear out. Third, when data collection requires interpretation of the clinical information (e.g., determining whether an adverse event has occurred), there can be substantial disagreement between reviewers (i.e., poor interrater reliability). Vague specification of variables and poorly designed abstraction tools can also compromise data quality.

The growing use of electronic health records (EHRs) sparked the hope—and perception—that clinical record-based quality of care data would become readily obtainable and of better quality. However, electronic quality measure reports show wide variation in accuracy because of processes of care being recorded in free text notes or scanned documents, where they are "invisible" to the automated reporting algorithm; different test results showing as "most recent" to the reporting algorithm versus a human reviewer; and poor capture of valid reasons for not providing recommended care. Between 15% and 81% of the "quality failures" identified in EHR-based reports satisfy the performance measures or exclusion criteria on manual review.

Another challenge to wide-scale use of EHR reporting is data incompatibility between sites and EHR systems because of differences in meaning and structure of data elements and the development of local glossaries for coded information; local documentation practices and data extraction methods also impact data quality and completeness, so one cannot assume comparability just because two sites use the same EHR product or belong to the same parent organization.

Direct observation: An alternative to clinical records is direct observation by a well-qualified observer. Although this preserves the benefit of providing detailed clinical information and avoids the reliance on the clinician's documentation of actions taken during a particular encounter, it adds to the expense and time required for data collection, does not solve the problem of data completeness with regard to information about the patient the clinician possesses from previous encounters, and introduces the additional complication of being likely to alter the clinician's behavior (the *Hawthorne* or *observer effect* in which study subjects alter their behavior because they know that they are being monitored.) Additionally, although direct observation may be a reasonable means of collecting data on process and structure measures, there are many outcome measures of interest in health care quality (e.g., 30-day postdischarge

readmission) that occur at unknown and unpredictable times and places and so will likely be missed.

Administrative data: Routine collection of data for insurance claims and enrollment make administrative databases readily available, inexpensive sources of quality measure data. This enables quality measurements to be done on large samples or even on all patients with the relevant condition treated by the provider during the measurement period and at more frequent intervals. Administrative data are frequently used for public reporting (e.g., CMS Hospital Compare measures for AMI, pneumonia, and heart failure) and value-based purchasing programs, for health care organizations' internal quality initiatives, and for studies evaluating the effectiveness of such initiatives. Because administrative databases and collection processes are designed primarily to support operations such as billing and reimbursement, however, they generally lack the clinical detail needed to determine whether a particular clinical action was necessary or appropriate; they may also be vulnerable to "upcoding" of the severity or complexity of a patient's illness or procedure when reimbursement is tied to these factors or underreporting of adverse events for which providers are not reimbursed.

In the United States, administrative data are a rich source for process measures because of the way health care charges are constructed. In contrast, the outcomes data routinely available tend to be limited to hospital readmissions or ED visits and in-hospital mortality rates. Postdischarge mortality data can sometimes be obtained through the National Death Index, CMS, or state vital statistics offices, but these sources typically have substantial time delays, apply only to selected populations (e.g., Medicare patients), or are available only for limited purposes (e.g., research). The AHRQ has also developed a set of tools (patient safety indicators) to identify complications and adverse events from hospital administrative data, although these show variable sensitivity and specificity for identifying the events they target. Use of administrative data to risk adjust outcomes is also problematic: failure to distinguish between preexisting conditions and complications that occur during the episode of care makes it difficult to assess the baseline risk factors.

Survey data: Survey data typically are used for quality measures related to patients' experiences of care, but surveys of clinicians or hospital administrators may also be used to collect data on frequency of use of certain treatments and procedures (process measures) or the availability of specific resources (structural measures). Strengths include the opportunity to elicit information from perspectives not typically captured in the routine delivery or administration of health care—specifically, those of patients, nurses, and consumers who make choices among health care plans or providers—and the variety of media through which they can be administered (in person or by phone, mail, or email). With the growing emphasis on patient-centered care, such data are becoming increasingly important to health care providers. Disadvantages to survey data include the expense involved in collecting them and the typically low response rates and associated nonresponse bias.

The most widely used patient surveys are the Consumer Assessment of Healthcare Providers and Systems (CAHPS) surveys, which are developed and maintained by the AHRQ. These surveys focus on aspects of quality of which patients are the best judges, such as the communication skills of providers and ease of access to health care services, and cover care provided in hospitals, nursing homes, home health care, dialysis facilities, and ambulatory care physician offices. They are used by commercial insurers, Medicaid, State Children's Health Insurance Program, and Medicare plans, and items from the Hospital CAHPS (HCAHPS) survey are among the quality measures that are reported publicly for hospitals participating in Medicare and used for the Medicare Hospital VBP program (see later discussion).

EXAMPLES OF QUALITY MEASURES

Hospital A in the Health Scenario is seeking to evaluate and improve the quality of care it provides to patients admitted for heart failure. **Table 15-2** provides examples of structure, process, and outcome measures within each of the six domains of quality identified by the IOM that Hospital A might consider.

Table 15-2. Example structure, process, and outcome measures in the six domains of quality.

	Structure	Process	Outcome
Safe	Does the hospital have an electronic medical record or computerized physician order entry system that provides drug–drug interaction and drug–allergy alerts?	Percentage of heart failure patients with medications reconciled at discharge	Percentage of patients admitted with heart failure who experience an adverse drug event
Timely	Does the hospital have a written process and defined standards to ensure each heart failure patient's physician or nurse explains the discharge instructions in person to the patient and a family member or caretaker before discharge?	Percentage of heart failure patients whose left ventricular systolic function is assessed before hospital discharge	Percentage of heart failure patients with a postdischarge appointment implemented within 1 week of hospital discharge
Effective	Does the hospital have a standardized evidence-based order set for the treatment of heart failure patients?	Percentage of heart failure patients with LVSD given a prescription for an ACEI and ARB at discharge	30-day mortality rate among patients discharged with heart failure
Efficient	Does the hospital use an electronic prescription system that alerts providers to generic alternatives?	Percentage use of generic drugs for appropriate heart failure patients	Average length of hospital stay (days) for heart failure patients
Equitable	Does the hospital provide interpretation or bilingual services to meet the language needs of its population?	Percentage of patient admissions in which preferred language for health care is screened and recorded	30-day mortality rate among patients discharged with heart failure, by race
Patient centered	Does the hospital conduct a survey to evaluate patient and family experiences with communication by physicians, nurses, and other hospital staff?	Percentage of patients who report on a survey that staff "always" explained about medicines before administering them	Percentage of patients who reported that their physicians "always" or "usually" communicated well

ACEI, angiotensin-converting enzyme inhibitor; ARB, angiotensin receptor blocker; LVSD, left ventricular systolic dysfunction

USES OF QUALITY MEASURES

Quality of care evaluations are used for a wide range of purposes. These include:

- Public reporting
- Pay-for-performance or value-based purchasing programs
- Informing health policy or strategy at the regional or national level
- Improving the quality of care provided within an organization
- Monitoring performance within an organization or across a region
- Identifying poor performing providers to protect public safety
- Providing information to enable patients or third-party payers to make informed choices among providers.

National Quality Measurement Initiatives

Quality measurement and evaluation play an important role in quality control regulation. They are prominent issues on the national health care agenda, largely through their incorporation into the criteria used by CMS for participation and reimbursement, but also through efforts of non-profit organizations such as the NQF, National Committee for Quality Assurance (NCQA) and the Institute for Healthcare Improvement (IHI).

The Joint Commission

The Joint Commission is an independent, not-for-profit organization that seeks to improve health care "by evaluating health care organizations and inspiring them to excel in providing safe and effective care of the highest quality and value." Health care organizations seeking to participate in and receive payment from Medicare or Medicaid must meet certain eligibility requirements, including obtaining a certification of compliance with the Conditions of Participation, which are specified in federal regulations. Under the 1965 Amendments to the Social Security Act, hospitals accredited by the Joint Commission were deemed to meet the Medicare Conditions of Participation; in 2008, this "deeming" authority was extended to other organizations CMS approves, but the Joint Commission still evaluates and accredits more than 20,000 health care organizations and programs in the United States.

In 2001, the Joint Commission adopted standardized sets of evidence-based quality measures, moving the focus of the accreditation process away from structural requirements and toward evaluating actual care

processes, tracing patients through the care and services they receive, and analyzing key operational systems that directly impact quality of care. The Joint Commission uses the quality measure data collected from accredited hospitals for a number of purposes intended to help improve quality. These include producing quarterly reports summarizing performance data for individual hospitals and health care organizations; highlighting measures showing poor performance issues; and reporting performance on Quality Check, a publicly available website. The Joint Commission's measures are further used internally by hospitals and health care organizations to drive quality improvement through goal-setting, audit-and-feedback, and executive pay-for-performance programs.

Centers for Medicare and Medicaid Services Quality Measurement and Reporting

CMS' quality measurement initiatives began in 1997 using the Healthcare Effectiveness Data Information Set (HEDIS) established by the NCQA to assess the performance of health maintenance organizations and physicians and physician groups. In 2001, DHHS announced The Quality Initiative, which aimed to assure quality health care for all Americans through published consumer information and quality improvement support from Medicare's Quality Improvement Organizations. Today, public reporting of quality measures is required of all nursing homes, home health agencies, hospitals, and dialysis facilities participating in Medicare, and physicians voluntarily report quality measures through the Physician Quality Reporting System (PQRS). As of 2015, physician reporting is required to avoid financial penalties, and performance is factored into physician reimbursement.

Hospital quality performance data are publicly reported on the Hospital Compare website (http://www.medicare.gov/hospitalcompare/search.html) for:

- Timely and effective care: Hospitals' compliance rates with evidence-based processes of care for patients with AMI, heart failure, pneumonia, stroke, and children's asthma, as well as for surgical care, pregnancy and delivery care, and blood clot prevention and management
- Readmissions, complications and deaths: 30-day readmission and mortality rates for AMI, heart failure, and pneumonia patients; 30-day readmission rate for elective hip/knee replacement patients; 30-day readmission rate for medical, surgical and gynecologic, neurologic, cardiovascular, and cardiorespiratory hospital patients are included in this measure; complication rates among hip and knee replacement patients; and rates (and mortality rates) of serious surgical complications

- Patient experience: Selected questions from the HCAHPS survey, mailed to a random selection of adult patients after their discharge from hospital, addressing such topics as how well nurses and doctors communicated, how responsive hospital staff were to patient needs, how well the hospital managed patients' pain, and the cleanliness and quietness of the hospital environment

- Use of outpatient medical imaging: Measures targeting common imaging tests that have a history of overuse (e.g., magnetic resonance imaging for low back pain) or underuse (e.g., follow-up imaging within 45 days of screening mammography)

Theoretically, such public reporting enables patients to influence quality of care through selective choice of the best available providers. There is little evidence that this occurs, however, partly because there is a lack of awareness, trust, and understanding of the reported quality data, and partly because patients' choices are often constrained by the insurance plans available to them.

The 2010 Patient Protection and Affordable Care Act (PPACA) brought a renewed focus on hospital quality measures: where, previously, hospitals had been required to report the quality measures above to receive payments from Medicare, PPACA authorized the use of these quality performance data to determine *how much* hospitals are paid by establishing the Hospital VBP Program and the Hospital Readmissions Reduction Program.

The Hospital VBP Program is a CMS initiative that rewards acute-care hospitals with incentive payments for the quality of care they provide to Medicare patients. Hospital VBP took effect in October 2012, initially placing 1% of hospital's base payments "at risk" according to their performance on measures in two areas: (1) clinical processes of care (drawn from those publicly reported for AMI, heart failure, pneumonia, and surgical care) and (2) patient experience (drawn from the HCAHPS survey), weighted 70:30 to obtain a total performance score. CMS evaluates hospitals for both *improvement* (relative to the hospital's own performance during a specified baseline period) and *achievement* (relative to the other hospitals' performance with the achievement threshold for points to be awarded being set at the median of all hospitals' performance during the baseline period) on each measure and uses the higher score toward the total performance score.

For the second year of the Hospital VBP program (i.e., starting October 2013), CMS added an Outcome Measures domain containing the 30-day mortality measures for AMI, heart failure, and pneumonia. Planned future revisions include adding an Efficiency domain and adjusting the included measures and weighting scheme more heavily toward outcomes, patient experience of care, and functional status measures. The amount of hospitals' reimbursement placed at risk according to their performance also changes each year, increasing 0.25 percentage point until it reaches a maximum of 2% in October 2016. As might be imagined, this amounts to significant amounts of money at the national level: in the program's first year, with only 1% placed at risk, almost $1 billion of Medicare reimbursement was tied to hospitals' performance.[77]

The Hospital Readmissions Reduction Program also took effect in October 2012, reducing Medicare payments to hospitals with "excess" readmissions within 30 days of discharge, defined in comparison with the national average for the hospital's set of patients with the applicable condition, looking at 3 years of discharge data and requiring a minimum of 25 cases to calculate a hospital's excess readmission ratio for each applicable condition. The initial list of "applicable conditions" was limited to those that have been reported publicly since 2009 (AMI, heart failure, and pneumonia) but will be expanded in the future. In the program's first year, the maximum penalty that applied was 1% of the hospital's base operating diagnosis-related group (DRG) payments, but in October 2014, this rose to 3%. In the program's first year, about 9% of hospitals incurred the maximum penalty, roughly 30% incurred none, and the total penalty across the more than 2200 hospitals receiving penalties was about $280 million (0.3% of total Medicare base payment to hospitals). From an individual hospital's perspective, Ohio State University's Wexner Medical Center estimated a loss of about $700,000 under a 0.64% penalty. Because the program is structured around performance relative to the national average (rather than a fixed performance target), roughly half the hospitals will *always* face a penalty, and the overall size of the penalty will remain much the same, even if, as it is hoped, the hospitals improve overall over time.

Proprietary Report Cards

In the past 2 decades, numerous quality "report cards" have entered the scene, many of them developed and conducted by for-profit companies. Examples include those issued by *Consumer Reports, US News & World Report*, Healthgrades, and Truven Health Analytics. Although hospital marketing departments frequently tout their facility's rankings in these reports, the methods by which they are produced typically do not bear scrutiny when examined for criteria such as transparent methodology, use of evidence-based measures, measure alignment, data sources, current data, risk adjustment, data quality, consistency of data, and preview by hospitals. Many of these report cards use a combination of claims-based and clinical measures (often representing data already reported on CMS' Hospital Compare website) and their own unique measures based on things like reputation or public opinion.

Local Quality Measurement and Improvement

Local quality measurement and monitoring became popular in the 1990s as health care organizations and providers adopted continuous quality improvement (also called total quality management) from the Japanese industrial setting. Key principles are:

1. "Quality" is defined in terms of meeting "customers'" needs, with customers including patients, clinicians, and others who consume the services of the institution.
2. Quality deficiencies typically result from faulty systems rather than incompetent individuals, so energy should be focused on improving the system.
3. Data, particularly outcomes data, are essential drivers and shapers of systems improvement, used to identify areas where improvements are needed and to determine whether the actions taken to address those areas are effective.
4. Management and staff at all levels of the organization must be involved in quality improvement, and a culture emphasizing quality must be created.
5. Quality improvement does not end; there is always room for further progress.

The Institute for Healthcare Improvement advocates use of the Model for Improvement (**Figure 15-1**) to guide implementation of these principles in health care. The model combines three simple questions with the plan, do, study, act (PDSA) cycle developed by W. Edwards Deming.

The PDSA cycle is an iterative process, repeating the following four steps until the desired improvement is achieved:

1. *Plan* a change aimed at quality improvement (including a plan for data collection and analysis to evaluate success).
2. *Do* the tasks required to implement the change, preferably on a pilot scale.
3. *Study* the results of the change, analyzing data collected to determine whether the improvement sought was achieved.
4. *Act* on results (alter the plan if needed or adopt more widely if it showed success).

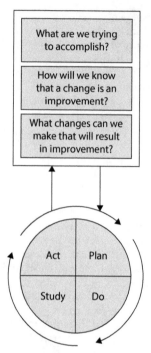

Figure 15-1. The model for improvement. (Reproduced with permission from Institute for Healthcare Improvement, Cambridge, MA; 2014; available at http://www.IHI.org.)

Hospital A from the Health Scenario applies this methodology to its efforts to improve the quality of heart failure care. Hospital A knows, from the penalties it received under the Medicare VBP and Readmissions Reduction Programs, that it needs to improve compliance with the publicly reported heart failure processes of care, to decrease its 30-day readmissions, and to improve patients' experiences of care.

Reviewing the literature, clinical quality leaders at Hospital A learn that adopting a standardized evidence-based order set for heart failure can significantly increase compliance with recommended practices for inpatient heart failure care. They also learn that involving pharmacists in medication reconciliation and patient education on discharge instructions for heart failure patients shows promise in reducing readmission rates. Finally, they find some evidence that providing language translation services for communications with physicians and nurses improves patients' experience of care. They decide to focus initially on improving performance on the publicly reported heart failure processes of care and documenting patients' language preferences to determine the translation services that are needed. Their chosen intervention is hospital-wide implementation of a standardized order set based on the current American College of Cardiology/American Heart Association clinical practice guidelines.

Quality measures chosen: (1) The proportion of eligible heart failure patients for whom physicians used the standardized order set, (2) performance on the publicly reported heart failure process measures, and (3) the proportion of patients with a documented language preference

Performance targets: (1) Physicians use the standardized order set for at least 80% of eligible heart failure patients; (2) performance on each of the publicly reported process of care measures is at or above the national average for that measure in the most recent period reported on the Hospital Compare website (April 2012–March 2013), and (3) all admitted patients have a language preference documented. Statisticians in the quality improvement department also develop an analytic plan to compare performance on the heart failure process measures for 12 weeks both before and after implementation of the order set.

Definition of the target population: For order set use and the publicly reported heart failure processes of care: all patients discharged with a final diagnosis of heart failure; for documentation of language preference: all patients

Data sources and collection: Hospital A obtains data on the publicly reported heart failure measures from the integrated outcomes, resource, and case management system it uses to collect the data needed to construct its billing charges. The information technology department adds a field to this system for patients with a heart failure diagnosis to record whether or not the standardized order set was used and, for all patients, to record language preference.

Evaluation of the improvement initiative: During the first 12 weeks of the improvement initiative, Hospital A sees documentation of a language preference reach 95% and use of the standardized order set reach 34% of eligible heart failure patients. The quality leaders do not see any noticeable changes in their performance on the process of care measures. They believe the low adoption rate of the order set explains this lack of improvement, so they initiate an intensive program to encourage physicians to use it, including education on the underlying scientific evidence, demonstrations on how to access and use it within the electronic medical record system, and fortnightly physician-specific reports showing what percentage of eligible heart failure

patients for whom they had used the order set compared with their peers.

After a further 12 weeks, Hospital A sees use of the standardized order set approach 60% of eligible patients and performance on all three of the evidence-based processes of care improve significantly from preintervention levels, reaching the targeted national average for left ventricular function assessment and prescription of ACEIs and ARBs for LVSD. Hospital A is pleased with the progress and decides to continue its efforts to increase adoption of the standardized order set, placing particular emphasis on the portion dealing with discharge instructions as they introduce a program to integrate pharmacists into the medication reconciliation and discharge instruction process. Having used the data collected on language preference to identify the predominant translation needs in Hospital A's patient population, the quality leaders next turn their attention to improving performance on the provider communication measures, initiating a new PDSA cycle to implement the chosen translation resources and increase awareness and use of them by physicians, nurses, and patients.

THE NATIONAL QUALITY STRATEGY

Section 3011 of PPACA required the Secretary of DHHS to establish a national strategy for quality improvement in health care that sets priorities to guide improvement efforts and provides a strategic plan for achieving the goal of increasing access to high-quality, affordable health care for all Americans.[87] The National Quality Strategy (NQS) was developed through a collaborative process that called on a wide range of health care stakeholders for contributions and comment, incorporated input from the National Priorities Partnership (52 public, private, for-profit, and nonprofit organizations working to improve the quality and value of health care in the United States) and culminated in public comment on a proposed approach, principles, and priorities. **Table 15-3** summarizes the NQS' resulting aims, priorities, and principles.

Building consensus on how to measure quality is a critical step in implementing the NQS to enable patients; providers; employers; health insurance companies; academic researchers; and local, state, and federal governments to align their efforts and maximize the gains in quality and efficiency. Agencies within DHHS are moving toward common performance measures across programs (reducing the reporting burden on providers), and groups such as the Measures Application Partnership, a public–private partnership that reviews performance measures being

Table 15-3. Aims, priorities, and principles of the National Quality Strategy.

Aims	Priorities	Principles
Better care: Improve the overall quality, by making health care more patient centered, reliable, accessible, and safe.	• Making care safer by reducing harm caused in the delivery of care • Ensuring that each person and family is engaged as partners in their care • Promoting effective communication and coordination of care	1. Person centeredness and family engagement, including understanding and valuing patient preferences, will guide all strategies, goals, and improvement efforts. 2. Specific health considerations will be addressed for patients of all ages, backgrounds, health needs, care locations, and sources of coverage. 3. Eliminating disparities in care, including but not limited to those based on race, color, national origin, gender, age, disability, language, health literacy, sexual orientation and gender identity, source of payment, socioeconomic status, and geography, will be an integral part of all strategies, goals, and health care improvement efforts.
Healthy people and healthy communities: Improve the health of the U.S. population by supporting proven interventions to address behavioral, social, and environmental determinants of health in addition to delivering higher quality care.	• Promoting the most effective prevention and treatment practices for the leading causes of death, starting with cardiovascular disease • Working with communities to promote wide use of best practices to enable healthy living	4. Attention will be paid to aligning the efforts of the public and private sectors. 5. Quality improvement will be driven by supporting innovation, evaluating efforts around the country, rapid-cycle learning, and disseminating evidence about what works. 6. Consistent national standards will be promoted while maintaining support for local, community, and state-level activities that are responsive to local circumstances.
Affordable care: Reduce the cost of quality health care for individuals, families, employers, and government.	• Making quality care more affordable for individuals, families, employers, and governments by developing and spreading new health care delivery models	7. Primary care will become a bigger focus, with special attention toward the challenges faced by vulnerable populations, including children, older adults, and those with multiple health conditions. 8. Coordination among primary care, behavioral health, other specialty clinicians, and health systems will be enhanced to ensure that these systems treat the "whole person." 9. Integration of care delivery with community and public health planning will be promoted. 10. Providing patients, providers, and payers with the clear information they need to make choices that are right for them will be encouraged.

considered for federal public reporting and performance-based payment programs are working more broadly to align measures used in public and private sector programs. The annual NQS progress reports have identified national tracking measures, goals, and target performance levels relevant to each of the six priority areas, providing some guidance for such alignment.

CURRENT HEALTH CARE QUALITY STATUS AND TARGETS

The United States' poor performance on health and health care quality measures relative to other industrialized nations is well-known, as is the much higher per capita health care spending. In 2011, the United States spent $8608 per capita on health care, an amount exceeded only by Norway, Luxembourg, and Switzerland. By comparison among other Western nations, the Netherlands and Australia each spent roughly $6000, Germany and France spent around $5000, and the United Kingdom and New Zealand spent approximately $3500. The United States' health care spending amounts to about 17% of its gross domestic product compared with the 12% or less of similarly industrialized nations.

Various theories have been advanced for the United States' disproportional spending—for example, the aging of the U.S. population, poorer health behaviors, racial and ethnic diversity and associated health disparities, and greater utilization or supply of health care resources. However, a 2012 comparison between the United States and 12 other industrialized Organization for Economic Cooperation and Development nations demonstrated that the United States has a comparatively young population and that adults were less likely to smoke than in the comparison nations; that although the health disadvantage is more pronounced in low-income minority populations, it persists in non-Hispanic whites and adults with health insurance, college education, high income, or healthy behaviors; and that it has fewer physicians, physician visits, and hospital beds and admissions per capita than was typical of the comparison nations. U.S. adults, however, were the most likely to be obese (a condition to which an estimated 10% of health care spending may be attributable), and U.S. hospitals stays (although shorter) were almost twice as expensive as those in other countries—a difference that could result from more resource-intensive hospital stays, higher prices for services, or a combination thereof. Fees for physician services, diagnostic imaging, procedures, and prescription medications are all higher in the United States, and the pervasive medical technology and associated prices appear to be potent drivers behind the "supersized" portion of resources devoted to health care in the United States.

The high spending might be justifiable if the United States had proportionately better health and health outcomes, but that is not the case—and the health disadvantage seems to be increasing. A 2013 report from the National Research Council and IOM found that individuals in the United States in all age groups up to 75 years have shorter life expectancies than their peers in 16 industrialized nations and that the United States has comparatively high prevalence and mortality rates for multiple diseases, faring worse than average across nine health domains: adverse birth outcomes; injuries, accidents, and homicides; adolescent pregnancy and sexually transmitted infections; HIV and AIDS; drug-related mortality; obesity and diabetes; heart disease; chronic lung

disease; and disability. To be fair, the United States did perform better than average on control of hypertension and serum lipids, cancer and stroke mortality rates, and life expectancy after 75 years. These "strengths," however, reflect what the U.S. health care system tends to reward (through payment), focusing on prolonging life as death encroaches rather than on promoting the healthy behaviors and preventive measures that, starting early in life, can avoid much subsequent loss of life and quality of life. Determinants underlying the United States' health disadvantage include:

1. The lack of universal health insurance coverage or a tax-financed system that ensures health care affordability (something every other industrialized nation provides)
2. A weaker foundation in primary care
3. Greater barriers to access and affordable care
4. Poor care coordination
5. Unhealthy behaviors, including high-calorie, low-nutrition diets; drug abuse; alcohol-involved motor vehicle crashes; and high rates of firearm ownership

We know, because other countries have achieved it, that a better health care system and a healthier population are realistic goals. The question is what are the people of the United States, particularly the stakeholders in the health care system, prepared to do to achieve them? Based on what we see in other countries, it will likely require health care to become less profit focused, bringing the costs and use of physician services, hospital stays, and procedures and imaging into line with international practice. It will also likely require resources to be shifted away from developing and adopting expensive technology that offers only incremental gains in health to a small number of people toward preventive care and public health initiatives with which the gains per dollar spent are much larger. These are unlikely to be popular changes, but they are what the data show the United States needs, and true scientists will not ignore that evidence. Nor will those who are serious about quality improvement.

Some steps are being taken in this direction. Several of the National Quality Strategy priorities (discussed earlier) address the determinants of the U.S. health disadvantage, targeting care coordination, prevention, and healthy living. Progress on these and the other priority areas is slow (**Table 15-4**), but at least relevant measures, baseline rates, and target performance levels have been identified. Further progress can be achieved if all health care stakeholders incorporate the National Quality Strategy priorities and associated measures into their own

Table 15–4. Measures, targets and progress identified for the National Quality Strategy Priority Areas.

Priority	Measure Focus	Measure Description	Baseline Rate*	Most Recent Rate*	Target
1. Making care safer by reducing harm caused in the delivery of care	HACs	Incidence of measurable HACs	145 HACs per 1000 admissions	142 HACs per 1000 admissions in 2011	Reduce preventable HACs by 40% by end of 2014
	Hospital readmissions	All-payer 30-day readmission rate	14.4% based on 32.9 million admissions	14.4% based on 32.7 million admissions in 2011	Reduce all readmissions by 20% by end of 2014
2. Ensuring that each person and family is engaged as partners in his or her care	Timely care	Adults who needed care right away for an illness, injury, or condition in the past 12 months who sometimes or never got care as soon as wanted	14.1%	N/A	Reduce to <10% by 2017
	Decision making	People with a usual source of care whose health care providers sometimes or never discuss decisions with them	15.9%	N/A	Reduce to <10% by 2017
3. Promoting effective communication and coordination of care	Patient-centered medical home	Percentage of children needing care coordination who receive effective care coordination	69%	66.1%	Increase to 90% by 2017
	Three-item Care Transition Measure	• During this hospital stay, staff took my preferences and those of my family or caregiver into account in deciding what my health care needs would be when I left. • When I left the hospital, I had a good understanding of the things I was responsible for in managing my health. • When I left the hospital, I clearly understood the purpose for taking each of my medications.	45%	N/A	Increase to 50% by 2017
4. Promoting the most effective prevention and treatment practices for the leading causes of death, starting with cardiovascular disease	Aspirin use	Outpatient visits at which adults with cardiovascular disease are prescribed or maintained on aspirin	47%	53%	Increase to 65% by 2017
	Blood pressure control	Adults with hypertension who have adequately controlled blood pressure	46%	53%	Increase to 65% by 2017
	Cholesterol management	Adults with high cholesterol who have adequate control	33%	32%	Increase to 65% by 2017
	Smoking cessation	Outpatient visits at which current tobacco users received tobacco cessation counseling or cessation medications	23%	22%	Increase to 65% by 2017

Table 15-4. Measures, targets and progress identified for the National Quality Strategy Priority Areas. (*Continued*)

Priority	Measure Focus	Measure Description	Baseline Rate[*]	Most Recent Rate[*]	Target
5. Working with communities to promote wide use of best practices to enable healthy living	Depression	Percentage of adults who reported symptoms of a major depressive episode in the past 12 months who received treatment for depression in the past 12 months	68.2%	68.1% for 2011	Increase to 78.2% by 2020
	Obesity	Proportion of adults who are obese	35.7%	N/A	Reduce to 30.5% by 2020
6. Making quality care more affordable for individuals, families, employers, and governments by developing and spreading new health care delivery models	Out-of-pocket expenses	Percentage of people younger than age 65 years with out-of-pocket medical and premium expenses >10% of income	18.5%	N/A	N/A
	Health spending per capita	Annual all-payer health care spending per person	$8,402	$8680 per person in 2011	N/A

[*]See the 2013 Annual Report to Congress for data sources and applicable measurement periods (http://www.ahrq.gov/workingforquality/nqs/nqs2013annlrpt.htm#improvequal).
HAC, hospital-acquired condition; N/A, not available.

daily operations and, applying the principles of quality improvement, enter into PDSA cycles within those unique contexts.

SUMMARY

In this chapter, the measurement and improvement of health care quality were illustrated using the example of inpatient heart failure care. *Quality* is defined in terms of six principal domains: safety, timeliness, effectiveness, equity, efficiency, and patient centeredness. Quality measures can be divided into three broad types—structure, process, and outcome—each of which is subject to particular strengths and weaknesses but that provides insights into different aspects of quality. The choice between structure, process, and outcome measures (or some combination thereof) depends on the purpose and context of the particular quality evaluation and from whose perspective quality is being assessed. Generally speaking, outcomes measures are most useful when the perspective is broad because they can reflect the influence of a wide range of factors. Process measures may be more appropriate for narrower perspectives (e.g., evaluating an individual provider's performance) because they are less subject to the influence of factors outside the provider's control. Structure measures provide little insight into the care that is actually provided but are useful when trying to elucidate differences among health care settings and contexts that contribute to variations in care that suggest opportunities for improvement.

Health care quality data can be derived from a variety of sources but are most typically obtained from clinical records, provider and payer administrative databases, and surveys. Particularly with the former two sources, it is important to keep in mind that the data have not been collected or recorded with the purpose of quality measurement in mind but rather to facilitate the provision of care and daily operations of the health care organization. As such, they may not contain the level of detail desirable for quality measurement or may contain inaccuracies that although not problematic for their primary purposes, distort the picture of the quality of care provided.

Quality measures have a variety of applications, ranging from internal efforts to improve the quality of care provided with an organization to informing national policies regarding health care policy. Recent public attention has mostly been focused on public reporting efforts and the integration of quality measures into pay-for-performance and value-based purchasing programs. However, much of the day-to-day application of quality measures comes in the context of continuous quality improvement initiatives implemented by or within individual practices, departments, hospitals, or health care organizations. Borrowed from industrial settings, continuous quality improvement relies on the PDSA cycle: *plan* a change aimed at quality improvement, *do* the tasks required to implement the change, *study* the results of the change, and *act* on the results. The National Quality Strategy, established by the DHHS under the PPACA, is intended to provide guidance that will help providers; payers; researchers; and local, state, and federal governments align their quality improvement initiatives to enable both more efficient and more effective improvement. Success in these areas is hoped to bring the United States' health care spending and outcomes into line with other industrialized nations, which it currently outspends and underperforms.

STUDY QUESTIONS

1. Compliance with evidence-based recommendations for venous thromboembolism prophylaxis in the intensive care unit is an example of a quality measure most connected with which of the IOM domains of quality?
   A. Effective
   B. Patient centered
   C. Equitable
   D. Efficient

2. The proportion of patients with low back pain who had magnetic resonance imaging without trying recommended treatments first, such as physical therapy, is an example of which type of measure within Donabedian's framework for measuring quality of care?
   A. Structure
   B. Efficiency
   C. Process
   D. Effective

3. The proportion of people who report being uninsured all year, by English proficiency and place of birth, is an example of a quality measure most connected with which of the IOM domains of quality?
   A. Equitable
   B. Patient centered
   C. Access to care
   D. Safety

4. A safety net hospital has a higher unadjusted 30-day readmission rate for heart failure than the private hospital in an affluent neighborhood across town despite showing better performance on the public-reported recommended processes of care for heart failure. The safety net hospital has a high volume of indigent patients, but the private hospital's patients typically have higher education levels, fewer comorbidities, and better access to care. A possible explanation for the unadjusted 30-day readmission result is

A. surveillance bias.

B. reporting bias.

C. information bias.

D. confounding bias.

5. In 1998, Hospital A, a large academic teaching hospital, had a 2.5% operative mortality rate among patients undergoing CABG. In 1999, Hospital A partnered with local cardiac and vascular surgeons to open a neighboring specialty heart and vascular hospital, equipped to perform percutaneous coronary intervention (PCI) but not open heart surgery. From then on, the vast majority of patients with single- or two-vessel disease underwent revascularization via PCI at the specialty hospital, and patients with multivessel disease or other factors making their condition more complex continued to be treated via CABG at Hospital A. In 1999 and 2000, Hospital A saw a sharp increase in its operative mortality rate. By focusing quality improvement efforts on surgical technique and postsurgical care, it was able to reduce the mortality rate somewhat in subsequent years but has not been able to equal or better the 2.5% achieved in 1998. An explanation for this result is

A. surveillance bias.

B. reporting bias.

C. selection bias.

D. confounding bias.

6. Looking at whether a physician practice routinely conducts a survey to assess patient experience related to access to care, communication with the physician and other practice staff, and coordination of care is a(n) _____ measure within Donabedian's framework, addressing the _____ domain of health care quality.

A. Outcome, patient-centered

B. Structure, timeliness

C. Process, timeliness

D. Structure, patient-centered

7. Administrative data sources (e.g., hospital billing data or health insurance claims data) are frequently used for quality measurement because

A. the data are routinely collected for operational purposes and can be obtained rapidly and at relatively low cost for large numbers of patients.

B. the data contain the comprehensive clinical detail needed to risk adjust outcome measures to enable fair comparisons among providers.

C. in the United States, thanks to the way health care charges are constructed, they are a rich source of outcomes data.

D. they provide insight into the health care system from the patient's perspective, enabling assessment of the patient-centered domain of quality.

8. Quality of care measures are useful for

A. patients or payers trying to choose among health care providers.

B. state or government agencies responsible for setting health care policies and priorities.

C. hospitals seeking to improve the care they provide their patients.

D. all of the above.

9. Which of the following quality measures is NOT typically assessed through patient surveys, such as the Consumer Assessment of Healthcare Providers and Systems?

A. Communication skills of providers

B. Technical skills of providers

C. Access to care

D. Understanding of medication instruction

10. Medical records are useful for all of the following purposes EXCEPT

A. assessing medical care processes.

B. monitoring quality improvement efforts.

C. assessing patient experience.

D. disease-specific registries.

FURTHER READING

Ballard DJ, Fleming NS, Allison JT, Convery PB, Luquire R, eds. *Achieving STEEEP Health Care*. Boca Raton, FL: CRC Press; 2013.

Bardach NS, Cabana MD. The unintended consequences of quality improvement. *Curr Opin Pediatr* 2009;21(6):777-782.

Corrigan JM, Donaldson MS, Kohn LT, Maguire SK, Pike KC. *Crossing the Quality Chasm: A New Health System for the 21st Century.* Washington, DC: National Academies Press; 2001

Klaber RE, Roland D. Delivering quality improvement: the need to believe it is necessary. *Arch Dis Child* 2014;99:175-749.

Lazar EJ, Fleischut P, Regan BK. Quality measurement in healthcare. *Annu Rev Med* 2013;64:485-496.

Ransom ER, Joshi MS, Nash DB, Ransom SB, eds. *The Healthcare Quality Book: Vision, Strategy and Tools*, 2nd ed. Chicago: Health Administration Press; 2008.

REFERENCES

Health Scenario and Clinical Background

Go AS, Mozaffarian D, Roger VL, et al. Heart disease and stroke statistics—2013 update: a report from the American Heart Association. *Circulation.* 2013;127(1):e6-e245.

Schwartz JB, Zipes DP. Cardiovascular disease in the elderly. In: Zipes DP, Libby P, Bonow PO, eds. *Braunwald's Heart Disease: A Textbook of Cardiovascular Medicine.* Philadelphia: Elsevier Saunders; 2005:1923–1953.

Vogeli C, Kang R, Landrum MB, Hasnain-Wynia R, Weissman JS. Quality of care provided to individual patients in US hospitals: results from an analysis of national Hospital Quality Alliance data. *Med Care.* 2009;47(5):591-599.

Epidemiology and Quality of Care

Forster M, dir. World War Z [Film]. Paramount Pictures. June 21, 2013.

Gordis L. *Epidemiology.* 2nd ed. Philadelphia: W.B. Saunders; 2000.

Petersen W, dir. Outbreak [Film]. Warner Bros. March 10, 1995.

Soderbergh S, dir. Contagion [Film]. Warner Bros. September 9, 2011.

What is "Quality of Care?"

About the National Quality Strategy (NQS). http://www.ahrq.gov/workingforquality/about.htm. Accessed December 20, 2013.

Advisory Commission on Consumer Protection and Quality in the Health Care Industry. Quality First: Better Health Care for All Americans. Published 1998. http://www.hcqualitycommission.gov/final. Accessed February 20, 2014.

Brook RH, McGlynn EA, Shekelle PG. Defining and measuring quality of care: a perspective from US researchers. *Int J Qual Health Care.* 2000;12(4):281-295.

Corrigan JM, Donaldson MS, Kohn LT, Maguire SK, Pike KC. *Crossing the Quality Chasm: A New Health System for the 21st Century.* Washington, DC: National Academies Press; 2001.

Chassin MR, Galvin RW. The urgent need to improve health care quality. Institute of Medicine National Roundtable on Health Care Quality. *JAMA.* 1998;280(11):1000-1005.

Hibbard JH, Greene J, Daniel D. What is quality anyway? Performance reports that clearly communicate to consumers the meaning of quality of care. *Med Care Res Rev.* 2010;67(3):275-293.

Pirsig RM. *Zen and the Art of Motorcycle Maintenance: An Inquiry Into Values.* New York: HarperCollins; 2005.

Rubin HR, Pronovost P, Diette GB. The advantages and disadvantages of process-based measures of health care quality. *Int J Qual Health Care.* 2001;13(6):469-474.

Schuster MA, McGlynn EA, Brook RH. How good is the quality of health care in the United States? *Milbank Q.* 1998;76(4):517-563, 509.

World Health Organization. *Quality of Care: A Process for Making Strategic Choices in Health Systems.* Geneva: World Health Organization; 2006.

Measuring Health Care Quality

Berenson RA, Provonost PJ, Krumholz HM. Achieving the Potential of Health Care Performance Measures. Timely Analysis of Health Policy Issues. Published 2013. http://www.rwjf.org/content/dam/farm/reports/reports/2013/rwjf406195. Accessed February 4, 2014.

Donabedian A. *The Definition of Quality and Approaches to its Assessment.* Vol 1. Ann Arbor, MI: Health Administration Press; 1980.

Epstein AM. The role of quality measurement in a competitive marketplace. *Baxter Health Policy Rev.* 1996;2:207-234.

Furrow BR, Greaney TL, Johnson SH, Jost TS, Schwarts RL. Quality control regulation of health care institutions. In: *The Law of Health Care Organization and Financing.* St. Paul, MN: Thomson West; 2008:140-175.

Furrow BR, Greaney TL, Johnson SH, Jost TS, Schwarts RL. Introduction to health law and policy. In: *The Law of Health Care Organization and Financing.* St. Paul, MN: Thomson West; 2008:1-95.

Iezzoni LI. The risks of risk adjustment. *JAMA.* 1997;278(19):1600-1607.

Krumholz HM, Brindis RG, Brush JE, et al. Standards for statistical models used for public reporting of health outcomes: an American Heart Association Scientific Statement from the Quality of Care and Outcomes Research Interdisciplinary Writing Group: cosponsored by the Council on Epidemiology and Prevention and the Stroke Council. Endorsed by the American College of Cardiology Foundation. *Circulation.* 2006;113(3):456-462.

Mant J. Process versus outcome indicators in the assessment of quality of health care. *Int J Qual Health Care.* 2001;13(6):475-480.

Marshall G, Shroyer AL, Grover FL, Hammermeister KE. Time series monitors of outcomes. A new dimension for measuring quality of care. *Med Care.* 1998;36(3):348-356.

National Committee for Quality Assurance. *Report Card Pilot Project, Key Findings and Lessons Learned: 21 Plans' Performance Profiles.* Washington, DC: National Committee for Quality Assurance; 1995.

Nigam A. Changing health care quality paradigms: the rise of clinical guidelines and quality measures in American medicine. *Soc Sci Med.* 2012;75(11):1933-1937.

Sackett D, Straus SE, Richardson W, Rosenburg W, Haynes R. *Evidence-based Medicine. How to Practise and Teach EBM.* 2nd ed. Edinburgh: Churchill-Livingstone; 2000.

U.S. General Accounting Office. *Report Cards: A Useful Concept but Significant Issues Need to be Addressed.* Washington, DC: GAO; 1994.

Werner RM, Bradlow ET, Asch DA. Does hospital performance on process measures directly measure high quality care or is it a marker of unmeasured care? *Health Serv Res.* 2008;43(5 Pt 1):1464-1484.

World Health Organization. *Quality of Care: A Process for Making Strategic Choices in Health Systems.* Geneva: World Health Organization; 2006.

Attributes of Quality Measures

Agency for Healthcare Research and Quality. Patient Safety Indicators Overview. http://qualityindicators.ahrq.gov/Modules/psi_resources.aspx. Accessed February 5, 2014.

Agency for Healthcare Research and Quality. About CAHPS. https://cahps.ahrq.gov/about-cahps/index.html. Accessed February 5, 2014.

Allison JJ, Wall TC, Spettell CM, et al. The art and science of chart review. *Jt Comm J Qual Improv.* 2000;26(3):115-136.

Ballard DJ, Bryant SC, O'Brien PC, Smith DW, Pine MB, Cortese DA. Referral selection bias in the Medicare hospital mortality prediction model: are centers of referral for Medicare beneficiaries necessarily centers of excellence? *Health Serv Res.* 1994;28(6):771-784.

Ballard DJ, Ogola G, Fleming NS, et al. Impact of a standardized heart failure order set on mortality, readmission, and quality and costs of care. *Int J Qual Health Care.* 2010;22(6):437-444.

Ballard DJ, Nicewander DA, Qin H, Fullerton C, Winter FD Jr, Couch CE. Improving delivery of clinical preventive services: a multi-year journey. *Am J Prev Med.* 2007;33(6):492-497.

Berenson RA, Provonost PJ, Krumholz HM. Achieving the Potential of Health Care Performance Measures. Timely Analysis of Health Policy Issues. Published 2013. http://www.rwjf.org/content/dam/farm/reports/reports/2013/rwjf406195. Accessed February 4, 2014.

Chan KS, Fowles JB, Weiner JP. Review: electronic health records and the reliability and validity of quality measures: a review of the literature. *Med Care Res Rev.* 2010;67(5):503-527.

Corrigan JM, Donaldson MS, Kohn LT, Maguire SK, Pike KC. *Crossing the Quality Chasm: A New Health System for the 21st Century.* Washington, DC: National Academies Press; 2001.

da Graca B, Filardo G, Nicewander D. Consequences for healthcare quality and research of the exclusion of records from the Death Master File. *Circ Cardiovasc Qual Outcomes.* 2013;6(1):124-128.

Davies SM, Geppert J, McClellan M, McDonald KM, Romano PS, Shojania KG. *Refinement of the HCUP Quality Indicators.* Rockville, MD: Agency for Healthcare Research and Quality; 2001.

Devoe JE, Gold R, McIntire P, Puro J, Chauvie S, Gallia CA. Electronic health records vs Medicaid claims: completeness of diabetes preventive care data in community health centers. *Ann Fam Med.* 2011;9(4):351-358.

Donabedian A. Evaluating the quality of medical care. 1966. *Milbank Q.* 2005;83(4):691-729.

Farmer SA, Black B, Bonow RO. Tension between quality measurement, public quality reporting, and pay for performance. *JAMA.* 2013;309(4):349-350.

Fishbein DB, Willis BC, Cassidy WM, et al. Determining indications for adult vaccination: patient self-assessment, medical record, or both? *Vaccine.* 2006;24(6):803-818.

Fitch K, Bernstein SJ, Aguilar MD, et al. *The RAND/UCLA Appropriateness Method User's Manual.* Santa Monica, CA: RAND; 2001.

Fleming NS, Masica A, McCarthy I. Evaluation of clinical and financial outcomes. In: Ballard DJ, Fleming NS, Allison JT, Convery PB, Luquire R, eds. *Achieving STEEEP Health Care.* Boca Raton, FL: CRC Press; 2013:85-92.

Gordis L. *Epidemiology.* 2nd ed. Philadelphia: W.B. Saunders; 2000.

Herrin J, da Graca B, Nicewander D, et al. The effectiveness of implementing an electronic health record on diabetes care and outcomes. *Health Serv Res.* 2012;47(4):1522-1540.

Herrin J, Nicewander D, Ballard DJ. The effect of health care system administrator pay-for-performance on quality of care. *Jt Comm J Qual Patient Saf.* 2008;34(11):646-654.

Hollander P, Nicewander D, Couch C, et al. Quality of care of Medicare patients with diabetes in a metropolitan fee-for-service primary care integrated delivery system. *Am J Med Qual.* 2005;20(6):344-352.

Iezzoni LI, ed *Risk adjustment for measuring health care outcomes.* 3rd ed. Chicago: Health Administration Press; 2003.

Kennerly DA, Valdes M, Nicewander D, Green RT. STEEEP analytics. In: Ballard DJ, Fleming NS, Allison JT, Convery PB, Luquire R, eds. *Achieving STEEEP Health Care.* Boca Raton, FL: CRC Press; 2013:75-80.

Kern LM, Malhotra S, Barron Y, et al. Accuracy of electronically reported "meaningful use" clinical quality measures: a cross-sectional study. *Ann Intern Med.* 2013;158(2):77-83.

Krumholz HM, Brindis RG, Brush JE, et al. Standards for statistical models used for public reporting of health outcomes: an American Heart Association Scientific Statement from the Quality of Care and Outcomes Research Interdisciplinary Writing Group: cosponsored by the Council on Epidemiology and Prevention and the Stroke Council. Endorsed by the American College of Cardiology Foundation. *Circulation.* 2006;113(3):456-462.

Lee GM, Kleinman K, Soumerai SB, et al. Effect of nonpayment for preventable infections in U.S. hospitals. *N Engl J Med.* 2012;367(15):1428-1437.

Mackin RS, Arean PA. Incidence and documentation of cognitive impairment among older adults with severe mental illness in a community mental health setting. *Am J Geriatr Psychiatry.* 2009;17(1):75-82.

Mant J. Process versus outcome indicators in the assessment of quality of health care. *Int J Qual Health Care.* 2001;13(6):475-480.

National Quality Forum. http://www.qualityforum.org. Accessed January 23, 2014.

Persell SD, Wright JM, Thompson JA, Kmetik KS, Baker DW. Assessing the validity of national quality measures for coronary artery disease using an electronic health record. *Arch Intern Med.* 2006;166(20):2272-2277.

Roth CP, Lim YW, Pevnick JM, Asch SM, McGlynn EA. The challenge of measuring quality of care from the electronic health record. *Am J Med Qual.* 2009;24(5):385-394.

Sclesselman JJ. *Case-Control Studies: Design, Conduct, and Analysis.* New York: Oxford University Press; 1982.

Sen AI, Morgan RW, Morris MC. Variability in the implementation of rapid response teams at academic American pediatric hospitals. *J Pediatr.* 2013;163(6):1772-1774.

Shekelle PG. Quality indicators and performance measures: methods for development need more standardization. *J Clin Epidemiol.* 2013;66(12):1338-1339.

Shekelle PG, Ortiz E, Rhodes S, et al. Validity of the Agency for Healthcare Research and Quality clinical practice guidelines: how quickly do guidelines become outdated? *JAMA.* 2001;286(12):1461-1467.

Shojania KG, Sampson M, Ansari MT, et al. *Updating Systematic Reviews.* Rockville, MD: Agency for Healthcare Research and Quality; 2007.

Steinbusch PJ, Oostenbrink JB, Zuurbier JJ, Schaepkens FJ. The risk of upcoding in casemix systems: a comparative study. *Health Policy.* 2007;81(2-3):289-299.

Stelfox HT, Straus SE. Measuring quality of care: considering conceptual approaches to quality indicator development and evaluation. *J Clin Epidemiol.* 2013;66(12):1328-1337.

Sutcliffe D, Lester H, Hutton J, Stokes T. NICE and the Quality and Outcomes Framework (QOF) 2009-2011. *Qual Prim Care.* 2012;20(1):47-55.

Timmermans S, Mauck A. The promises and pitfalls of evidence-based medicine. *Health Aff (Millwood).* 2005;24(1):18-28.

Uses of Quality Measures

42 C.F.R. §§ 412.154. http://www.ecfr.gov/cgi-bin/text-idx?c=ecfr&tpl=/ecfrbrowse/Title42/42cfr412_main_02.tpl. Accessed January 20, 2014.

42 C.F.R. § 412.160. http://www.ecfr.gov/cgi-bin/text-idx?c=ecfr&tpl=/ecfrbrowse/Title42/42cfr412_main_02.tpl. Accessed January 22, 2014.

Berenson RA, Provonost PJ, Krumholz HM. Achieving the Potential of Health Care Performance Measures. Timely Analysis of Health Policy Issues. Published 2013. http://www.rwjf.org/content/dam/farm/reports/reports/2013/rwjf406195. Accessed February 4, 2014.

Centers for Medicare & Medicaid Services. Physician Quality Reporting System (PQRS) Overview. http://www.cms.gov/Medicare/Quality-Initiatives-Patient-Assessment-Instruments/PQRS/Downloads/PQRS_OverviewFactSheet_2013_08_06.pdf. Accessed January 20, 2014.

Centers for Medicare & Medicaid Services. Hospital Compare: what information can I get about hospitals? http://www.medicare.gov/hospitalcompare/About/Hospital-Info.html. Accessed January 20, 2014.

Centers for Medicare & Medicaid Services. Readmissions Reduction Program. http://www.cms.gov/Medicare/Medicare-Fee-for-Service-Payment/AcuteInpatientPPS/Readmissions-Reduction-Program.html. Accessed January 20, 2014.

Centers for Medicare & Medicaid Services and the Joint Commission. Introduction. *Specifications Manual for National Hospital Quality Measures*, Version 4.2b. 2013; i-viii. http://www.jointcommission.org/specifications_manual_for_national_hospital_inpatient_quality_measures.aspx. Accessed March 12, 2014.

Department of Health and Human Service, Centers for Medicare and Medicaid Services. Medicare and Medicaid programs: hospital outpatient prospective payment; ambulatory surgical center payment; hospital value-based purchasing program; physician self-referral; and patient notification requirements in provider agreements. Final rule with comment period. *Fed Regist.* 2011;76(230):74122, 74527-74531, 74543-74544.

Faber M, Bosch M, Wollersheim H, Leatherman S, Grol R. Public reporting in health care: how do consumers use quality-of-care information? A systematic review. *Med Care.* 2009;47(1):1-8.

Goodrich K, Garcia E, Conway PH. A history of and a vision for CMS quality measurement programs. *Jt Comm J Qual Patient Saf.* 2012;38(10):465-470.

Health Policy Brief: Medicare Hospital Readmissions Reduction Program. Published November 12, 2013. http://healthaffairs.org/healthpolicybriefs/brief_pdfs/healthpolicybrief_102.pdf. Accessed January 20, 2014.

Herrin J, Nicewander D, Ballard DJ. The effect of health care system administrator pay-for-performance on quality of care. *Jt Comm J Qual Patient Saf.* 2008;34(11):646-654.

Holtz K, DeVol E. Alignment, goal-setting, and incentives. In: Ballard DJ, Fleming NS, Allison JT, Convery PB, Luquire R, eds. *Achieving STEEEP Health Care.* Boca Raton, FL: CRC Press; 2013:23-28.

Hospital Association of New York State. HANYS Report Card on hospital report cards. Published 2013. http://www.hanys.org/quality/data/report_cards/2013/. Accessed February 4, 2014.

Institute for Healthcare Improvement. How to improve. http://www.ihi.org/resources/Pages/HowtoImprove/default.aspx. Accessed February 10, 2014.

Jost TS. Oversight of the quality of medical care: regulation, management, or the market? *Ariz L Rev.* 1995;37:825-869.

Mant J. Process versus outcome indicators in the assessment of quality of health care. *Int J Qual Health Care.* 2001;13(6):475-480.

Panzer RJ, Gitomer RS, Greene WH, Webster PR, Landry KR, Riccobono CA. Increasing demands for quality measurement. *JAMA.* 2013;310(18):1971-1980.

Rau J. Medicare Discloses Hospitals' Bonuses, Penalties Based on Quality. http://www.kaiserhealthnews.org/stories/2012/december/21/medicare-hospitals-value-based-purchasing.aspx. Accessed January 22, 2014.

The Advisory Board Company. How much will readmission penalties cost? Hospitals do the math. http://www.advisory.com/Daily-Briefing/2012/08/24/How-much-will-readmission-penalties-cost. Accessed October 26, 2012.

The Joint Commission. History of the Joint Commission. http://www.jointcommission.org/about_us/history.aspx. Accessed January 10, 2014.

The Joint Commission. Facts about federal deemed status and state recognition. http://www.jointcommission.org/assets/1/18/Federal_Deemed_Status.pdf. Accessed January 10, 2014.

Thompson DN, Wolf GA, Spear SJ. Driving improvement in patient care: lessons from Toyota. *J Nurs Adm.* 2003;33(11):585-595.

The National Quality Strategy

Patient Protection and Affordable Care Act, 124 Stat. 119, §3011 (2010).

U.S. Department of Health and Human Services. 2012 Annual Progress Report to Congress: National Strategy for Quality Improvement in Health Care. Published 2012. http://www.ahrq.gov/workingforquality/nqs/nqs2012annlrpt.pdf. Accessed February 6, 2014.

U.S. Department of Health and Human Services. 2013 Annual Progress Report to Congress: National Strategy for Quality Improvement in Health Care. Published 2013. http://www.ahrq.gov/workingforquality/nqs/nqs2013annlrpt.pdf. Accessed February 6, 2014.

Working for Quality. About the National Quality Strategy. http://www.ahrq.gov/workingforquality/about.htm. Accessed February 6, 2014.

Working for Quality. Principles for the National Quality Strategy. http://www.ahrq.gov/workingforquality/nqs/principles.htm. Accessed February 6, 2014.

Current Health Care Quality Status and Targets

Finkelstein EA, Trogdon JG, Cohen JW, Dietz W. Annual medical spending attributable to obesity: payer-and service-specific estimates. *Health Aff (Millwood).* 2009;28(5):w822-831.

International Federation of Health Plans. *2011 Comparative Price Report: Medical and Hospital Fees by Country*. London: IFHP;2011

Laugesen MJ, Glied SA. Higher fees paid to US physicians drive higher spending for physician services compared to other countries. *Health Aff (Millwood)*. 2011;30(9):1647-1656.

Squires DA. *Explaining High Health Care Spending in the United States: An International Comparison of Supply, Utilization, Prices, and Quality*. New York: The Commonwealth Fund; 2012.

U.S. Health in International Perspective: Shorter Lives, Poorer Health: The National Academies Press; 2013.

The World Bank. Health Expenditure per Capita. http://data.worldbank.org/indicator/SH.XPD.PCAP. Accessed February 10, 2014.

Thomson S, Osborn R, Squires DA, Reed SJ. *International Profiles of Health Care Systems*. New York: The Commonwealth Fund; 2011.

U.S. Department of Health and Human Services. 2013 Annual Progress Report to Congress: National Strategy for Quality Improvement in Health Care. Published 2013. http://www.ahrq.gov/workingforquality/nqs/nqs2013annlrpt.pdf. Accessed February 6, 2014.

Woolf SH, Aron LY. The US health disadvantage relative to other high-income countries: findings from a National Research Council/Institute of Medicine report. *JAMA*. 2013;309(8):771-772.

Variations in Care

16

David J. Ballard, Briget da Graca and David Nicewander

HEALTH SCENARIO

Hospital A from the Health Scenario described in Chapter 15 is pleased with the progress it has made in improving performance on the publicly reported Heart Failure Core Measures but is concerned that the improved delivery of these processes of care does not seem to be reducing the 30-day readmission rate for heart failure patients. Hospital A is concerned about the high readmission rate because it suggests there is substantial room for further improvement in the care provided to heart failure patients and because currently the hospital is paying a penalty under the Medicare Readmissions Reduction Program. To learn more about heart failure readmissions and identify effective strategies to reduce them, Hospital A's clinical and quality leaders turn to the published research literature. They learn that there is substantial variation in risk-adjusted heart failure readmission rates among hospitals across the United States, which suggests that the hospitals with higher rates can likely achieve performances closer to those demonstrated by the hospitals with lower rates if they can identify the ways in which their practices, communities, and patient populations differ, enabling revision of the former and appropriate risk adjustment for the latter.

CLINICAL BACKGROUND

Data released by the Centers for Medicare and Medicaid Services (CMS) in 2013 show a median national risk-standardized 30-day unplanned heart failure readmission rate of 22.9% (95% confidence interval [CI], 17.1, 30.7) for Medicare patients. Risk-standardized heart failure readmission rates show distinct geographic patterns: areas with the highest rates are located almost exclusively in Eastern, Southeastern, and Midwestern states, and the majority of areas with rates in the lowest quintile are found in Western states (**Figure 16-1**). Almost 60% of the national variation in publicly reported

risk-standardized 30-day readmission rates (i.e., for heart failure, acute myocardial infarction, and pneumonia) is at the county level, and approximately half of that 60% is explained by county characteristics, including demographic and socioeconomic factors, access to care factors, and nursing home quality factors. County characteristics associated with lower readmission rates include greater numbers of primary care physicians and nursing homes per capita and classification of the county as a rural or retirement area. Characteristics associated with higher readmission rates include greater numbers of specialists and hospital beds per capita and higher proportions of the population that never married, are Medicare beneficiaries, or have low education status and higher percentages of long-stay nursing home patients with pressure ulcers or with an increased need for help. Other research shows higher heart failure readmission rates among patients discharged from public (vs. private nonprofit) hospitals, hospitals without cardiovascular services, hospitals with low levels of nurse staffing, and small hospitals. However, hospitals that partner with community physicians or local hospitals to decrease readmission, that have processes in place to ensure patients' discharge summaries are sent to their primary care physicians, and that assign staff to follow up on test results after discharge have been found to have lower 30-day readmission rates. The variation seen in risk-standardized heart failure readmission rates among hospitals in the United States is evidence of room for improved quality of care; the evidence regarding the sources of this variation indicates that although some improvement may be achieved by a hospital simply changing its own practices (e.g., following up on postdischarge test results), meaningful improvement will require efforts directed broadly toward access to primary care and nursing homes providing good-quality care, as well as greater coordination and collaboration between hospitals and primary care and postacute providers.

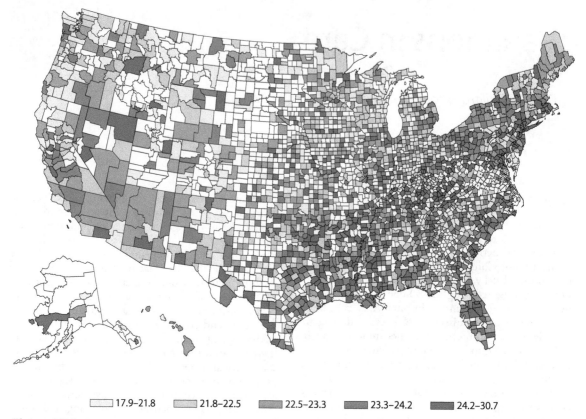

17.9–21.8   21.8–22.5   22.5–23.3   23.3–24.2   24.2–30.7

Figure 16-1. County-level risk-standardized 30-day heart failure readmission rates (%) in Medicare patients by performance quintile for July 2009 to June 2012. (Data from Centers for Medicare & Medicaid Services; available at https://data.medicare.gov/data/hospital-compare.)

HISTORY AND DEFINITIONS

Variation in clinical care, and what it reveals about that care, is a topic of great interest to researchers and clinicians. It can be divided broadly into **outcome variation**, *which occurs when the same process produces different results in different patients*, and **process variation**, *which refers to different usage of a therapeutic or diagnostic procedure among organizations, geographic areas, or other groupings of health care providers.* Studies of outcome variation can provide insight into patient characteristics and care delivery that predispose patients to either a successful or an adverse outcome and help identify patients for whom a particular treatment is likely to be effective (or ineffective). Process variation, in contrast, can provide insight into such things as the underuse of effective therapies or procedures and the overuse of ineffective therapies or procedures.

Study of the variation in clinical care dates back to 1938, when Dr. J. Allison Glover published a study revealing geographic variation in the incidence of tonsillectomy in school children in England and Wales that could not be explained by anything other than variation in medical opinion on the indications for surgery. Since then, research has revealed variation among countries and across a range of medical conditions and procedures, including prostatectomy, knee replacement, arteriovenous fistula dialysis, and invasive cardiac procedures. Actual rates of use of procedures, different variability in supply of health care services, and the system of health care organization and financing (health maintenance organizations [HMOs], fee-for-service [FFS], and national universal health care) do not necessarily determine or even greatly affect the degree of variation in a particular clinical practice. Rather, the degree of variation in use relates more to the characteristics of the procedure. Important characteristics include:

• The degree of professional uncertainty about the diagnosis and treatment of the condition the procedure addresses

- The availability of alternative treatments
- Controversy versus consensus regarding the appropriate use of the procedure
- Differences among physicians in diagnosis style and in belief in the efficacy of a treatment

When studying variation in medical practice—or interpreting the results of someone else's study of variation—it is important to distinguish between **warranted variation**, *which is based on differences in patient preference, disease prevalence, or other patient- or population-related factors*; and **unwarranted variation**, *which cannot be explained by patient preference or condition or the practice of evidence-based medicine.* Whereas warranted variation is the product of providing appropriate and personalized evidence-based patient care, unwarranted variation typically indicates an opportunity to improve some aspect of the quality of care provided, including inefficiencies and disparities in care.

John E. Wennberg, MD, MPH, founding editor of the Dartmouth Atlas of Health Care and a leading scholar in clinical practice variation, defines three categories of care and the implications of unwarranted variation within each of them:

1. *Effective care* is that for which the evidence establishes that the benefits outweigh the risks and the "right rate" of use is 100% of the patients defined by evidence-based guidelines as needing such treatment. In this category, variation in the rate of use within that patient population indicates underuse.

2. *Preference-sensitive care* consists of those areas of care in which there is more than one generally accepted diagnostic or therapeutic option available, so the "right rate" of each depends on patient preference.

3. *Supply-sensitive care* is care for which the frequency of use relates to the capacity of the local health care system. Typically, this is viewed in the context of the delivery of care to patients who are unlikely to benefit from it or whose benefit is uncertain; in areas with high capacity for that care (e.g., high numbers of hospital beds per capita) more of these patients receive the care than in areas with low capacity, where the resources have to be reserved for (and are operating at full capacity with) patients whose benefits are more certain. Because studies have repeatedly shown that regions with high use of supply sensitive care do not perform better on mortality rates or quality of life indicators than regions with low use, variation in such care may indicate overuse. Local health care system capacity can influence frequency of use in other ways, too. For example,

the county-level association between fewer primary care physicians and higher 30-day hospital readmission rates suggests that inadequate primary care capacity may result in preventable hospitalizations.

Table 16-1 provides examples of warranted and unwarranted variation in each of these categories of care.

A second important distinction that must be made when considering variation in care is between **common cause** and **special cause variation**. Common cause variation (*also referred to as "expected" or "random" variation) cannot be traced to a root cause* and as such may not be worth studying in detail. Special cause variation (*or "assignable" variation) arises from a single or small set of causes that can be traced and identified and then implemented or eliminated through targeted quality improvement initiatives*). Statisticians have a broad range of tests and criteria to determine whether variation is assignable or random and with the increasing sensitivity and power of numerical analysis can measure assignable variation relatively easily. The need for statistical expertise in such endeavors must be emphasized, however; the complexity of the study designs and interpretation of results (particularly in distinguishing true variation from artifact or statistical error) carries a high risk of misinterpretation in its absence.

LOCAL VARIATION

Although variation in care processes and outcomes frequently is examined and discussed in terms of large-scale geography (among countries, states, or hospital referral regions, as, for example, was shown in the heart failure readmissions national map in **Figure 16-1**), it can be examined and provide equally useful information on a much smaller scale. For example, **Figure 16-2** shows variation in 30-day risk-adjusted heart failure readmission rates for hospitals within a single county (Dallas, Texas), ranging from 20% below to 25% above the national average and with three hospitals showing readmission rates that were statistically significantly lower than the national average. Although no hospitals had readmission rates that were statistically significantly higher than the national rate, the poorer performing hospitals might nevertheless be interested in improving. Cooperation among the quality and clinical leaders of the hospitals within Dallas County would enable investigation of differences in practices and resources among the hospitals, which might identify areas to be targeted for improvement for those hospitals with higher readmission rates.

Local between-provider variation is often encountered in the form of quality reports or scorecards. Such tools seek to identify high versus low performers

Table 16-1. Examples of warranted and unwarranted variations in heart failure care.

	Warranted Variation	Unwarranted Variation
Effective care	Only 49% of heart failure patients with reduced ejection fraction in Cardiology Practice A are prescribed beta-blockers (which the evidence shows reduce risk of death and hospitalization) compared with 76% in Cardiology Practice B, where 51% of heart failure patients in Practice A and 24% in Practice B had documented contraindications to beta-blockers.	Only 49% of heart failure patients with reduced ejection fraction and no documented contraindications in Cardiology Practice A are prescribed beta-blockers (which the evidence shows reduce risk of death and hospitalization) compared with 100% in Cardiology Practice B.
Preference-sensitive care	Among advanced heart failure patients treated by Dr. X. and Dr. Y. respectively in 2013, 33% and 57% received ICDs. A survey of patient preferences shows that these proportions reflected the fact that more of Dr. X.'s patients preferred the risk of sudden cardiac death associated with not having an ICD implanted to the risks of increased hospitalization and a lingering death with an ICD, but the opposite was true for Dr. Y.'s patients.	Among advanced heart failure patients treated by Dr. X. and Dr. Y. respectively in 2013, 33% and 57% received ICDs. A survey of patient preferences shows that in both physicians' patient populations, 50% of patients preferred the risk of sudden cardiac death (reduced by ICDs) to the risk of increased hospitalizations and a lingering death (increased by ICDs).
Supply-sensitive care	None	Hospitalization rates of Medicare patients with congestive heart failure vary by a factor of 4 across geographic regions of the United States, with approximately half of this variation being explained by the number of staffed hospital beds in the region. The greater resource use in regions with higher hospitalization rates does not translate into better survival.

ICD, implantable cardiac defibrillator.

among hospitals, practices, or physicians to create incentives for high performance either by invoking providers' competitive spirit or by placing a portion of their compensation at risk according to their performance through value-based purchasing or pay-for-performance programs. In other words, they show unwarranted variation in the delivery of care. Care must be taken in presenting and interpreting such variation data, however. For example, league tables (or their graphical equivalent, caterpillar charts), which order providers from the lowest to highest performers on a chosen measure and use CIs to identify providers with performance that is statistically significantly different from the overall average, are both commonly used to compare provider performance on quality measures and easily misinterpreted. One's instinct on encountering such tables or figures is to focus on the numeric ordering of the providers and assume, for example, that a provider ranked in the 75th percentile provides much higher quality care than one in the 25th percentile. This, however, is not necessarily the case: league tables do not capture the degree

of uncertainty around each provider's point estimate, so much of the ordering in the league table reflects random variation, and the order may vary substantially from one measurement period to another, without providers making any meaningful changes in the quality of care they provide. As such, there may not be any statistically significant or meaningful clinical difference among providers even widely separated in the ranking.

Forest plots, such as **Figure 16-2**, for hospitals in Dallas County are a better, although still imperfect, way of comparing provider performance. Forest plots show both the point estimate for the measure of interest (e.g., risk-adjusted heart failure 30-day readmission rates) and its CI (represented by a horizontal line) for each provider, as well as a preselected norm or standard (e.g., national average; represented by a vertical line). By looking for providers for whom not only the point estimate but the *entire* CI falls to either the left or right of the vertical line, readers can identify those whose performance was either significantly better or significantly worse than the preselected standard.

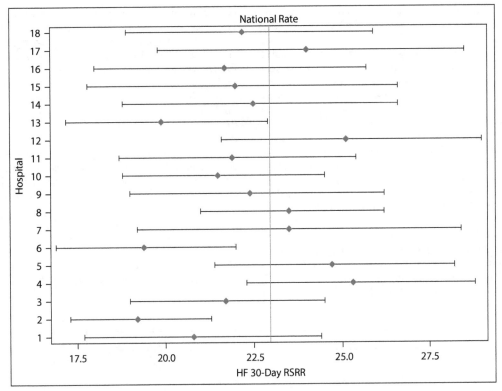

Figure 16-2. Forest plot showing variation in heart failure 30-day risk-standardized readmission rates (HF 30-day RSRR, %) in Medicare patients for hospitals in Dallas County, Texas for July 2009 to June 2012. Hospitals were assigned random number identifiers in place of using names. (Data from Centers for Medicare & Medicaid Services; available at https://data.medicare.gov/data/hospital-compare.)

Although Forest plots may be ordered so that hospitals are ranked according to the point estimates, that ranking is vulnerable to the same misinterpretation as in league tables. An easy way to avoid this problem is to order the providers according to something other than the point estimate—for example, alphabetically by name. Because Forest plots are easy to produce without extensive statistical knowledge or programming skills, such an approach can be very useful in situations in which experienced statisticians are not available to assist with the performance comparisons.

The funnel plot is probably the best approach for presenting comparative performance data, but it does require more sophisticated statistical knowledge to produce. In a funnel plot, the rate or measure of interest is plotted on the y axis against the number of patients treated on the x axis; close to the origin, the CI bands drawn on the plot are wide (where the numbers of patients are small) and narrow as the numbers of patients increase. The resulting funnel shape gives

its name to the plot. Providers with performance falling outside the CI bands are outliers, with performance that may be statistically significantly better or worse than the overall average. Those that excel can be examined as role models to guide others' improvement. Those that lag behind their peers can be considered as opportunities for improvement, which might benefit from targeted interventions. And because the funnel plot does not attempt to rank providers (beyond identifying the outliers), it is less open to misinterpretation by readers who fail to consider the influence of random variation.

Control charts (discussed later in detail in the context of examining variation over time) can be used in a manner similar to funnel plots to compare provider performance. In such control charts, the CI bands of the funnel plot are replaced with upper and lower control limits (typically calculated as ±3 standard deviations [SDs] from the mean [or other measure of central tendency]), and providers need not be ordered according to decreasing number of patients in the denominator of the measure of interest. As in the funnel plot, however, the providers whose performance is statistically significantly higher (or lower) than the mean are identified as those for whom the point estimate falls above the upper (or below the lower) control limit. **Figure 16-3** shows an example of such a control chart for the risk-adjusted 30-day heart failure readmission rates for the hospitals in Dallas County, Texas. Unlike the forest plot in **Figure 16-2**, which compares each hospital's performance with the national average, **Figure 16-3** considers only the variation among the hospitals located in Dallas County. As can be seen, no data points fall outside the control limits. Interpretation of control charts is discussed in greater detail later, but this suggests that all the variation in the readmission rates among these hospitals is explained by common cause variation (not attributable to any specific cause) rather than by any specific difference in the hospitals' characteristics or practices. This is interesting in light of the **Figure 16-2** results, which show that three hospitals' readmission

rates differed significantly from the national average. However, it should be kept in mind, first, that the CIs used to make this determination in **Figure 16-2** are set at 95% compared with the control limits in **Figure 16-3** which are set at 3 SDs (corresponding to 99.73%) for reasons explained in the following section. Second, **Figure 16-3** draws only on the data for 18 hospitals, which is a much smaller sample than the national data, and the smaller number of observations results in relatively wide control limits.

Finally, variation can be studied at the most local level: within a provider—even within a single physician—over time. Such variation is best examined using control charts, discussed in detail in the next section.

QUANTITATIVE METHODS OF STUDYING VARIATION

Data-driven practice-variation research is an important diagnostic tool for health care policymakers and clinicians, revealing areas of care where best practices

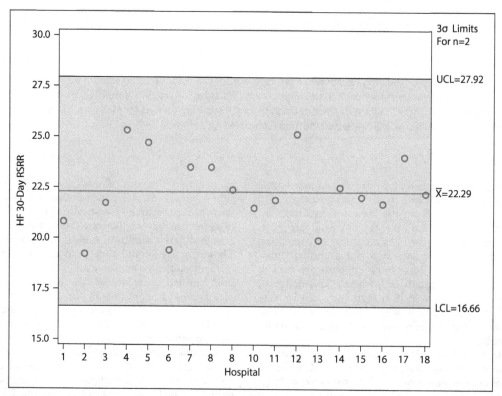

Figure 16-3. Control chart showing variation in heart failure 30-day risk-standardized readmission rates (HF 30-day RSRR, %) in Medicare patients for hospitals in Dallas County for July 2009 to June 2012). Hospitals were assigned random number identifiers in place of using names. LCL, lower control limit; UCL, upper control limit. (Data from Centers for Medicare & Medicaid Services; available at https://data.medicare.gov/data/hospital-compare.)

may need to be identified or—if already identified—implemented. It compares utilization rates in a given setting or by a given provider with an average utilization rate; in this it differs from appropriateness of use and patient safety studies, which compare utilization rates with an identified "right rate" and serve as ongoing performance management tools.

A good framework to investigate unwarranted variation should provide:

1. A scientific basis for including or excluding each influencing factor and to determine when the factor is applicable or not applicable
2. A clear definition and explanation of each factor suggested as a cause
3. An explanation of how the factor is operationalized, measured, and integrated with other factors

Statistical Process Control and Control Charts

Statistical process control (SPC), similar to continuous quality improvement, is an approach originally developed in the context of industrial manufacturing for the improvement of systems processes and outcomes and was adopted into health care contexts only relatively recently. The basic principles of SPC are summarized in **Table 16-2**. Particularly in the United States, SPC has been enthusiastically embraced for quality improvement and applied in a wide range of health care settings and specialties and at all levels of health care delivery, from individual patients and providers to entire hospitals and health care systems. Its appeal

Table 16-2. Basic principles of statistical process control.

1. Individual measurements of any process or outcome will show variation.
2. If the process or outcome is stable (i.e., subject only to common cause variation), the variation is predictable and will be described by one of several statistical distributions (e.g., normal [or bell-shaped], exponential, or Poisson distribution).
3. Special cause variation will result in measured values that deviate from these models in some observable way (e.g., fall outside the predicted range of variation).
4. When the process or outcome is in control, statistical limits and tests for values that deviate from predictions can be established, providing statistical evidence of change.

and value lie in its integration of the power of statistical significance tests with chronological analyses of graphs of summary data as the data are produced. This enables similar insights into the data that classical tests of significance provide but with the time sensitivity so important to pragmatic improvement. Moreover, the relatively simple formulae and graphical displays used in SPC are generally easily understood and applied by nonstatistician decision makers, making this a powerful tool in communicating with patients, other clinicians, and administrative leaders and policymakers. **Table 16-3** summarizes important benefits and limitations of SPC in health care contexts.

Table 16-3. Benefits and limitations of statistical process control in health care.

Benefits	Limitations
• Easy to use • Typically requires smaller volumes of data than traditional statistical analysis • Helps describe and quantify variability in clinical processes and outcomes • Helps distinguish special from common cause variation • Helps identify opportunities for improvement • Helps assess the impact of quality improvement interventions on health care processes • Provides a common language for communication between clinicians and managers (or clinicians and patients) working to improve the same health care process or outcome. • Enables patients with chronic conditions to become active partners in clinical management	• Ease of use can be deceptive—the ability of stakeholders to *correctly* apply SPC may be limited • Statistical control does not necessarily equate to clinical control or desired performance • Identification of a change with statistical significance does not typically identify the specific cause of the change • When used to examine health care outcomes, patient risk factors must be adequately adjusted for • Typically not well suited to analyzing rare events • Because SPC relies on the assumption of independence of data collected over time, the autocorrelation (in which the preceding observation predicts the next observation) present in many health care measures limits the ability to apply SPC or requires the application of special purpose control charts

SPC, statistical process control.

Tools used in SPC include control charts, run charts, frequency plots, histograms, Pareto analysis, scatter diagrams, and flow diagrams, but control charts are the primary and dominant tools.

Control charts are time series plots that show not only the plotted values but also upper and lower reference thresholds (calculated using historical data) that define the range of the common cause variation for the process or outcome of interest. When all the data points fall between these thresholds (i.e., only common cause variation is present), the process is said to be "in control." Points that fall outside the reference thresholds may indicate special cause variation due to events or changes in circumstances that were not typical before. Such events or changes may be positive or negative, making control charts useful both as a warning tool in a system that usually performs well and as a tool to test or verify the effectiveness of a quality improvement intervention deliberately introduced in a system with historically poor performance.

The specific type of control chart needed for a particular measure depends on the type of data being analyzed, as well as the behavior and assumed underlying statistical distribution. The choice of the correct control chart is essential to obtaining meaningful results. **Table 16-4** matches the most common data types and characteristics for the appropriate control chart(s).

After the appropriate control chart has been determined, further issues include (1) how the upper and lower control limit thresholds will be set, (2) what statistical rules will be applied to separate special cause variation from common cause variation, and (3) how many data points need to be plotted and at what time intervals.

Broadly speaking, the width of the control limit interval must balance the risk between falsely identifying special cause variation where it does not exist (type I statistical error) and missing it where it does (type II statistical error). Typically, the upper and lower control limits are set at ±3 SDs from the estimated mean of the measure of interest. This range is expected to capture 99.73% of all plotted data compared with the 95% captured by the 2 SDs criterion typically used in traditional hypothesis testing techniques. This difference is important because, unlike in the traditional hypothesis test in which the risk of type I error (false positive) applies only once, in a control chart, the risk applies to *each* plotted point. Thus, in a control chart with 25 plotted points, the cumulative risk of a false positive is $1 - (0.9973)^{25} =$ 6.5% when 3 SD control limits are used compared with $1 - (0.95)^{25} = 72.3\%$ when 2 SD limits are used.

The primary test for special cause variation, then, is a data point that falls outside the upper or lower control limit. Other common tests are listed in **Table 16-5**. Although applying these additional tests does slightly increase the false-positive rate from that inherent in the control limit settings, they greatly increase the control chart's sensitivity to improvements or deteriorations in the measure. The statistical "trick" here lies in observing special cause patterns and accumulating

Table 16-4. Appropriate control charts according to data type and distribution.

Data type	Assumed Distribution	Control Chart
Continuous variable[a]		
Multiple samples collected during each time period	Normal[b]	x̄-Chart (mean) and s-chart (SD)
Individual measure for each time period	Normal[b]	x-Chart
Discrete (attribute) variable		
Count	Poisson	c-Chart (count)
Rate[c]	Poisson	u-Chart (rate)
Proportion	Binomial	p-Chart (proportion)
Bernoulli random variable[d]	Geometric	g-Chart

[a]The temptation to collect continuous data as, or convert it into, discrete (attribute) data (categories, or a count of how frequently a particular standard was met) should be resisted; this causes unnecessary loss of information, which in turn causes loss of ability to detect important changes.

[b]For skewed continuous data (e.g., lognormal or exponential distribution) x̄- and x-charts may not perform well, particularly if the sample taken at each time point is small. In such situations, consult a statistician to calculate the limits from the appropriate distribution or, if appropriate, apply a normalizing transformation that will allow use of an x̄- or x-chart.

[c]Rates are generally more informative than counts, particularly when the opportunity for the event varies over time (e.g., number of central line infections per 1000 device-use days is more informative than just the number of central line infections).

[d]The outcome of interest is known for each individual patient (e.g., whether or not each surgery patient developed a surgical site infection), so that each case can be considered a binomial variable with a sample size of 1. The g-chart assumes an underlying geometric distribution and would plot the total number of surgery patients until an infection occurs.

SD, standard deviation.

Table 16-5. Common control chart tests for special cause variation.

- 1 point outside the upper or lower control limit
- 2 of 3 successive points more than 2 SDs from the mean on the same side of the center line
- 4 of 5 successive points more than 1 SD from the mean on the same side of the center line
- 8 successive points on the same side of the center line
- 6 successive points increasing or decreasing
- Obvious cyclic behavior

SD, standard deviation.

information while waiting for the total sample size to increase to the point where it has the power to detect a statistically significant difference. The volume of data needed for a control chart depends on:

1. The type of control chart used
2. How the data have been organized and collected
3. The distributional characteristics of the data (determining these may require collection of preliminary data points, prior to the calculation of the control limits)
4. How rapidly a change needs to be detectable (larger sampler sizes will enable more rapid detection)

It should also be kept in mind that 20 to 30 data points are generally needed for the initial calculation of the control limits.

Ultimately, the quality of information that can be obtained from a control chart depends on the quality of the data collection (including sampling and risk adjustment) and correct application of the methods (including selection of the appropriate type of control chart and application of appropriate tests for special cause variation). Both of these aspects are frequently more challenging in the health care context than in the industrial manufacturing setting for which SPC was developed. As discussed in Chapter 15, health care outcomes are influenced by a wide range of demographic, clinical, societal, and environmental factors that need to be adjusted for to enable identification of special cause variation (or, alternatively, that need to be considered as the special causes of variation). However, with process measures, it is essential that the population in which the delivery of the health care process is being measured is defined accurately to include patients who will benefit and exclude patients who will not. Likewise, with respect to the correct application of the statistical methods, many important health care measures do not behave as "tidily" as their manufacturing counterparts, making them more likely to violate

the assumptions on which control charts depend and therefore require special treatment. Autocorrelation—which violates the control chart's assumption that all data collected over time are independent—is a common characteristic of many health care clinical and quality measures, particularly when the measurements are being taken in the same patient or for the same provider over time. Positive autocorrelation (in which large values tend to follow large values and small values follow small values) causes some types of control charts (e.g., x-charts with limits based on moving ranges) to have high false-positive rates for special cause variation. Systematic seasonal variation (e.g., day-of-the-week effect) likewise causes problems. If the autocorrelation or seasonal variation is not considered part of the "natural" process, it should be removed if possible—for example, by sampling the data less frequently. When this is not the case (or is not possible), more advanced statistical methods are needed to construct an appropriate control chart. One recommended approach for dealing with autocorrelation illustrates how complicated the "easy-to-use" SPC approach can become under these circumstances. It requires the development of a time series model to predict values one step ahead of each measurement, so that the one-step-ahead forecast errors (or residuals) can be calculated from the observed values and then plotted on a control chart.

Finally, having identified apparent incidents of special cause variation from a control chart, it remains necessary to investigate the underlying causes. When the purpose of the investigation of variation is to verify the effectiveness of a deliberate quality improvement intervention, this may be a relatively simple matter of comparing timing of the special cause variation with that of the implementation, and checking that no simultaneous changes were made that could affect the measure in question. When the investigation was done to identify opportunities for improvement, underlying causes may be harder to determine, and after they have been determined require characterization as either warranted variation (indicating the need for better risk adjustment in the measure of interest) or unwarranted variation (indicating the need for quality improvement action).

Figure 16-4 shows a control chart for Hospital A's performance on the publicly reported heart failure process of care measure "angiotensin converting enzyme inhibitor or angiotensin receptor blocker for left ventricular systolic dysfunction" before and after implementing the standardized order set for heart failure care as part of its quality improvement efforts (see Chapter 15). Early during the preimplementation phase (July 2006–December 2007), this process of care was not "in control" (as shown by the September 2006 data point falling below the lower control limit) and showed substantial room for improvement. Although the later months of the preimplementation period

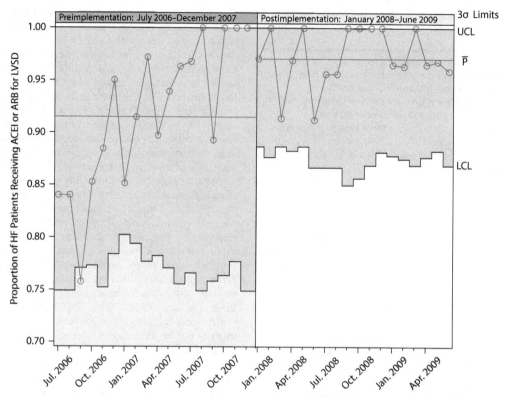

Figure 16-4. p-Chart showing the proportion of heart failure patients with left ventricular systolic dysfunction (LVSD) who were prescribed an angiotensin converting enzyme inhibitor (ACEI) or angiotensin receptor blocker (ARB) before and after Hospital A (from the Health Scenario in Chapters 15 and 16) deployed a standardized heart failure order set. LCL, lower control limit; UCL, upper control limit.

show generally better performance and no evidence of special cause variation, there was nonetheless still room for improvement and for consistency in good performance. After implementation of the heart failure order set (January 2008–June 2009), Hospital A shows not only statistical control for this process of care but also evidence of successful quality improvement: the mean performance line has risen closer to 100%, and the control limit range has narrowed, indicating reduced variability around that higher performance.

FACTORS INFLUENCING VARIATION

Variation in clinical practice has been studied from the perspective of multiple frameworks, which have identified diverse factors that appear to underlie unwarranted variation. These include:

- Inadequate patient involvement in decision making
- Inequitable access to resources
- Poor communication, role confusion, and misinterpretation or misapplication of relevant clinical evidence

- Clinician uncertainty in defining disease, making a diagnosis, selecting a procedure, observing outcomes, assessing probabilities, and assigning preferences
- Providers' economic incentives

In frameworks that focus on economic incentives as drivers of unwarranted variation, physicians are seen as taking advantage of their dual role as the seller of a service and the agent for the buyer (patient) to influence demand for a service. Support for this hypothesis is found in such evidence as the significantly higher rate of negative findings in magnetic resonance images of the knee among those ordered by physicians with a financial interest in the imaging equipment compared with those without. When the images were interpreted by the same radiologists, the actual numbers and distributions of subtypes and severities of abnormalities in the positive findings were similar between the groups, and the ordering physicians practiced within the same community and had similar training. Such models have, however, been criticized as misinterpreting physician behavior by underestimating the market implications of uncertainty in diagnosing and treating disease.

An alternative point of view characterizes variation as the product of differences in "belief sets" held by individual physicians. Factors influencing these belief sets, and thus potential sources of variation, are both endogenous (e.g., education and ability) and exogenous (e.g., reimbursement structures, role models, organizational policies, patients' economic constraints), with the exogenous forces having the ability to overcome the endogenous, to produce conformity with local practice. In this context, physicians are viewed as demanding resources consistent with patients' clinical needs, as determined by their educational and experiential backgrounds but modified by local exogenous influences, including the patient's financial resources and access to care, the policies and protocols of the hospital or health care organization within which the physician practices, and environmental constraints such as the number of hospital beds or other facilities per capita.

Reimbursement mechanisms have substantial influence on practice patterns. For example, a Medicare demonstration project conducted in the 1990s showed that switching from a reimbursement structure that applied fixed-dollar amount, diagnosis-related group payments to hospitals but fee-for-service payments to physicians providing care to patients during hospitalization to one that pooled the physician and institutional payments into a single, fixed-dollar amount per admission for coronary artery bypass graft surgery (CABG) resulted in several significant changes in practice, including (1) introduction of same-day admissions, (2) use of less expensive contrast media, (3) standardization of materials used during surgery, (4) shorter operating room times and turnovers, (5) reductions in both intensive care unit and total hospital length of stay, and (6) reductions in the numbers of medical consultations. Importantly, these changes, which generated substantial cost savings, did not result in any increases in either short-term or 1-year mortality rates.

Exogenous factors can influence variation in more ways than just the direct impact on individual clinical decisions. For example, physicians might choose the community or organization they practice within to match their aggressive or nonaggressive intervention style, perpetuating that style in both the individual physician and the community, or they might adapt their practice style to the expectations of the local community or to maintain their income in response to local market forces. Practice intensity is undeniably correlated with local health care spending. Although research shows little variation in the likelihood that physicians will recommend guideline-supported interventions during any particular encounter, those in high-spending areas see patients more frequently, recommend more tests of uncertain benefit, and opt for more resource-intensive interventions without achieving better patient outcomes.

APPLYING EVIDENCE OF VARIATION TO IMPROVE QUALITY OF CARE

Evidence based medicine is the conscientious, explicit, and judicious use of current best evidence in making decisions about the care of individual patients. The practice of evidence based medicine means integrating individual clinical expertise with the best available external clinical evidence from systematic research. (Sacket and colleagues, 1996).

Evidence-based medicine and variations in clinical practice thus inform one another. The "clinical evidence from systematic research" (and particularly from comparative effectiveness research) that underlies evidence-based medicine also is what enables classification of processes of care as effective, preference sensitive, or supply sensitive and what underlies the identification of warranted versus unwarranted variations in care. With these distinctions in place, evidence of variation in clinical practice provides information on how truly evidence based the delivery of care is and can help identify opportunities for improvement—either for individual providers or for geographic regions.

In **effective care**, *best practices have been identified and the goal is delivery of that care to 100% of the patients who fall within the population for which the procedure or treatment is known to be effective and who do not have any contraindications.* This is frequently assessed in terms of compliance with clinical guidelines. However, the popularity of the "evidence-based bandwagon" has led to numerous individuals, organizations, and insurers producing overlapping, sometimes poorly constructed, guidelines such that the benefits of consistency are often lost in the resulting confusion. As such, the source and quality of any guideline needs to be assessed before it is implemented or used as a standard to assess the quality of care provided. When a well-constructed evidence-based guideline is identified, physicians, hospitals, and other health care organizations can use it as the basis for a variety of quality improvement tools in their efforts to reduce unwarranted variation in effective care, including benchmarking and report cards, academic detailing, and pay-for-performance programs. However, the ability to monitor variation patterns and relate them to outcomes is limited to health care providers with the necessary patient volume and infrastructure (e.g., electronic medical records, data analysts) to collect and analyze these data on an ongoing basis.

In **preference-sensitive care**, *evidence of unwarranted variation calls first for comparative effectiveness research to uncover and elucidate differences between available treatment options that will enable selection of the option that best meets the individual patient's concerns and priorities, complemented by greater involvement of patients in their treatment decisions.* Such efforts fall squarely within the "patient-centeredness" domain of health care quality improvement, and increasingly hospitals report initiatives to increase patient engagement and education among their quality improvement strategies. Progress on reducing unwarranted variation is harder to measure than for effective care because the "right rate" depends on patient preference, which is neither easily known nor independent of contextual factors that can change rapidly and without warning. Ironically, although increasing informed patient involvement will decrease *unwarranted* variation in preference-sensitive care by bringing utilization rates into line with patient preferences, it might increase *total* variation because patients, coming from varied backgrounds and contexts, might have more diverse preferences than their physicians, who share a generally similar educational background and training.

With respect to **supply-sensitive care,** *evidence of unwarranted variation suggests the need for quality improvement strategies that target the elimination of overuse.* Such efforts must be supported by evidence from outcomes research that demonstrates equivalent patient outcomes (e.g., mortality, morbidity, and quality of life) between areas of high and low use. Furthermore, to ensure that efforts to eliminate overuse do not drive practice too far in the opposite direction (toward underuse), effectiveness or comparative effectiveness research is needed to better define the population that truly benefits from the care in question and the patient preferences that need to be considered in defining those benefits.

VARIATION DATA AND NATIONAL HEALTH CARE POLICY

Variation data play important roles in designing and maintaining national health care policies intended to improve quality of care and to reduce costs. For example, the evidence that practice patterns can be strongly influenced simply by the way providers' compensation is structured (discussed earlier in the context of physician and hospital compensation for care provided to CABG patients) has sparked interest in the potential that bundled payments—which provide a fixed dollar amount per patient for an "episode of care"—have to inspire providers along the continuum of care to maximize the coordination and efficiency of their services. (An episode of care is defined by Section 3023 of the Patient Protection and Affordable Care Act to cover all care from 3 days before hospitalization through 30 days after discharge, including all acute care inpatient services, all inpatient and outpatient physician services, all outpatient and emergency department hospital services, and postacute care.) Currently, the CMS is testing four bundled payment models covering a variety of specific medical and surgical diagnosis-related groups. Although the obvious

target of bundled payments is the reduction of ineffective or duplicative care (i.e., overuse of supply-sensitive care), they should also discourage underuse of effective care because this can cause greater costs to be incurred further down the continuum of care.

A second area of national health policy in which the use of variation data can be seen in Medicare's public reporting, Hospital Value-Based Purchasing (VBP), and Readmissions Reductions Programs described in Chapter 15. First, variation is important in the selection of the quality measures required for public reporting and used for the Hospital VBP program. As discussed in Chapter 15, quality measures used for improvement initiatives need to be "current" in the sense that they are defined to reflect both the recent evidence regarding effective care and a current opportunity (and priority) for improvement. In other words, they represent an area of care with unwarranted variation—generally either underuse of effective care or overuse of supply-sensitive care. When measures "top out" with almost all providers routinely achieving near optimal performance (i.e., little or no remaining unwarranted variation), the measure needs to be replaced with one representing a new priority for improvement. For example, when the measures to be used to determine hospitals' quality scores for Medicare's Hospital VBP program in fiscal year 2015 were being selected, two of those included in the set publicly reported on the Hospital Compare website ("surgery patients with perioperative temperature management" and "acute myocardial infarction patients with statins prescribed at discharge") were omitted specifically because all but a few hospitals have achieved a similarly high level of performance on them. Variation data drive these selection and retirement decisions. Second, the Hospital VBP and Readmissions Reduction Programs rely (albeit not rigorously) on variation in the structure of the incentive awards and penalties. In the Hospital VBP Program, hospitals' performance scores are calculated according to how much they improved on a particular measure from a baseline period (i.e., essentially looking for special cause variation that indicates successful quality improvement efforts) or how far their performance during the measurement period exceeds the threshold set at the 50th percentile of all hospitals' performance during the baseline period (i.e., trying to identify and reward the hospitals that are not underusing effective care or overusing supply-sensitive care). Similarly, the Readmissions Reduction Program penalizes hospitals with "excess" 30-day risk-adjusted readmissions relative to the national average, using variation among the hospitals to divide them into good and poor performers. Among the criticisms of these programs is the concern that, similar to lending too much weight to the ranking assigned to providers in league tables, these methods do not adequately consider the influence of common cause variation on providers' relative performance in any given measurement period. Better approaches might be along the lines of the funnel plots suggested earlier for provider performance comparisons, which limit themselves to identifying the statistical outliers—those whose high or low performance can almost certainly not be explained by common cause variation.

SUMMARY

Patient outcomes and the use of various diagnostic and therapeutic procedures or treatments can vary greatly over time, among providers, and among geographic regions. To the extent that *variation is explained by differences in patient preference, disease prevalence, or other patient- or population-related factors*, it is **warranted** and reflects the delivery of personalized, evidence-based care. **Unwarranted** variation is *that which cannot be explained by such factors and may indicate opportunities to improve the quality of care provided.*

When unwarranted variation is observed in risk-adjusted patient outcomes, it may indicate disparities in the care patients have access to or receive or may indicate that additional research is needed to identify the patient-related risk factors for which the outcome needs to be adjusted.

When unwarranted variation is observed in processes of care, its interpretation depends on the type of care to which that process belongs:

1. Unwarranted variation in **effective care** (*that for which the evidence establishes that the benefits outweigh the risks*) may indicate underuse when the rate of use is less than 100% among the eligible patient population.

2. Unwarranted variation in **preference-sensitive care** (*that in which there is more than one generally accepted diagnostic or therapeutic option available*) indicates a need for greater patient involvement in the decision-making process to ensure the option selected best meets the individual patient's concerns and priorities.

3. Unwarranted variation in **supply-sensitive care** (*that for which the frequency of use relates to the capacity of the local health care system*) may indicate overuse when rates of use are high.

When considering variation from the perspective of monitoring or improving quality of care, **common cause variation** (*which cannot be traced to a root cause*) needs to be distinguished from **special cause variation** (*which arises from a single or small set of causes that can be traced and identified*). Identification of the latter and tracing the underlying causes can form the basis for targeted quality improvement interventions, either seeking to eliminate underlying causes that have negative effects

on quality or to standardize and disseminate underlying causes that have positive effects. Statistics offers a variety of tools to help identify incidents of special cause variation, the primary one being the control chart.

Control charts are time series plots showing the plotted values together with upper and lower reference thresholds that define the range of the natural variation for the measure. When all the data points fall between these thresholds, the measure is "in control," meaning that only common cause variation is present. Data points that fall outside the reference thresholds may indicate occurrences of special cause variation. These occurrences may be either unintentional or the result of a deliberate intervention, such as the implementation of a quality improvement intervention. As such, control charts are useful both as a warning tool in a system that typically performs well and as a tool to test the effectiveness of a quality improvement intervention.

Factors that underlie unwarranted variation—and that can therefore be targeted in quality improvement efforts—are diverse, ranging from inadequate patient involvement in decision making and inequitable access to care to clinician uncertainty and economic incentives. As such, meaningful improvements in achieving desirable rates of use across the spectrum of effective, preference-sensitive, and supply-sensitive care will likely require coordinated cooperation across all stakeholders in the health care system, including patients; individual clinicians; health care organizations; payers; and local, state, and federal government entities.

Reflecting these diverse causes and the need to address them, the uses of variation data are not limited to health services research and local quality improvement efforts; they also underlie the selection of quality measures for national public reporting initiatives, the Medicare Hospital VBP and Readmissions Reduction Programs, and the demonstration projects currently underway to investigate the potential for bundled payments to influence clinical practice patterns toward greater efficiency and coordination across the full continuum of care a patient accesses during a care episode.

STUDY QUESTIONS

1. *Variation in clinical practice is evidence of poor-quality care.*

   A. *Always*

   B. *Never*

   C. *Only if the clinical practice is preference sensitive*

   D. *None of the above*

2. The three categories of care Wennberg defined for the purpose of studying variation in clinical processes are

A. warranted, unwarranted, and preference sensitive.

B. variably used, underused, and overused.

C. effective, preference sensitive, and supply sensitive.

D. preference sensitive, supply sensitive, and provider sensitive.

3. Variation in a clinical process or outcome is warranted when

A. it is explained by differences in patient preference, disease prevalence, or other patient- or population-related factors.

B. it occurs within a provider's patient population over time but not when it occurs among providers in different geographic regions.

C. it is explained by physicians' preferences and habits developed during clinical training.

D. a control chart plotted for the clinical process or outcome measure shows it to be in statistical control.

4. Unwarranted variation in an effective clinical process suggests

A. the correct rate of use is equal to the average rate of use among all providers.

B. underuse where this process of care is provided to less than 100% of the patient population in which the evidence shows its benefits outweigh the risks.

C. there is a need for greater patient involvement in decisions about care.

D. there is a need for better risk adjustment in the statistical model.

5. Which of the following is true?

A. Special cause variation arises from a single or small set of causes that can be traced and identified

B. Incidents of special cause variation can be useful in identifying opportunities and targets for quality improvement

C. Common cause variation cannot be traced to root causes

D. All of the above are true

6. Factors that can contribute to unwarranted variation in use of clinical processes include

A. patients' preferences and risk factors.

B. physicians' belief sets and economic incentives.

C. both of the above.

D. none of the above.

Questions 7 to 10 refer to the following control chart:

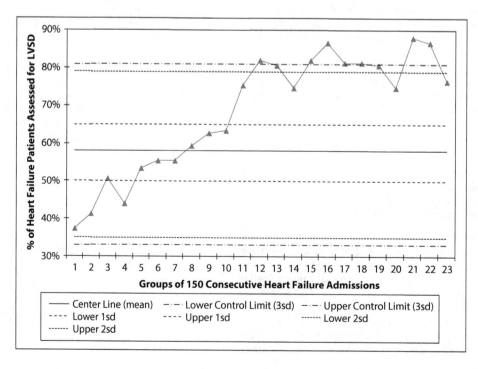

7. In the control chart above, the upper and lower control limits (3 standard deviation [SDs])

    A. represent the hospital's baseline performance and quality improvement target for this heart failure quality measure.

    B. define the range of the common cause variation for the hospital's performance on this heart failure quality measure.

    C. represent the best and worst performance on this heart failure quality measure by individual physician who treated patients admitted for heart failure during the measurement period.

    D. none of the above.

8. Applying all the tests for special cause variation listed in **Table 16-5**,

    A. for groups 1 to 11, the process is in statistical control.

    B. for groups 12 to 23, the evidence of special cause variation indicates poor quality of care.

    C. both of the above.

    D. neither of the above.

9. Assume the control chart above is for Hospital A and that the heart failure order set developed to help improve its performance on the publicly reported heart failure quality measures was implemented between the last admission included in group 4 and the first admission included in group 5. Also, that no other intentional or unintentional changes were made related to the delivery of heart failure processes of care thereafter. Applying all of the tests for special cause variation from **Table 16-5**, what is the earliest point at which the control chart suggests the order set was effective in improving performance on the "Assessment of heart failure patients for left ventricular systolic dysfunction [LVSD]" measure? Note that performance in groups 6 and 7 is identical (neither increases nor decreases).

    A. Group 10 because this is the sixth successive point after group 4 without any decreases, and no other test for special cause variation was met first

    B. Group 14 because groups 10 to 14 make up five successive points more than 1 SD from the mean above the center line, and no other test for special cause variation was met first

    C. Group 12 because it is the first point outside the upper control limit (set at 3 SDs from the

mean), and no other test for special cause variation was met first

    D. Nowhere because at no point are there more points above the upper control limit than below it

10. In the control chart above, the upper and lower control limits were set at ±3 SDs from the mean, a range expected to catch 99.73% of all plotted data, assuming a normal distribution. As such, the cumulative risk of a false positive for an occurrence of special cause variation (applying only the test of whether of point falls outside the control limits or not) was _____. If the control limits had been set at ±2 SDs, this cumulative risk would have been _____

    A. 6.5%; 72.3%.

    B. 6.0%; 69.3%.

    C. 1.3%; 37.0%.

    D. Unable to determine.

FURTHER READING

Center for the Evaluative Clinical Sciences. Effective Care: A Dartmouth Atlas Project Topic Brief. http://www.dartmouthatlas.org/downloads/reports/effective_care.pdf.

Center for the Evaluative Clinical Sciences. Preference Sensitive Care: A Dartmouth Atlas Project Topic Brief. http://www.dartmouthatlas.org/downloads/reports/preference_sensitive.pdf.

Center for the Evaluative Clinical Sciences. Supply Sensitive Care: A Dartmouth Atlas Project Topic Brief. http://www.dartmouthatlas.org/downloads/reports/supply_sensitive.pdf.

Provost LP, Murray SK. Case studies using Shewart charts. In: *The Health Care Data Guide: Learning from Data for Improvement.* San Francisco: Jossey-Bass; 2011:371-434.

van Dishoeck AM, Looman CW, van der Wilden-van Lier EC, Mackenbach JP, Steyerberg EW. Displaying random variation in comparing hospital performance. *BMJ Qual Saf.* 2011;20:651-657.

REFERENCES

Clinical Background

Bradley EH, Curry L, Horwitz LI, et al. Hospital strategies associated with 30-day readmission rates for patients with heart failure. *Circ Cardiovasc Qual Outcomes.* 2013;6(4):444-450.

Herrin J, St Andre J, Kenward K, Joshi MS, Audet AM, Hines SC. Community factors and hospital readmission rates. *Health Serv Res.* 2014 Apr 9. doi:10.1111/1475-6773.12177. [Epub ahead of print].

Joynt KE, Jha AK. Who has higher readmission rates for heart failure, and why? Implications for efforts to improve care using financial incentives. *Circ Cardiovasc Qual Outcomes.* 2011;4(1):53-59.

Suter LG, Li SX, Grady JN, et al. National patterns of risk-standardized mortality and readmission after hospitalization for acute myocardial infarction, heart failure, and pneumonia: update on publicly reported outcomes measures based on the 2013 release. *J Gen Intern Med.* 2014;29(10):1333-1340.

History and Definitions

Gauld R, Horwitt J, Williams S, Cohen AB. What strategies do US hospitals employ to reduce unwarranted clinical practice variations? *Am J Med Qual.* 2011;26(2):120-126.

Glover JA. The incidence of tonsillectomy in school children: (Section of Epidemiology and State Medicine). *Proc R Soc Med.* 1938;31(10):1219-1236.

Katz BP, Freund DA, Heck DA, et al. Demographic variation in the rate of knee replacement: a multi-year analysis. *Health Serv Res.* 1996;31(2):125-140.

Lu-Yao GL, Greenberg ER. Changes in prostate cancer incidence and treatment in USA. *Lancet.* 1994;343(8892):251-254.

McPherson K, Wennberg JE, Hovind OB, Clifford P. Small-area variations in the use of common surgical procedures: an international comparison of New England, England, and Norway. *N Engl J Med.* 1982;307(21):1310-1314.

Peterson PN, Chan PS, Spertus JA, et al. Practice-level variation in use of recommended medications among outpatients with heart failure: Insights from the NCDR PINNACLE program. *Circ Heart Fail.* 2013;6(6):1132-1138.

Powell AE, Davies HT, Thomson RG. Using routine comparative data to assess the quality of health care: understanding and avoiding common pitfalls. *Qual Saf Health Care.* 2003;12(2):122-128.

Rayner HC. Tackling practice variation. Lessons from variation can help change health policy. *BMJ.* 2011;342:d2271.

Samsa G, Oddone EZ, Horner R, Daley J, Henderson W, Matchar DB. To what extent should quality of care decisions be based on health outcomes data? Application to carotid endarterectomy. *Stroke.* 2002;33(12):2944-2949.

Sejr T, Andersen TF, Madsen M, et al. Prostatectomy in Denmark. Regional variation and the diffusion of medical technology 1977-1985. *Scand J Urol Nephrol.* 1991;25(2):101-106.

Wennberg J. Time to tackle unwarranted variations in practice. *BMJ.* 2011;342:d1513.

Wennberg JE. Variation in use of Medicare services among regions and selected academic medical centers: is more better? Published 2005. http://www.commonwealthfund.org/~/media/files/publications/fund-report/2005/dec/variation-in-use-of-medicare-services-among-regions-and-selected-academic-medical-centers--is-more-b/874_wennberg_variation_medicaresvcs-pdf.pdf. Accessed July 10, 2014.

Wennberg JE, Barnes BA, Zubkoff M. Professional uncertainty and the problem of supplier-induced demand. *Soc Sci Med.* 1982;16(7):811-824.

Wennberg DE, Kellett MA, Dickens JD, Malenka DJ, Keilson LM, Keller RB. The association between local diagnostic testing intensity and invasive cardiac procedures. *JAMA.* 1996;275(15):1161-1164.

Westert GP, Faber M. Commentary: the Dutch approach to unwarranted medical practice variation. *BMJ.* 2011;342:d1429.

Westert GP, Groenewegen PP, Boshuizen HC, Spreeuwenberg PM, Steultjens MP. Medical practice variations in hospital care; time trends of a spatial phenomenon. *Health Place.* 2004;10(3):215-220.

Wheeler DJ. *Understanding Variation: The Key to Managing Chaos.* 2nd ed. Knoxville, TN: SPC Press; 2000.

Local Variation and Performance Comparisons

van Dishoeck AM, Looman CW, van der Wilden-van Lier EC, Mackenbach JP, Steyerberg EW. Displaying random variation in comparing hospital performance. *BMJ Qual Saf.* 2011;20(8):651-657.

Woodall WH, Adams BM, Benneyan JC. The Use of control charts in healthcare. In: Faltin F, Kenett R, Ruggeri F, eds. *Statistical Methods in Healthcare.* Chichester, England: Wiley; 2012:253-265.

Quantitative Methods for Studying Variation

Benneyan JC, Lloyd RC, Plsek PE. Statistical process control as a tool for research and healthcare improvement. *Qual Saf Health Care.* 2003;12(6):458-464.

Mercuri M, Gafni A. Medical practice variations: what the literature tells us (or does not) about what are warranted and unwarranted variations. *J Eval Clin Pract.* 2011;17(4):671-677.

Parente ST, Phelps CE, O'Connor PJ. Economic analysis of medical practice variation between 1991 and 2000: the impact of patient outcomes research teams (PORTs). *Int J Technol Assess Health Care.* 2008;24(3):282-293.

Thor J, Lundberg J, Ask J, et al. Application of statistical process control in healthcare improvement: systematic review. *Qual Saf Health Care.* 2007;16(5):387-399.

Woodall WH, Adams BM, Benneyan JC. The use of control charts in healthcare. In: Faltin F, Kenett R, Ruggeri F, eds. *Statistical Methods in Healthcare.* Chichester, England: Wiley; 2012:253-265.

Factors Influencing Variation

Cromwell J, Dayhoff DA, Thoumaian AH. Cost savings and physician responses to global bundled payments for Medicare heart bypass surgery. *Health Care Financ Rev.* 1997;19(1):41-57.

Davis P, Gribben B, Scott A, Lay-Yee R. The "supply hypothesis" and medical practice variation in primary care: testing economic and clinical models of inter-practitioner variation. *Soc Sci Med.* 2000;50(3):407-418.

Eddy DM. Variations in physician practice: the role of uncertainty. *Health Aff (Millwood).* 1984;3(2):74-89.

Fisher ES, Wennberg DE, Stukel TA, Gottlieb DJ, Lucas FL, Pinder EL. The implications of regional variations in Medicare spending. Part 2: health outcomes and satisfaction with care. *Ann Intern Med.* 2003;138(4):288-298.

Lee AJ. The role of financial incentives in shaping clinical practice patterns and practice efficiency. *Am J Cardiol.* 1997;80(8B):28H-32H.

Long MJ. An explanatory model of medical practice variation: a physician resource demand perspective. *J Eval Clin Pract.* 2002;8(2):167-174.

Lungren MP, Amrhein TJ, Paxton BE, et al. Physician self-referral: frequency of negative findings at MR imaging of the knee as a marker of appropriate utilization. *Radiology.* 2013;269(3):810-815.

Sepucha K, Ozanne E, Mulley AG Jr. Doing the right thing: systems support for decision quality in cancer care. *Ann Behav Med.* 2006;32(3):172-178.

Sirovich B, Gallagher PM, Wennberg DE, Fisher ES. Discretionary decision making by primary care physicians and the cost of U.S. Health care. *Health Aff (Millwood).* 2008;27(3):813-823.

Wennberg J. Time to tackle unwarranted variations in practice. *BMJ.* 2011;342:d1513.

Wennberg JE, Barnes BA, Zubkoff M. Professional uncertainty and the problem of supplier-induced demand. *Soc Sci Med.* 1982;16(7):811-824.

Applying Evidence of Variation to Improve Quality of Care

Gauld R, Horwitt J, Williams S, Cohen AB. What strategies do US hospitals employ to reduce unwarranted clinical practice variations? *Am J Med Qual.* 2011;26(2):120-126.

Greer AL, Goodwin JS, Freeman JL, Wu ZH. Bringing the patient back in Guidelines, practice variations, and the social context of medical practice. *Int J Technol Assess Health Care.* 2002;18(4):747-761.

Ham C. Review of the Week. A roadmap for health system reform. *BMJ.* 2011;342:d1757.

Sackett DL, Rosenberg WM, Gray JA, Haynes RB, Richardson WS. Evidence based medicine: what it is and what it isn't. 1996. *Clin Orthop Relat Res.* 2007;455:3-5.

Timmermans S, Mauck A. The promises and pitfalls of evidence-based medicine. *Health Aff (Millwood).* 2005;24(1):18-28.

Variation Data and National Health Policy

Centers for Medicare and Medicaid. Bundled Payments for Care Improvement (BPCI) Initiative: General Information. Published 2013. http://innovation.cms.gov/initiatives/bundled-payments. Accessed September 16, 2013.

Centers for Medicare and Medicaid. Fact Sheet: Bundled Payments for Care Improvement Initiative. Published 2013. http://www.cms.gov/apps/media/press/factsheet.asp?Counter=4515&intNumPerPage=10&checkDate=&checkKey=&srchType=1&numDays=3500&srchOpt=0&srchData=&keywordType=All&chkNewsType=6&intPage=&showAll=&pYear=&year=&desc=&cboOrder=date. Accessed September 16, 2013.

Department of Health and Human Service, Centers for Medicare and Medicaid Services. Medicare program; hospital inpatient prospective payment systems for acute care hospitals and the long-term care hospital prospective payment system and fiscal year 2014 rates; quality reporting requirements for specific providers; hospital conditions of participation; payment policies related to patient status. *Fed Regist.* 2013;78(160):50496, 50678-50704.

Hussey PS, Ridgely MS, Rosenthal MB. The PROMETHEUS bundled payment experiment: slow start shows problems in implementing new payment models. *Health Aff (Millwood).* 2011;30(11):2116-2124.

Implementation Science

Cathy L. Melvin and Kathleen T. Brady

CASE STUDY: IMPLEMENTATION OF HUMAN PAPILLOMAVIRUS VACCINE: MISSED OPPORTUNITIES

Approximately 80% of individuals will become infected with human papillomavirus (HPV) during their lifetimes. Infection occurs at various sites in both sexes and may result in anogenital and oropharyngeal condyloma, precancers, or cancers. HPV causes more than 750,000 cases of cancer and 275,128 deaths worldwide per year. Comprehensive cancer screening, diagnosis, and treatment programs have reduced the incidence of HPV-related cancers where implemented, but these secondary cancer prevention efforts are associated with tremendous expense ($8 billion/year in the United States), complicated logistics, and significant morbidity. HPV vaccine offers an amazing opportunity to prevent the adverse outcomes associated with HPV infection. HPV vaccine is a safe, evidence-based intervention to prevent certain cancers and reduce health care costs.

Despite its great potential, HPV vaccination is not widely accepted by health care providers and the public. HPV vaccination rates are much lower in the United States (33% for all three doses in 2012) than in many other countries (**Figure 17-1**). A robust body of literature indicates that vaccine uptake is influenced by both parental and provider knowledge and attitudes about the vaccine. Parents have unfounded worries about vaccine safety and the stigma associated with a vaccine to prevent a sexually transmitted infection. Some primary health care providers (PHCPs) are reluctant to strongly recommend HPV vaccines for their patients despite provider recommendation being the best predictor of vaccine initiation. Providers may be unfamiliar with the burden of disease and deterred in their recommendation of the vaccine in anticipation of difficult parental discussions about sexual issues. These perceived and actual barriers to the uptake of HPV vaccination can be addressed using evidence-based dissemination and implementation (D & I) strategies.

Systematic reviews and dissemination research show that active, multifaceted dissemination strategies are more effective than passive strategies for changing provider behavior. Educational outreach, academic detailing, and the use of local opinion leaders are the most consistently effective interventions reported. *Implementation strategies* likely to work best in primary care and among PHCP include academic detailing and quality improvement approaches. **Table 17-1** describes evidence-based goals and strategies for both D & I approaches to address deficits in HPV vaccination rates.

OVERVIEW: IMPLEMENTATION SCIENCE

This chapter is structured to acquaint the reader with the growing and emerging field of implementation sciences (IS), the study of methods to promote the integration of research findings and evidence into health care policy and practice. IS seeks to understand the behavior of health care professionals and other stakeholders as a key variable in the sustainable uptake, adoption, and implementation of evidence-based interventions.

As a newly emerging field, the definition of IS and the type of research encompassed by it may vary according to setting and sponsor. However, the intent of IS and related research is to investigate and address major bottlenecks (e.g., social, behavioral, economic, management) that impede effective implementation, test new approaches to improve health programming, and determine a causal relationship between the implementation intervention and its impact.

We present the rationale and need for IS along with definitions, outcomes, and constructs that place IS within both the translational continuum and the broader framework of D & I research. We also present

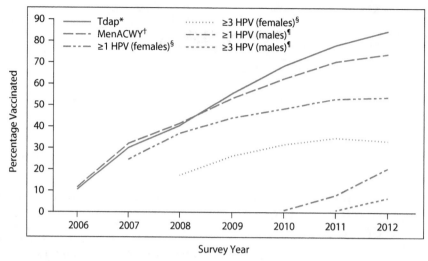

Figure 17-1. National immunization survey of teens, United States, 2006 to 2013. ACIP, Advisory Committee on Immunization Practices; HPV, human papillomavirus; MenACYW, meningococcal conjugate; Tdap, tetanus toxoid, reduced diphtheria toxoid, and acellular pertussis. (Reproduced from Centers for Disease Control and Prevention (CDC). National and state vaccination coverage among adolescents aged 13-17 years—United States, 2012. *MMWR Morb Mortal Wkly Rep.* 2013;62(34):685-706.)

theories and models used in D & I research. The earlier scenario presents an example of how D & I and especially IS can be applied to a pressing public health concern: increasing delivery of the HPV vaccine among adolescent females and males.

INTRODUCTION: RATIONALE AND NEED FOR IMPLEMENTATION SCIENCE

Over the past 25 years, we witnessed great strides in biomedical knowledge, including our understanding of basic biologic processes and the pathophysiology of disease, the development of interventions to prevent and treat disease, and the creation of evidence-based guidelines to support health and health care practice. Despite these efforts and the possibility of even more exciting discoveries in the near term, we have not realized the tremendous potential for impact and benefit of these dramatic therapeutic innovations on the management and cure of previously fatal diseases and

on the prevention of conditions contributing to serious health consequences.

American health care falls short of care in other developed countries based on measures of quality, outcomes, costs, and equity. One reason for this paradox is that the results of many research studies are never translated into meaningful changes in patient care. By some estimates, it takes 15 to 20 years for many new interventions to become part of usual care, and this "implementation gap" prevents the public from experiencing timely benefits from the resources invested in research and can needlessly prolong suffering. A report by the Institute of Medicine commented on the remarkable disconnect between medical research and practice, noting that scientific knowledge about best care is not systematically applied. The report estimated an average of 17 years for 14% of knowledge generated by clinical trials to be incorporated into practice, and even then application is not uniform. The committee recommended that the U.S. government establish a comprehensive program aimed at making scientific evidence more useful and more accessible to clinicians and patients.

Table 17-1. Dissemination and implementation goals and strategies for increasing human papillomavirus vaccination rates.

Dissemination Goal: Adoption by Practices	Implementation Goal: HPV Vaccine Uptake and Reach

• Focus on poorly performing practices
• Conduct audience research with providers
• Identify barriers and enablers
• Develop tailored, evidence-based communication strategies, materials, and products
• Distribute through credible channels
• Repeat exposure
	• Develop an implementation team in each practice
	• Foster supportive organizational and community-wide climate and conditions
	• Develop an implementation plan
	• Receive tailored training
	• Evaluate the effectiveness of the intervention
	  • Increased series completion
	  • Decreased missed opportunities

HPV, human papillomavirus.
Data from Rogers EM. *Diffusion of Innovations.* New York: Simon and Schuster; 2010.

Delays in assembling, disseminating, and implementing scientific evidence to support the use of proven health and health care interventions and practices and the discontinuation of interventions with little or no evidence of efficacy are particularly problematic for the U.S. health care system given increasing financial and regulatory incentives and mandates promoting a shift toward evidence-based practice. Findings from clinical, health services, and comparative effectiveness studies—especially as assembled for systematic reviews and similar documents—need to be communicated and disseminated effectively to influence optimal and timely practice and health policy implementation. A growing emphasis on effective D & I science is developing in response to this evidence-to-practice gap.

D & I science seeks to understand how to systematically facilitate the utilization of evidence-based approaches to improve the quality and effectiveness of health promotion, health services, and health care. Barriers to D & I can arise at multiple levels in our complex health care delivery system, including the patient, health care provider, organization, market, and policy levels.

DEFINITIONS, OUTCOMES, AND CONSTRUCTS

There are no fixed and universally accepted definitions of *evidence, IS, implementation,* or *implementation research.* Furthermore, these terms are often combined or confused with *diffusion, dissemination,* and *dissemination research.* This ambiguity creates confusion among health care providers and other users of scientific evidence as well as challenges for D & I researchers seeking to expand the evidence base for this emerging field.

We present definitions for selected terms from widely recognized and accepted sources and recent reviews of D & I research. We suggest that intention and outcome-based constructs for choosing among these terms depends on the purpose of the work, the intended audience, and expected outcome(s) (**Table 17-2**). Regardless of the specifics associated with each definition of D & I, the expected outcome or intent of the activities described for each definition distinguishes it from the other. We further define constructs of D & I approaches used primarily with health and health care stakeholders in various settings to advance the awareness, adoption, use, and impact of health and health care evidence, information, and interventions (**Table 17-3**).

Evidence

We use a recently suggested definition of *evidence:* data that have been assembled, reviewed, and presented by evidence developers and that have been used to make recommendations. Evidence may be assembled from the peer-review literature, gray literature, or a combination of both. Included studies may be randomized controlled trials (RCT), observational studies, or practice-based evidence reported in the peer reviewed literature or elsewhere (e.g., gray literature). Evidence about nonclinical interventions often derives from the social, behavioral, and management sciences. Because findings from single research studies are usually insufficient to guide practice and behavior change, most evidence is created using systematic review processes, including meta-analysis.

Systematic reviews are undertaken on a wide range of health and health care topics by a number of organizations and groups including the United States Preventive Services Task Force (USPSTF), The Community Guide to Preventive Services (Community Guide), the Agency for Healthcare Research and Quality (AHRQ) Evidence-based Practice Center (EPC), the Cochrane Collaborative, and professional and other organizations. Evidence resulting from these reviews may be biased by the type

Table 17-2. Dissemination and implementation definitions and outcomes.

Construct	Definition(s)	Intention or Expected Outcome(s)
Diffusion	The *passive process* by which a program or product is absorbed into more widespread use (Rogers, 2010)	Adoption: The decision of an organization or a community to commit to and initiate an evidence-based intervention (Brownson et al., 2012; Rabin et al., 2008)
Dissemination	The *active and targeted* distribution of information and interventions to a specific public health or clinical practice audience via determined channels using planned strategies (Brownson et al., 2012; Rabin et al., 2008)	Increase reach of evidence to a variety of audiences Increase motivation to use and apply evidence Increase ability to use and apply evidence (McCormack et al., 2013)
Dissemination research	Addresses how information about health promotion and care interventions is created, packaged, transmitted, and interpreted among a variety of important stakeholder groups	
Implementation science or research	The study of methods to promote the integration of research findings and evidence into health care policy and practice	To understand the behavior of health care professionals and other stakeholders as a key variable in the sustainable uptake, adoption, and implementation of evidence-based interventions

of review method(s) used, by the framing of specific key questions to be answered by the review, by the types of literature included in the review, by conflict of interest among those undertaking and endorsing or soliciting the review, and by temporal effects.

The most robust evidence is based on comparisons of two or more approaches designed and tested via RCT to achieve the same goal although current practice or usual care is often one of these approaches. For example, information about the efficacy of one drug compared with another drug for a specific indication such as pain relief may be evaluated based on studies evaluating harm (e.g., adverse events, addictive properties) and benefit (e.g., magnitude of expected effect or pain relief) associated with each drug. Because systematic review findings are often unequivocal or hampered by inconsistent study designs and outcomes, most review processes include a means of achieving consensus among experts and stakeholders about review findings and how those findings inform our understanding of intervention(s) to affect change in health or health care. Mechanisms for involvement of experts and stakeholders vary depending on the sponsor of the review but generally include periodic involvement of these individuals in all phases of a systematic review and, in particular, phases requiring decisions about review design, specification of key questions for the review, review findings, and interpretation of findings.

Dissemination

Dissemination is described in many ways (see **Table 17-2**) but in most instances refers to the active and targeted distribution of evidence, information, or interventions via determined channels using planned strategies to a specific public health or clinical practice audience. In contrast to *diffusion*, which is a passive, informal process, dissemination is a formal, planned process with the intent of spreading knowledge and associated evidence-based interventions to stimulate adoption and enhance the integration of the evidence, information, or intervention (or combinations of these) into routine practice. Dissemination has been characterized as a necessary but not sufficient antecedent of adoption and implementation of evidence.

Dissemination Outcomes

Existing dissemination models and approaches identify several very broad goals or outcomes for the dissemination of evidence and information. We focus on three intended goals of dissemination:

1. *Increase reach to a variety of audiences: Reach* is defined as the absolute number, proportion, and representativeness of individuals who are willing to participate in a given initiative. Approaches for increasing reach include distributing evidence, information, or interventions widely to intended

Table 17-3. Constructs and definitions.

Construct	Definition
Approach	An explicit set of techniques or activities for achieving spread (D & I) of interventions or strategies
Audience	
Delivery settings or sites	Any location where health care services are delivered or received, including, but not limited to, hospitals, long-term care facilities, doctors' offices, primary care clinics, pharmacies, school or community health clinics, and home care
Initiative	A comprehensive approach or set of approaches for spread (D & I) undertaken in a coordinated fashion across multiple sites and among groups of stakeholders
Intervention	A specific activity, action, or technique that can be used individually or in combination in support of a broader strategy
	Interventions are generally thought of as including any or all of the following: evidence-based interventions, practice findings, and care delivery improvements. Evidence and research findings about practices or interventions for improving clinical outcomes, care delivery, or the performance of delivery systems cover both broad improvement strategies and specific interventions or techniques. These strategies and interventions may aim for outcomes at the individual, group (or team), organizational, population, delivery system, local community, or regional level. The objectives can focus on clinical, behavioral, or organizational change. Objectives for change may be broadly defined or narrowly focused.
Network	An established, broad-based association, coalition, or partnership of clinical practitioners; provider practices or organizations; or other groups, entities, or organizations playing an influential role in health care delivery, with a history of collaborative relationships directed at improving health care quality. Relationships among these linked actors can be formal or informal; capacities must include at a minimum established channels for communication and data sharing and an infrastructure that has proven to be capable of supporting joint actions to improve care and collaborations for improvement or shared learning.
Provider	Any individual or organization that provides care to patients (including, but not limited to, physicians, nurses, other health care practitioners, group practices, hospitals, ambulatory care centers, integrated delivery systems)
Stakeholder group	Any group, entity, or organization involved in providing, receiving, or paying for health care; any group that represents or advocates on behalf of those who provide, receive, or pay for care
Strategy	Sets of practices, techniques, or interventions with an underlying logic for improving the quality of clinical care or care delivery (e.g., introducing decision-support systems, fostering patient self-management, developing cross-disciplinary care teams)

D & I, dissemination and implementation.

audiences and across many settings using appropriate channels of communication and dissemination, including postal and electronic mail and electronic or digital, social, and mass media. Common metrics to measure increased reach among members of a target audience include increases in:

a. The proportion of audience members indicating awareness of the evidence or able to adequately describe the evidence, its components and source(s)

b. The range of media and other exposure to the evidence within geographic or certain population groups or practice settings

2. *Increase motivation to use and apply such information:* Motivation is defined as increasing audience member interest in using and applying the evidence, information, or interventions in their practice settings. Frequent strategies to increase motivation to use and apply evidence include the use of experts, champions (also known as a cheerleader), opinion or thought leaders, or social networks.

3. *Increase ability to actually use and apply evidence:* This includes providing additional resources in terms of the evidence, information, or interventions, such as how it can be incorporated into current practice or specific suggestions for change, to enhance a traditional dissemination strategy (e.g., by also providing additional resources or information; skills-building efforts).

It is also common practice to combine multiple dissemination strategies (often labeled as *multicomponent* strategies) to address a combination of reach, ability, or motivation goals. Several recent reviews indicate that multicomponent strategies are in fact the most efficacious and effective approaches to achieve dissemination goals and outcomes. For example, to alleviate the health effects of secondhand smoke exposure, the Centers for Disease Control and Prevention (CDC), the Legacy Foundation, and other professional and advocacy organizations use multicomponent dissemination strategies such as small and mass media, testimony, and in-person presentations by opinion leaders and celebrities and skills-building activities to increase the numbers of individuals and organizations who are aware of the dangers of secondhand smoke exposure and who are motivated to use and apply this evidence to change smoke-free environment policy and legislation in a variety of settings.

Dissemination Research

Dissemination research addresses how evidence, information, and interventions to promote and improve health and health care are created, packaged, transmitted, and interpreted among a variety of important stakeholder groups. For example, a study might explore the effectiveness of various combinations of strategies to deliver tailored and targeted messages about evidence. Strategies could include different media channels (e.g., print, Internet, radio or TV or other mass media, face-to-face interactions, or social media). Effectiveness could be evaluated via comparisons of outcomes associated with each dissemination strategy such as intervention reach, adoption, or use in the target audience.

Implementation

Implementation has been defined as the use of strategies to integrate evidence-based health interventions and change practice patterns within specific settings. Alternate forms of this definition (see **Table 17-2**) offer slight variations on this theme by asserting that implementation also involves adoption or integration of evidence-based interventions and strategies by individuals, sites, and organizations within specific settings. Implementation is often seen as a step after successful completion of dissemination strategies. The intent of implementation strategies is to address major, identified bottlenecks (e.g., social, behavioral, economic, management) that impede effective implementation and test new approaches to improve health programming, as well as determine a causal relationship between the implementation intervention and its impact. The evidence base for implementation strategies and interventions is empirical documentation of sufficient strength, clarity, and technical merit to produce strong expectations as to the likelihood of success in achieving improvement goals.

Implementation Outcomes

Implementation outcomes include the actual, documented use or integration of the intervention or innovation by the intended users into their practice, community, or academic setting. For example, the Treating Tobacco Use and Dependence Guidelines from the USPSTF have been widely disseminated and support the efficacy of pharmacologic and behavioral approaches for helping patients to quit using tobacco. Treatments are specified for all smokers and for different categories of smokers, such as pregnant women, hospitalized patients, and those with multiple comorbidities. Although physicians may be aware of efficacious treatment options recommended for smoking cessation, recommended approaches for assessing and treating patient tobacco use are often not undertaken for a variety of reasons specific to their organizations or sites and to individual practitioners such as not being aware of the evidence, time constraints affecting use of the evidence, or self-efficacy regarding implementation of evidence. Successful implementation of methods to assess tobacco use status could be established via electronic health record (EHR)–based practitioner prompts to assess and record tobacco use status for each patient at every visit. This achievement would establish tobacco use as a vital sign on par with other practices such as blood pressure measurement and indicate successful, universal implementation of one part of a treatment guideline. Continuing to pursue other components of the recommended tobacco treatment strategy such as assessing willingness to quit using tobacco, offering assistance in quitting, and arranging appropriate referral and follow-up might require the use of different implementation strategies to achieve universal delivery of each component.

Implementation Science

Implementation science (or *research*) is the study of methods and strategies to promote the integration of research findings and evidence into health care policy and practice. It seeks to understand the behavior of health care professionals and other stakeholders as a key variable in the sustainable uptake, adoption, and implementation of evidence-based interventions. For example, primary care clinicians generally have little time available to help their patients quit smoking cigarettes. To reduce the barrier associated with clinician time, several options are recommended by the current guidelines, including the use of reminders, EHR prompts, and less time-intensive approaches such as the 3 As + R method (ask, advise, assess, and refer). In addition to assessing differences in "effect" of each of these strategies, IS would also attempt to determine if one approach compared with another would be more likely to (1) be implemented (e.g., process outcome), (2) achieve cessation for tobacco users (e.g., behavioral or clinical outcome), or (3) to be preferred by either practitioners or patients.

Implementation science and research tools and approaches often used to undertake the development and assessment of alternate implementation strategies include qualitative research methods to identify bottlenecks and underlying determinants from varying perspectives, continuous quality improvement measures and methods, performance monitoring, and assessments of patient and clinician satisfaction.

DISSEMINATION AND IMPLEMENTATION RESEARCH THEORIES AND MODELS

Although this discussion focuses on health promotion, health services and health care, much of the work to date in D & I science and practice stems from other industries and disciplines, including agriculture, public health, organizational behavior, psychology, political science, and marketing. Because of the interdisciplinary nature of implementation research, it is important to organize and synthesize models and frameworks from a broad perspective to better understand overlapping constructs and establish a framework for moving the field forward.

A recent review of the use of theory in D & I research found that only 53 of 252 studies reviewed

used theories, and a small number of theories accounted for the majority of theory or model use, including PRECEDE (Predisposing, Reinforcing, and Enabling Constructs in Educational Diagnosis and Evaluation), diffusion of innovations, information overload, and social marketing (academic detailing). All models acknowledge the complex variables that can influence D & I. Greenhalgh and colleagues (2004) emphasize characteristics of the innovation itself and of the adopters of the innovation (either as individuals or as a system) along with the adoption process as critical in determining implementation success. As such, the interaction among the innovation, the proposed adopter(s), and the context determines the success of dissemination and implementation strategies (see **Figure 17-2**).

In terms of innovation or intervention characteristics, those more likely to be adopted and implemented have a clear and unambiguous advantage for the individual and system and are compatible with adopter values and norms; are feasible, workable, and easy to use; have proximal, observable benefits; and can be tried on a limited basis before adoption. Important prerequisites for adoption include awareness of the intervention or innovation by intended adopters, the availability of sufficient information or training in its use, and clarity about how the intervention or innovation will impact users personally. Because successful individual adoption is only one component of implementation in organizations, critical advances are also needed in the field to understand and evaluate system readiness and specific implementation strategies and processes. Studies to date suggest that if a large organization is mature,

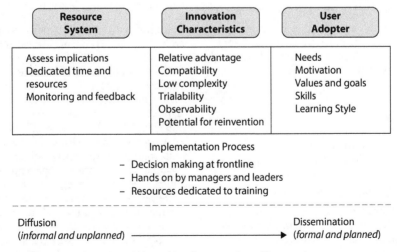

Figure 17-2. Factors impacting dissemination and implementation of innovation.

functionally differentiated (divided into departments or units) with decentralized decision-making structures and dedicated time and resources for innovation, it is more likely to be successful in implementing interventions. Nonstructural determinants of organizational readiness include the absorptive capacity for new knowledge (i.e., do the staff have the skills and time available to consider and use the innovation or intervention?) and the receptive context for change, including strong leadership, strategic vision, and good managerial relationships.

Other systematic reviews and dissemination research show that active dissemination strategies are more effective than passive strategies, and active multifaceted approaches are most effective for changing provider behavior. Educational outreach, academic detailing, and the use of local opinion leaders are the most consistently effective interventions reported. Interventions that are theory based, that incorporate two or more distinct strategies (i.e., that are multicomponent), or that do both are consistently more likely to work than single interventions. Moreover, the Internet, technologic platforms for social networking, and Web 2.0 applications can serve as important dissemination channels, allowing users to create and actively interact with information in ways that support intervention adoption, use, and implementation.

A recent narrative review of D & I research models identified 61 models. Models were sorted into three author-defined categories based on:

1. *Construct flexibility:* Rated on a scale of 1 to 5, where 1 was broad (loosely outlined and defined constructs) and 5 was operational (detailed, step-by-step actions for completion of the D & I research process) and with models falling in between scored as 2, 3, or 4.
2. *Dissemination or implementation focus:* defined as
   a. Dissemination only (D-only): Focus on active approach of spreading evidence-based interventions to the target audience via determined channels using planned strategies
   b. Dissemination = Implementation (D=I): equal focus on D & I
   c. Implementation only (I-only): Focus on putting to use or integrating evidence-based interventions within a setting
3. *Socioecologic framework:* The level(s) of the socioecologic framework at which the model operates: individual, organization, community, or system.

The review identified 11 D-only models, 16 were combined dissemination and implementation models with a predominant focus on dissemination

(D >I), 17 were D = I, five were combined dissemination and implementation models with a predominant focus on implementation (I >D), and 12 were I-only. The socioecologic level targeted by each model was variable and ranged from a systemwide orientation to community, organizational, individual, or policy levels. We present an example of a broad D = I model and an operational I-only model to illustrate construct choices available for researchers and practitioners in choosing a model to frame their work.

The Interactive Systems Framework (ISF) for Dissemination and Implementation is an integrated model developed by Wandersman and colleagues (2008) focused on the infrastructure and systems (e.g., practitioners, organizations that provide support to practitioners) needed for D & I to take place at multiple levels (e.g., system, community, organization, individual, and policy). The ISF is a broad model (score of 2) designed to accommodate multiple perspectives (e.g., the perspective of the funder, researcher) and includes the activities or functions carried out by people in multiple types of roles, highlighting the need for communication among different stakeholders in the system for D & I to be successful. Focused on prevention, ISF consists of three systems:

1. The *Prevention Synthesis and Translation System (PSTS)* is conceptualized as distilling information about innovations and preparing them for implementation by end users.
2. The *Prevention Support System (PSS)* is conceptualized as supporting the work of those who will put the innovations into practice.
3. The *Prevention Delivery System (PDS)* is focused on the implementation of innovations (e.g., delivery of programs) in the field.

Individuals and organizations using the ISF framework may conduct systematic reviews and meta-analyses as described in the PSTS to create evidence along with related tools and materials that translate evidence findings into key concepts and actionable messages that may be tailored for a particular audience. Examples include clinical practice guidelines issued by the AHRQ (http://www.ahrq.gov), CDC (http://www.cdc.gov), USPSTF (http://www.uspreventiveservicestaskforce.org), or Cochrane Collaboration (http://www.cochrane.org), professional organizations and societies representing a specific area of clinical practice. These organizations conduct a systematic review process, publish their findings, and design and disseminate tools and materials to inform patients, practitioners, and researchers about their findings. A recent example includes the 2014 publication of *The Health*

Consequences of Smoking—50 Years of Progress: A Report of the Surgeon General along with its accompanying *Executive Summary, Consumer Booklet, Fact Sheets, Video and Podcast Series and list of Partner Resources* (http://www.surgeongeneral.gov/library/reports/50-years-of-progress/).

Other organizations may use alternative methods such as expert testimony and existing resources to define a major clinical or public health problem and present consensus recommendations detailing opportunities for improving practice and conducting research. *The President's Cancer Panel Annual Report 2012–2013: Accelerating HPV Vaccine Uptake: Urgency for Action to Prevent Cancer* (http://deainfo.nci.nih.gov/advisory/pcp/annualReports/HPV/Acknowledgements.htm#sthash.7LHOnm9S.dpbs) was released in April 2014. The report is based on expert testimony and advice gathered in four U.S. cities in 2012 and 2013. The report makes the case for HPV vaccination using available evidence, describes the urgent need for action and details four goals for accelerating HPV vaccine uptake in the United States, and outlines high-priority research to advance prevention of HPV related cancers.

PSS activities could focus on either the creation or use of efficacious or effective strategies to build capacity and skills among individuals or organizations attempting to put research into practice. Evidence creators, program developers, or practice champions may provide either general capacity building such as learning about how evidence is created or found in a particular field or intervention-specific capacity building such as toolkits describing evidence-based approaches to increasing practitioner self-efficacy in offering HPV vaccines to young adults or their parents.

Activities in the PDS focus on overcoming implementation barriers or building on implementation strengths of individuals or organizations. These activities may be designed within the ISF or as part of an I-only framework such as the Consolidated Framework for Implementation Research (CFIR). The CFIR combines constructs across published theories with redundant or overlapping definitions into an overarching typology designed to promote both implementation theory development and a context for evaluation of implementation efforts.

The CFIR is an operational model (score = 4) composed of five major domains: intervention characteristics, inner and outer setting, characteristics of the individuals involved, and the process by which the implementation is accomplished. Eight characteristics of an intervention, including evidence strength and quality, are specified. The outer setting includes the economic, political, and social context within which

an organization resides, and the inner setting includes features of structural, political, and cultural contexts through which the implementation process will proceed. Four constructs relate to outer setting (e.g., patient needs and resources), 12 constructs to the inner setting (e.g., culture, leadership engagement), and 5 relate to individual characteristics. Successful implementation involves an active change process aimed to achieve individual and organizational level use of the intervention as designed (e.g., fidelity) and eight constructs related to process (e.g., plan, evaluate, and reflect). For example, the President's Cancer Panel recommends implementation strategies such as changing policy to allow pharmacists to administer the HPV vaccine and to remove financial barriers to vaccination. Within practices, changes are recommended to provide adequate reimbursement for HPV vaccines and administration, expand Healthcare Effectiveness Data and Information Set (HEDIS) measure regarding HPV vaccination to include adolescent males, and development of centralized immunization information systems that are interoperable and integrated with office-based EHRs.

SUMMARY

Evidence-based D & I approaches exist, should be used and evaluated when possible if practice or individual practitioner or patient change is desired. Research designed to compare the effectiveness of alternate D & I strategies is needed to both assess the relative advantage of one evidence-based strategy over another or the relative advantage of a new strategy compared with an existing evidence-based strategy. Care should be taken to determine and specify the desired endpoint or primary outcome, to choose and consistently use a known model and its constructs to frame the research question and evaluate relative effectiveness, and to engage the intended audience in the design and conduct of the research.

In summary, a greater focus on implementation and dissemination of scientific findings and evidence-based medical practices is essential to realizing potential gains from biomedical research and improving the quality and efficiency of health care. Recent developments to guide D & I science include the development and use of theories, frameworks, and models along with associated methods and metrics. Although great progress has been made, there is much work to be done. In particular, more consistency in terminology and better definition of outcome measures will be important to systematic progress in this area of incredible importance to public health and well-being.

STUDY QUESTIONS

1. Implementation science
   A. seeks to understand the behavior of health care professionals and other stakeholders.
   B. is the study of methods to promote the integration of research findings and evidence into health care policy and practice.
   C. is an emerging field of growing importance to health care delivery.
   D. is all of the above.

2. Issues most likely to interfere with implementation of effective health care interventions include
   A. economic and behavioral issues.
   B. spatiotemporal issues.
   C. geopolitical issues.
   D. mathematical probabilities.

3. Dissemination is:
   A. a passive, informal approach to communication.
   B. a formal, planned process with the intent of spreading knowledge.
   C. a mechanism of reviewing an evidence base.
   D. the preparatory phase before diffusion of information.

4. Implementation outcomes generally would NOT include
   A. use of an intervention by an individual practitioner.
   B. integration of an intervention within established practice.
   C. citation index of an article.
   D. use of an innovation within a community setting.

5. An intervention or innovation is more likely to be adopted if
   A. it is easy to use.
   B. it is based on credible evidence.
   C. it has a clear, unambiguous advantage for the individual and system.
   D. it can be tried on a limited basis before widespread adoption.

6. Organizational characteristics of large organizations that predict successful implementation of interventions or innovations include all but
   A. absorptive capacity for new knowledge.
   B. strong leadership and strategic vision.

   C. decentralized decision-making structures.
   D. well-designed data systems.

7. The Interactive Systems Framework describes three systems. Which system is not part of the ISF?
   A. Prevention Synthesis and Translation System
   B. Prevention Awareness and Communication System
   C. Prevention Support System
   D. Prevention Delivery System

8. HPV vaccination rates lag behind those in other countries for which reasons?
   A. Parental and provider knowledge and attitudes about the vaccine
   B. Parental concerns about vaccine safety
   C. Providers' lack of familiarity with burden of disease associated with HPV-related cancers
   D. Documented side effects of the vaccine

9. Recent developments to guide dissemination and implementation science include all but which of the following?
   A. The development of theories, frameworks, and models
   B. Creation of model-driven methods and metrics
   C. Compilations of data from D & I studies
   D. Head-to-head comparisons of methods and metrics

10. Which of the following is not an intended outcome of dissemination?
    A. Promote the integration of research findings and evidence into health care policy and practice
    B. Increase motivation to use and apply evidence
    C. Increase reach to a variety of audiences
    D. Increase ability to actually use and apply evidence

FURTHER READING

Bernhardt JM, Mays D, Kreuter MW. Dissemination 2.0: closing the gap between knowledge and practice with new media and marketing. *J Health Commun.* 2011;16(suppl 1):32-44.

Brownson RC, Colditz GA, Proctor EK. *Dissemination and Implementation Research in Health.* New York: Oxford University Press; 2012.

Tabak RG, Khoong EC, Chambers DA, Brownson RC. Bridging research and practice: models for dissemination and implementation research. *Am J Prev Med.* 2012;43(3):337-350.

REFERENCES

Case Study: Implementation of Human Papillomavirus Vaccine: Missed Opportunities

Centers for Disease Control and Prevention (CDC). National and state vaccination coverage among adolescents aged 13-17 years—United States, 2012. *MMWR Morb Mortal Wkly Rep.* 2013;62(34):685-706.

Centers for Disease Control and Prevention (CDC). Human papillomavirus-associated cancers—United States, 2004-2008. *MMWR Morb Mortal Wkly Rep.* 2012;61:258-261.

Davis K, Dickman ED, Ferris D, Dias JK. Human papillomavirus vaccine acceptability among parents of 10- to 15-year-old adolescents. *J Low Genit Tract Dis.* 2004;8(3):188-194.

Ferris DG, Cromwell L, Waller JL, Horn L. Most parents do not think receiving human papillomavirus vaccine would encourage sexual activity in their children. *J Low Genit Tract Dis.* 2010;14(3):179-184.

Friedman AL, Shepeard H. Exploring the knowledge, attitudes, beliefs, and communication preferences of the general public regarding HPV: findings from CDC focus group research and implications for practice. *Health Educ Behav.* 2006;34(3):471-485.

Grimshaw JM, Shirran L, Thomas R, et al. Changing provider behavior: an overview of systematic reviews of interventions. *Med Care.* 2001;39(8 suppl 2):II2-II45.

Rosenthal SL, Weiss TW, Zimet GD, Ma L, Good MB, Vichnin MD. Predictors of HPV vaccine uptake among women aged 19-26: importance of a physician's recommendation. *Vaccine.* 2011;29(5):890-895.

World Health Organization/ICO (Institut Català d'Oncologia). Information Center on HPV and Cancer. United States of America: Human Papillomavirus and Related Cancers Fact Sheet. December 15, 2014. Barcelona, Spain.

Overview: Implementation Science

Fogarty International Center, National Institutes of Health (producer). Implementation Science Information and Resources. Published May 7, 2014. http://www.fic.nih.gov/researchtopics/pages/implementationscience.aspx.

Introduction: Rationale and Need for Implementation Science

Fogarty International Center, National Institutes of Health (producer). Implementation Science Information and Resources. Published May 7, 2014. http://www.fic.nih.gov/researchtopics/pages/implementationscience.aspx.

Helfand M, Tunis S, Whitlock EP, et al. A CTSA agenda to advance methods for comparative effectiveness research. *Clin Transl Sci.* 2011;4(3):188-198.

Institute of Medicine. *Crossing the Quality Chasm: A New Health System for the 21st Century.* Washington, DC: Author; 2001.

National Research Council and the Institute of Medicine. Woolf SH, Aron L, eds. *Shorter Lives, Poorer Health.* Washington, DC: National Academies Press; 2013.

Proctor EK, Landsverk J, Aarons G, Chambers D, Glisson C, Mittman B. Implementation research in mental health services: an emerging science with conceptual, methodological, and training challenges. *Adm Policy Ment Health.* 2009;36(1):24-34.

Definitions, Outcomes, and Constructs

Brownson RC, Colditz GA, Proctor EK. *Dissemination and Implementation Research in Health.* New York: Oxford University Press; 2012.

Fiore MC, Jaen CR, Baker TB, et al. *Treating Tobacco Use and Dependence 2008 Update. Clinical Practice Guideline.* Rockville, MD: U.S. Department of Health and Human Services. Public Health Service; 2008.

Fogarty International Center, National Institutes of Health (producer). Implementation Science Information and Resources. Published May 7, 2014. http://www.fic.nih.gov/researchtopics/pages/implementationscience.aspx.

Glasgow RE, Vogt TM, Boles SM. Evaluating the public health impact of health promotion interventions: the RE-AIM framework. *Am J Public Health.* 1999;89(9):1322-1327.

Lomas J. Diffusion, dissemination, and implementation: who should do what? *Ann N Y Acad Sci.* 1993;703:226-235; discussion 235-227.

McCormack L, Sheridan S, Lewis M, et al. *Communication and Dissemination Strategies to Facilitate the Use of Health-Related Evidence.* Rockville, MD: University of North Carolina Evidence-based Practice Center under Contract No. 290-2007-10056-1; 2013.

Rabin BA, Brownson RC, Haire-Joshu D, Kreuter MW, Weaver NL. A glossary for dissemination and implementation research in health. *J Public Health Manag Pract.* 2008;14(2):117-123.

Rogers EM. *Diffusion of Innovations.* New York: Simon and Schuster; 2010.

Dissemination and Implementation Research Theories and Models

Bernhardt JM, Mays D, Kreuter MW. Dissemination 2.0: closing the gap between knowledge and practice with new media and marketing. *J Health Commun.* 2011(16 suppl 1):32-44.

Bero LA, Grilli R, Grimshaw JM, Harvey E, Oxman AD, Thomson MA. Closing the gap between research and practice: an overview of systematic reviews of interventions to promote the implementation of research findings. The Cochrane Effective Practice and Organization of Care Review Group. *BMJ.* 1998;317(7156):465-468.

Damschroder LJ, Aron DC, Keith RE, Kirsh SR, Alexander JA, Lowery JC. Fostering implementation of health services research findings into practice: a consolidated framework for advancing implementation science. *Implement Sci.* 2009;4:50.

Davies P, Walker AE, Grimshaw JM. A systematic review of the use of theory in the design of guideline dissemination and implementation strategies and interpretation of the results of rigorous evaluations. *Implement Sci.* 2010;5:14.

Greenhalgh T, Robert G, Macfarlane F, Bate P, Kyriakidou O. Diffusion of innovations in service organizations: systematic review and recommendations. *Milbank Q.* 2004;82(4):581-629.

Majumdar SR, Soumerai SB. Why most interventions to improve physician prescribing do not seem to work. *CMAJ.* 2003;169(1):30-31.

Sales A, Smith J, Curran G, Kochevar L. Models, strategies, and tools. Theory in implementing evidence-based findings into health care practice. *J Gen Intern Med.* 2006;21(suppl 2):S43-S49.

Tabak RG, Khoong EC, Chambers DA, Brownson RC. Bridging research and practice: models for dissemination and implementation research. *Am J Prev Med.* 2012;43(3):337-350.

Wandersman A, Duffy J, Flaspohler P, et al. Bridging the gap between prevention research and practice: the interactive systems framework for dissemination and implementation. *Am J Community Psychol.* 2008;41(3-4):171-181.

Answers to Study Questions

CHAPTER 1

1. A
2. D
3. D
4. B
5. D
6. A
7. C
8. C
9. D
10. B

CHAPTER 2

1. B
2. E
3. A
4. C
5. D
6. C
7. A
8. D
9. C
10. D

CHAPTER 3

1. B
2. A
3. C
4. A
5. D
6. B
7. C

8. D
9. C
10. D

CHAPTER 4

1. D
2. B
3. C
4. A
5. C
6. A
7. B
8. D
9. A
10. C

CHAPTER 5

1. B
2. D
3. C
4. C
5. A
6. D
7. B
8. A
9. B
10. C

CHAPTER 6

1. G
2. B
3. A

4. H
5. A
6. F
7. G
8. A
9. A
10. F

CHAPTER 7

1. A
2. D
3. D
4. C
5. D
6. A
7. A
8. A
9. A
10. C

CHAPTER 8

1. A
2. D
3. B
4. C
5. C
6. B
7. A
8. E
9. E
10. B

CHAPTER 9

1. C
2. F
3. E
4. F
5. C
6. E
7. D
8. B
9. A
10. C

CHAPTER 10

1. B
2. C
3. A
4. D
5. C
6. B
7. B
8. E
9. C
10. D

CHAPTER 11

1. C
2. B
3. C
4. B
5. D
6. A
7. D
8. B
9. D
10. C

CHAPTER 12

1. A
2. C
3. D
4. C
5. D
6. C
7. D
8. D
9. A
10. C

CHAPTER 13

1. D
2. B
3. C
4. E

5. D
6. A
7. C
8. B
9. E
10. E

CHAPTER 14

1. A
2. C
3. A
4. D
5. B
6. D
7. D

CHAPTER 15

1. A
2. C
3. A
4. D
5. C
6. D
7. A
8. D
9. B
10. C

CHAPTER 16

1. D
2. C
3. A
4. B
5. D
6. B
7. B
8. A
9. C
10. B

CHAPTER 17

1. D
2. A
3. B
4. C
5. B
6. D
7. B
8. D
9. C
10. A

Glossary

Access to health care: having the timely use of personal health services to achieve the best health outcomes

Accuracy: the extent to which a measurement or study result correctly represents the characteristic or relationship that is being assessed

Acquired immunodeficiency syndrome (AIDS): a disease characterized by a marked reduction in $CD4^+$ T lymphocytes and associated defects in immune response caused by the human immunodeficiency virus (HIV)

Active surveillance: a system of data collection in which those responsible for collecting the information go into the community under observation (typically defined by geographic boundaries) to gather data from various sources

Acute: a disease of short duration

Adaptive randomized controlled clinical trial: an experimental study in which the collected data are used to guide predefined design adaptations when the trial is in progress

Adjustment: a procedure for overall comparison of two or more populations in which background differences in the distribution of covariables are removed (see also **Standardization**)

Administrative data: billing data or hospital discharge data that can be used for research on health-related questions, including costs of care

Age adjustment: a procedure used to calculate summary rates for different populations in which underlying differences in the age distributions are removed (see also **Age standardization**)

Age-specific rate: a rate (usually incidence or mortality) for a particular age group

Age standardization (direct): a procedure for obtaining a weighted average of age-specific rates in which the weights are selected on the basis of a standard age distribution (e.g., the population of the United States in 2000)

Alpha error: see **Type I error**

Analytic epidemiology: activities related to the identification of possible determinants of disease occurrence

Analytic study: a research investigation designed to test a hypothesis, often used in reference to a study of an exposure-disease association

Antibody: a protein, often produced in response to exposure to an antigen that binds to the antigen and thereby stimulates its inactivation by the immune system

Antigen: a protein, usually foreign in origin, that is capable of generating an immune response in a host animal

Arithmetic mean: see **Mean**

Arteriosclerosis: hardening of the arteries

Association: the extent to which the occurrence of two or more characteristics is linked either through a causal or noncausal relationship

Asymptomatic persons: individuals who have a particular disease but do not manifest abnormalities of function, appearance, or sensation typically associated with that disease

Attack rate: the proportion of persons within a population who develop a particular outcome within a specified period of time

Attributable risk percent: the percentage of the overall risk of a disease outcome within exposed persons, related to the exposure of interest

Benign: a mild illness; when applied to an abnormal growth of cells (i.e., a neoplasm), it connotes a slowly progressing defect that is not invading adjacent tissues (in contrast to the rapid growth and invasive behavior of a malignant neoplasm)

Beta error: see **Type II error**

Bias: a nonrandom error in a study that leads to a distorted result

Biologic marker (or biomarker): a measurable characteristic that helps to classify either level of exposure to a risk factor or susceptibility to (or presence of) a disease

Birth cohort effect: an unusual age-specific rate (either incidence or mortality) within cross-sectional data that reflects the shared experience of persons born in specific years (birth cohort)

Blinding: assignment of treatment to individual subjects in a way such that subjects only (**single**

blinding) or both subjects and treating physicians (**double blinding**) do not know the actual treatment allocation

Cancer: a heterogeneous group of diseases characterized by the abnormal, uncontrolled growth of cells, which are capable of crossing normal anatomic boundaries to invade other tissues and even spread to remote anatomic sites

Case: a person who has a disease of interest (see also **Incident case** and **Prevalent case**)

Case-control study: an observational study in which subjects are sampled based on the presence (cases) or absence (controls) of the disease of interest; information is collected about earlier exposure to risk factors of interest

Case fatality: the proportion of persons with a particular disease who die from that disease within a specified period of time

Case-mix/risk adjustment: in comparing provider performance, using statistical methods to minimize the potential influence of differing distributions of severity of illness among patients treated

Causality: the extent to which the occurrence of a risk factor is responsible for the subsequent occurrence of a disease outcome

Cerebrovascular accident: a deficit in the delivery of oxygenated blood to the brain that may occur because of a blood clot or a hemorrhage; a synonym for a stroke

Chance node: an element in a decision analysis that represents a point at which specified outcomes are determined on the basis of probability

Cholesterol: a steroid that is abundant in animal tissues and is necessary for normal function; elevated levels of total cholesterol circulating in the blood of a host are associated with increased risks of cardiovascular disease

Chronic: a disease of long duration

Clinical scenario: one of two or more alternative paths of management available in a decision analysis

Clinical trial: an experimental study that is designed to compare the therapeutic benefits of two or more treatments

Cluster: a group of cases of a disease closely linked in time, place of occurrence, or both

Cluster randomization: a randomized controlled clinical trial in which groups of individuals (e.g., those within a particular clinical facility) are randomized to either receive a particular intervention or control

Cochrane Collaboration: an international organization dedicated to promoting well-informed health care decisions by preparing, maintaining, and ensuring accessibility to current, rigorous, systematic reviews of the benefits and risks of health care interventions; the organization is named in memory of Archie Cochrane, a physician epidemiologist who advocated using the best available evidence to guide health care decisions

Coefficient of determination: the square of the correlation coefficient; it represents the proportion of total variability in an outcome that can be explained by the predictors in a regression model

Cohort: a group of persons that shares a common attribute, such as birth in a particular year or residence in a particular town, and is followed over time

Cohort study: an observational study in which subjects are sampled based on the presence (exposed) or absence (unexposed) of a risk factor of interest; these subjects are followed over time for the development of a disease outcome of interest (see also **Prospective cohort study** and **Retrospective cohort study**)

Common cause (also expected or random) variation: differences in the delivery of health care that cannot be traced to a root cause

Common-source exposure: contact with a risk factor that originates in the shared environment of multiple persons

Comparative effectiveness research: rigorous evaluation of the impact of different options that are available for treating a medical condition for a particular set of patients

Concordant results: the same outcome status for two or more individuals, as in a pair-matched case-control study in which both the case and the control are exposed (or unexposed)

Confidence interval: a range of values for a measure that is believed to contain the true value within a specified level (e.g., 95%) of certainty

Confounder: a variable that distorts the apparent relationship between an exposure and a disease of interest

Confounding: a systematic error in a study that arises from mixing of the effect of the exposure of interest with other associated correlates of the disease outcome

Confounding by indication bias: a distortion of results in an observational study related to the fact that practicing clinicians tend to use the newest or best treatment available for their more severely ill or difficult-to-treat patients

Contamination: persons not intended to have an experimental treatment in a randomized controlled clinical trial end up receiving it anyway because of proximity to or sharing with the experimental subjects

Control: in a case-control study, a subject without the disease of interest (see also **Adjustment**)

Control chart: a tool used in statistical process control that provides a graphical display to help separate out common cause variation in health care delivery from special cause variation

Control group: a population of comparison subjects in an analytic investigation

Coronary artery (or heart) disease: complete or partial blockage of the blood vessels that bring oxygenated blood to the heart muscle (myocardium), usually arising from atherosclerosis; if the reduction in blood flow is severe, a myocardial infarction may result

Correlation coefficient: a statistical measure of the relatedness of two variables; it can range from −1 (perfectly related inversely to each other) to +1 (perfectly related in the same direction to each other); when the variables are unrelated to each other, the correlation coefficient has a value of zero

Correlation study: a hypothesis-generating investigation in which the values of two or more summary characteristics are associated across different population groups

Cross-over design: a randomized controlled clinical trial in which each subject serves as their own control, but subjects are randomized to the sequences of treatment

Cross-sectional study: an analytic investigation in which subjects are sampled at a fixed point or period of time, and the associations between the concurrent presence or absence of risk factors and diseases are then investigated

Crude mortality rate: the rapidity with which persons within a given population die from a particular disease, without adjustment for the underlying age distribution of the population

Cumulative effects: the accumulation of social advantage or disadvantage over time, which manifests in health status

Cumulative incidence: the risk of developing a particular disease within a specified period of time

Cutoff point: a value on an ordinal or a continuous scale of measurement used to distinguish categories; for example, values above this threshold may be classified as "abnormal," and values below this point may be classified as "normal"

Death rate: see **Mortality rate**

Decision analysis: a formal probabilistic process for making clinical decisions that incorporates information on medical options, anticipated likelihoods of various outcomes, and the uncertainty associated with clinical information

Decision diagram: a flow chart used in decision analysis that identifies the clinical management choices, probabilities of events, and likelihoods of outcomes

Decision node: an element of a decision tree that represents a choice between two or more competing alternative management approaches

Decision tree: see **Decision diagram**

Dependent variable: see **Outcome variable**

Descriptive epidemiology: activities related to characterizing patterns of disease occurrence

Diabetes mellitus: a disorder of carbohydrate regulation caused by either a markedly reduced or absent production of insulin by the pancreas (**type I**) or a decreased sensitivity to the effects of insulin in the peripheral tissues (**type II**)

Differential misclassification: incorrect categorization of the status of subjects with regard to one variable (e.g., exposure) that is influenced by other characteristics of interest (e.g., disease status)

Diffusion: the passive process by which a program or product is absorbed into more widespread use

Disability-adjusted life years (DALYs): a summary measure of a population's health status combining years of life lost because of premature death and years lived with disability

Discordant results: different outcome status for two or more individuals, as in a pair-matched case-control study, when one subject in a pair is exposed and the other individual is unexposed to the risk factor of interest

Disease outbreak: a sudden, unexpected increase in the occurrence of a disease within a relatively limited geographic area

Disparities in health care: racial or ethnic differences in the quality of health care that are not due to access-related factors or clinical needs, preferences, and appropriateness of treatment intervention

Dissemination: the active and targeted distribution of information and interventions to a specific public health or clinical practice audience via determined channels using planned strategies

Dissemination research: the study of how information about health promotion and care interventions is created, packaged, transmitted, and interpreted among a variety of important stakeholder groups

Dose-response relationship: an exposure-disease association in which the risk of developing a disease varies with respect to the intensity or duration of exposure

Ecologic fallacy: an association between summary characteristics across populations without actual linkage of the characteristics within individual persons

Ecologic study: see **Correlation study**

Effective care: health care for which the evidence establishes that the benefits outweigh the risks; all patients who meet the guidelines for the care should receive it

Eligibility (or inclusion/exclusion) criteria: a set of characteristics (e.g., age, sex, severity of illness) that determine whether a person is appropriate to serve as a study participant

Endemic rate: the usual rate of occurrence of particular events within a population

Epidemic: a dramatic increase above the usual or expected rate of occurrence of particular events within a population

Epidemiologic transition: improvements in nutrition, sanitation, immunization, and medical care in developing nations, leading to a reduction in mortality from infectious diseases, with consequent growth and aging of the population and a rise in degenerative and human-made diseases

Epidemiology: the study of the distribution and determinants of disease within human populations

Equitable health care: the lack of variation in quality of care because of personal characteristics such as gender, race, ethnicity, geographic location, and socioeconomic status

Equivalency (noninferiority) trial: a randomized controlled clinical trial in which the objective is to test whether a new intervention is as good as, or no worse than, an established one

Ethnicity: a sociopolitical construct for grouping individuals on the basis of shared culture, language, religion, and traditions

Etiology: the cause(s) of a disease or the study of disease causation

Evidence: data that have been assembled, reviewed, and presented by developers and that have been used to make recommendations

Evidence-based medicine: the integration of current best evidence from research with clinical expertise, pathophysiologic knowledge, and patient preferences used to make health care decisions

Excess risk: the extra risk of the occurrence of a particular disease among persons exposed to a risk factor of interest (see also **Risk difference**)

Exclusions: persons who are eliminated from an analytic study because they do not satisfy the eligibility (inclusion) criteria

Expected utility: a numerical value that represents the average result if the decision maker follows a particular path in a decision analysis

Exposure: contact with or possession of a characteristic that is suspected to influence the risk of developing a particular disease

External validity: the extent to which the conclusions of a study can be correctly applied to persons beyond those who were investigated (see also **Generalize**)

Face validity: in the context of comparative effectiveness research, a model for informing decisions that seems reasonable to experienced clinicians

Factorial design: a randomized controlled clinical trial in which two interventions are compared with a control within a single trial

False negative: a test result that is normal (negative) despite the true presence of the disease of interest or a study result that incorrectly fails to identify a true effect (see also **type II error**)

False positive: a test result that is abnormal (positive) despite the true absence of the disease of interest or a study result that incorrectly suggests an effect, when in truth, the purported effect does not exist (see also **type I error**)

Fixed effects model: a statistical approach to combining information from multiple sources in which it is assumed that the investigated relationship is constant across sources and any differences in individual results are attributable entirely to random variation

Follow-up study: see **Cohort study**

Forest plot: a graphical display of either treatment effects across multiple studies in a meta-analysis or provider variation in comparative performance evaluations in health care

Framingham Heart Study: a landmark prospective cohort study of risk factors for cardiovascular disease initiated in 1950 among residents of Framingham, Massachusetts

Funnel plot: a graphical display of data in which the measure of interest is plotted against the number of observations (patients) creating a funnel shape with wider confidence interval bands where there are fewer observations; often used for comparative performance evaluations in health care

Generalize: the ability to extrapolate study results from the study subjects to other persons who were not investigated

Genetic epidemiology: the use of epidemiologic techniques to study hereditary determinants of disease in human populations

Genome: the full complement of genes on all chromosomes

Glucosuria: an abnormally elevated level of glucose in the urine, as may occur in diabetes mellitus

Gray (or grey) literature: evidence, such as manuscripts, clinical trial registries, conference papers and posters, evaluation reports, and grant close-out reports, that is prepared by investigators but does not appear in the peer-reviewed published literature

Healthy life expectancy: the number of years a person can be anticipated to live in good health beyond a specified baseline age

Hematologic: of or relating to the blood or blood-forming tissues

Heterogeneity: the statistical property of variation in an investigated relationship across individual studies or across subgroups within a particular study

Historical cohort study: see **Retrospective cohort study**

Historical controls: subjects in a clinical study who were previously treated with the standard therapy before the new experimental treatment was introduced

HIV: see **Human immunodeficiency virus**

Homogeneity: the statistical property of lack of variation of an investigated relationship across individual studies or across individual subgroups within a particular study

Human immunodeficiency virus: the cause of the acquired immunodeficiency syndrome (AIDS) and other HIV-related disorders

Hyperglycemia: an abnormally high level of glucose in the blood, as may occur in untreated patients with diabetes mellitus

Hypertension: an abnormal elevation in blood pressure

Hypoglycemia: an abnormally low level of glucose in the blood, as may result from an overly aggressive administration of insulin in patients with diabetes mellitus

Hypothesis-generating study: an exploratory investigation designed to formulate questions that are evaluated in subsequent analytic studies

Hypothesis-testing study: an analytic investigation in which one or more specific refutable suppositions are evaluated

Immunity: a state in which a host is not susceptible to a particular infection or disease

Implementation science: the study of methods to promote the integration of research findings and evidence into health care policy and practice

Incidence density: see **Incidence rate**

Incidence rate: the rapidity with which new cases of a particular disease arise within a given population

Incident case: a person who is newly diagnosed with a disease of interest

Incubation period: the time interval between contact with a risk factor (often an infectious agent) and the first clinical evidence of the resulting illness

Independent variable: a factor that is suspected to influence the outcome of an analytic study

Information (or observation) bias: a systematic error in a study that arises from the manner in which data are collected from participants

Informed consent: the process of providing a patient with information about the risks and benefits of a proposed treatment plan and then securing the patient's (or if the patient is a child, the guardian's) agreement to undergo the planned intervention recognizing the risks and benefits

Insulin: a peptide hormone produced in the pancreas and secreted into the blood, which delivers it to target organs to help regulate glucose utilization, protein synthesis, and formation and storage of lipids

Intention to treat: analysis of the results of a clinical trial based on initial treatment assignment regardless of whether the subjects completed the full course of treatment

Internal validity: the extent to which the conclusions of a study are correct for the subjects under investigation

Latent effects: biologic or developmental early life experiences that impact health later in life

Latent period: the time between exposure to a risk factor and subsequent development of clinical manifestations of a particular disease

Lead-time bias: an apparent increase in the length of survival of patients with a disease as a result of earlier detection of the disease through the use of a screening procedure

Length-biased sampling: preferential detection of less aggressive forms of a disease through the use of a screening procedure

Life expectancy: the expected, or average, duration of life for persons in a particular population, under the assumption that current age-specific mortality patterns continue to apply

Likelihood: the probability of the occurrence of a specified event within a particular timeframe

Likelihood ratio: the probability of a particular test result for a person with the disease of interest divided by the probability of that test result for a person without the disease of interest

Likelihood ratio for a negative test result: the probability of a negative test result for a person with the disease of interest divided by the probability of a negative test result for a person without the disease of interest

Likelihood ratio for a positive test result: the probability of a positive test result for a person with the disease of interest divided by the probability of a positive test result for a person without the disease of interest

Longitudinal study: see **Cohort study**

Malignancy: the property of being malignant; often used interchangeably with the term *cancer*

Malignant: a severe disease that is resistant to treatment (e.g., severe hypertension); the term often is used in relation to the behavior of cancers

Markov model: see **State transition (Markov) model**

Matching: a procedure for sampling comparison subjects based on whether key attributes (i.e., **matching factors**) are similar to those of subjects in the index group

Materialist theory (of social determinants of health): access to resources is the most basic driving force in determining the quality of health of both individuals and populations

Mean: the arithmetic average of a distribution of values; calculated as the sum of the individual values divided by the number of observations

Median: a measure of central tendency of a distribution; calculated as the midpoint of the distribution when individual values are ordered from the smallest to the largest

Median survival time: the duration of time from diagnosis to death that is exceeded by exactly 50% of subjects with a particular disease

Medical outcome: see **Outcome**

Medical Subject Heading (MeSH) browser: detailed taxonomy of keywords developed by the National Library of Medicine to cover all the topics of biomedicine and used to search for relevant literature

Meta-analysis (quantitative systematic review): a statistical combination or integration of the results of several independent research studies that are considered to be combinable

Metabolic acidosis: an abnormally high level of acid and low level of bicarbonate in the blood and other tissues resulting either from an accumulation of acids from metabolic processes (as in diabetes mellitus) or from an abnormally high loss of bases from the body (as in diarrhea or renal disease)

Misclassification bias: incorrect characterization of the status of subjects with regard to a study variable, leading to a distorted conclusion (see also **Information [or observation] bias**)

Mode: a measure of central tendency of a distribution; it is the value that occurs most frequently within the distribution

Morbidity: a state of illness produced by a disease

Mortality: death, usually in reference to death caused by a particular disease (viz, **cause-specific mortality**)

Mortality rate: the rapidity with which persons within a given population die from a particular disease

Multicomponent dissemination strategies: dissemination of evidence that uses multiple approaches to better address reach, ability, or motivation

Multivariable models: statistical approaches used for deductive purposes to analyze data to identify patterns of relationships between or among variables and to test hypotheses

Myocardial infarction: a sudden diminution in the delivery of oxygenated blood to the heart muscle (viz, **myocardium**), most commonly caused by partial or complete blockage of one or more of the coronary arteries

Natural history: the progression of a disease through successive stages, often used to describe the course of an illness for which no effective treatment is available

Negative predictive value: the probability that a person with a negative (normal) test result actually does not have the disease of interest

Neomaterialist theory (of social determinants of health): production of health is related to the relative distribution of material resources within a population, not just the absolute level of resources available to the population

Neoplasm: a new growth that arises from the abnormal proliferation of cells; the proliferation may be benign or malignant (viz, **cancer**)

Nephropathy: a disorder of the kidney; among people with diabetes, the disorder arises because of damage to the small blood vessels of the kidney, which can lead to failure of the kidneys in an advanced stage

Nondifferential misclassification: incorrect categorization of the status of subjects with regard to one variable (e.g., exposure) that is unrelated to another characteristic of interest (e.g., disease status)

Nosocomial infection: an illness caused by exposure to a pathogen during hospitalization of the host

Notifiable disease: a disease for which regular, frequent, and timely information on individual cases is considered necessary for the prevention and control of the disease

Null value: the point on the scale of a measure of association that corresponds to no association (e.g., 1 for the risk ratio and the odds ratio and 0 for the risk difference and the attributable risk percent)

Observation bias: see **Information bias**

Observational study: a nonexperimental analytic study in which the investigator monitors, but does not influence, the exposure status of individual subjects and their subsequent disease status

Odds: the probability that a particular event will occur divided by the probability that the event will not occur

Odds ratio: the odds of a particular exposure among persons with a specific disease divided by the corresponding odds of exposure among persons without the disease of interest

Outbreak: see **Disease outbreak**

Outcome: clinical events that result from patient management decisions (e.g., morbidity, complications, quality of life, or mortality)

Outcome of care: a patient's current or future health status (including psychosocial functioning and patient attitudes and behavior) that can be attributed to antecedent care delivered

Outcome variable: in an analytic study, the response of interest (e.g., development of disease)

Outcome variation: differences in clinical care which occur when the same process produces different results in different patients

Pandemic: an elevated occurrence of a disease across a wide geographic area, affecting a substantial proportion of the population

Passive surveillance: a system of data collection in which those responsible for collecting information rely upon voluntary reporting by other individuals or groups without entering the community to gather data

Pathogen: an agent responsible for the development of a particular disease

Pathophysiology: derangement of function associated with a disease process

Pathway effects: experiences that set individuals onto trajectories that influence health and well-being over the course of a lifetime

Patient-centered care: health care that is respectful and responsive to individual patient preferences, needs, and values, thereby assuring that patient values guide all clinical decisions

PDSA cycle: a quality improvement model developed by statistician W. Edwards Deming that entails four sequential steps: **p**lan a change, **d**o the tasks required for the change, **s**tudy the results, and **a**ct on the findings

Person-time: a unit of measurement used in the estimation of rates that reflects the amount of time observed for persons at risk of a particular event

Person-to-person spread: propagation of a disease within a population by transfer from an affected person to susceptible persons

Person-years: a common unit for measuring person-time; 1 person-year corresponds to one person being followed for 1 year, or alternatively, two persons each followed for 1 half year, and so forth

Person-years of life lost: a measure of total life expectancy lost within a particular population because of premature death

Phase I clinical trial: a study in which the experimental compound is administered to human subjects for the first time to determine basic safety and pharmacokinetic information

Phase II clinical trial: a study in which subjects with the condition of interest are exposed to an experimental treatment to assess safety and initial evidence of efficacy

Phase III clinical trial: an experimental study in which subjects with the condition of interest are randomized to either receive the experimental treatment or a control for the purpose of assessing therapeutic benefit

Phase IV clinical trial (postmarketing study): a study designed to determine the risks, benefits and optimal use of an approved drug, often requiring large study groups followed over long periods of time

Placebo: a biologically inactive substance that is identical in appearance to the medicine under investigation

Placebo effect: occurs when persons affected with a specific illness demonstrate clinical improvement when treated with an inert substance

Population at risk: persons who are susceptible to a particular disease but who are not yet affected

Population-based study: an analytic study in which subjects are sampled from the general population

Positive predictive value: the probability that a person with a positive (abnormal) test result actually has the disease of interest

Posttest odds of disease: the estimated probability, after the administration of a diagnostic test, that a patient has the disease of interest divided by the probability that the patient does not have the disease of interest

Posttest probability of disease: the estimated likelihood, after the administration of a diagnostic test, that a patient has the disease of interest

Power: see **Statistical power**

Pragmatic (or practical) clinical trial: an experimental study that is designed to answer a question faced by clinicians in real world delivery of patient care

Precision: the extent to which a measurement is narrowly characterized; **statistical precision** is inversely related to the variance of the measurement

Predictive validity: in the context of comparative effectiveness research, a model's ability to predict the prevalence of key conditions and costs for populations other than those on which it was designed

Predictor variable: see **Independent variable**

Preference-sensitive care: health care for which there is more than one generally accepted diagnostic or therapeutic option available and patient preference determines the relative utilization of options

Premature death: a death that occurs earlier than would be expected in the absence of a particular disease

Pretest odds of disease: the estimated probability, before the administration of a diagnostic test, that a patient has the disease of interest divided by the probability that the patient does not have the disease of interest

Pretest probability of disease: the estimated likelihood, before the administration of a diagnostic test, that a patient has the disease of interest

Prevalence: the proportion of persons in a given population that has a particular disease at a point or interval of time

Prevalent case: a person who has a disease of interest that was diagnosed in the past

Process of care: activities occurring within or between practitioners and patients that can be directly observed or reviewed through recorded information

Process variation: differences in clinical care resulting from dissimilar use of a therapeutic or diagnostic procedure among organizations, geographic regions, or other groupings of health care providers

Prognosis: the predicted rate of progression of a disease process and its likely outcome(s)

Prognostic factor: an attribute anticipated to be related to the progression and outcome of a disease process

Propensity score: the probability of receiving a particular treatment given personal characteristics of the patient

Proportion: one quantity divided by another quantity in which the population in the numerator is a subset of the population in the denominator; the possible values of a proportion range from 0 to 1

Prospective cohort study: a cohort study in which exposure status and subsequent occurrence of disease both occur after the onset of the investigation

Pseudo-randomization: in observational research, the use of techniques to attempt to eliminate bias from the inability to randomize subjects to the exposure or treatment of interest

Publication bias: a distortion in conclusions derived from published studies because of the selective factors associated with the likelihood of publication, including whether the findings were positive and statistically significant and the potential proprietary interests of sponsors

Quality of health care: approaches to assessing the benefits and risks of care, as well as delivery in a manner that is culturally appropriate, humane, and patient participatory

Quantitative systematic review: see **Meta-analysis**

Race: a grouping of individuals based on phenotypic attributes (e.g., skin color), as well as social and cultural constructs and ancestry

Random effects model: a statistical approach to combining information from multiple sources in which it is assumed that the investigated relationship varies across individual sources in addition to the influences of random variation in estimates

Randomization: procedure for assigning treatments to patients by chance

Rate: the rapidity with which health events such as new diagnoses or deaths occur (see also **Incidence rate** and **Mortality rate**)

Rate ratio: the rate of occurrence of a specified health event among persons exposed to a particular risk factor divided by the corresponding rate among unexposed persons

Ratio: one quantity divided by another quantity in which the population in the numerator is not a part of the population in the denominator; the possible values of a ratio range from zero to positive infinity

Relapse: the return of the manifestations of a disease after a period of diminished manifestations

Relative risk: see **Risk ratio**

Reliability: the extent to which multiple measurements of a characteristic are in agreement

Remission: elimination or reduction in the number or severity of the manifestations of a disease, which may be transient or permanent

Response variable: see **Outcome variable**

Retinopathy: a disorder of the retina of the eye; among people with diabetes, the disorder arises from damage to the small blood vessels of the retina and can lead to blindness

Retrospective cohort study: a cohort study in which exposure status and subsequent development of disease both occur prior to the onset of the investigation

Risk difference: the risk of the occurrence of a particular disease among persons exposed to a given risk factor minus the corresponding risk among unexposed persons

Risk: the probability that an event (e.g., development of disease) will occur within a specific period of time

Risk factor: an attribute or agent suspected to be related to the occurrence of a particular disease

Risk ratio: the likelihood of the occurrence of a particular disease among persons exposed to a given risk factor divided by the corresponding likelihood among unexposed persons

Sample: a subset of a target population that is chosen for investigation

Screening: the use of tests to detect the presence of a particular disease among asymptomatic persons before the time that the disease would be recognized through routine clinical methods

SEER Program: The Surveillance, Epidemiology and End Results Program of the National Cancer Institute; it consists of 18 population-based cancer registries in various locations within the United States

Selection bias: a systematic error in a study that arises from the manner in which subjects are sampled

Sensitivity: the probability that a person who actually has the disease of interest will have a positive (abnormal) test result

Sensitivity analysis: (1) in systematic reviews, including meta-analyses, the evaluation of the pattern of results across subgroups of studies to characterize possible sources of heterogeneity and their respective influences on the overall summary effect; (2) in decision analysis, use of different values for an uncertain likelihood to determine whether the preferred course of action remains unchanged

Social determinants of health: societal and economic conditions (beyond biomedical and behavioral risk factors) that influence the health of individuals and populations

Special cause (or assignable) variation: differences in health care delivery that arise from a single or small number of causes that can be traced and identified and then can be reduced or eliminated through targeted quality improvement efforts

Specificity: the probability that a person who actually does not have the disease of interest will have a negative (normal) test result

Standardization: an analytic procedure for obtaining a summary measure for a population by applying standard weights to the measures within subgroups of the population

State transition (Markov) model: an approach to decision modeling in which the disease process is presented as a set of mutually exclusive, time-limited health states with transition between states based on observed progression rates in observational or experimental studies

Statistical power: the ability of a study to detect a true effect of a specified magnitude. The statistical power corresponds to 1 - type II error

Statistical process control: a technique developed in the context of industrial manufacturing but adapted to health care for the purpose of improving quality that applies statistical methods to distinguish special cause variation from common cause variation

Statistical significance: the likelihood that a difference as large as or larger than that observed between study groups could have occurred by chance alone in a sample of the size investigated; usually, the level of statistical significance is stated as a p value (e.g., $p < 0.05$)

Stochastic (decision) models: mathematical structures that are used for inductive purposes to link evidence from multiple sources to predict outcomes, such as effectiveness, costs, or cost effectiveness

Stroke: a sudden derangement in function, as in sunstroke or heat stroke; often used in relation to a sudden neurologic deficit that occurs because of insufficient delivery of oxygenated blood to the brain, as may occur after a blood clot or hemorrhage

Structure of health care: the characteristics of providers, the tools and resources at their disposal, and the physical and organizational settings where care is provided

Subacute: a rate of progression of a condition that is intermediate between acute and chronic

Supply-sensitive care: health care that varies based upon the delivery capacity of the local health care system

Surveillance: ongoing observation of a population for rapid and accurate detection of changes in the occurrence of particular diseases

Survival: the likelihood of remaining alive for a specified period of time after the diagnosis of a particular disease

Systematic error: see **Bias**

Systematic review: a synthesis of medical evidence on a topic, in which the synthesis has been prepared using strategies to minimize errors

Terminal node: in a decision tree, an element that represents the outcome for a particular clinical scenario

Transmission: the process by which a pathogen passes from one source of infection to a new host

Triple aim (for health care improvement): to achieve: (1) better quality care, (2) improvement in the health of the U.S. population by supporting proven interventions, and (3) reducing the cost of quality care thereby making it more affordable

True negative: a test result that is normal (negative) when the disease of interest is actually absent

True positive: a test result that is abnormal (positive) when the disease of interest is actually present

Tumor: a swelling that may occur from an inflammatory process or a benign or malignant neoplasm

Type I error: rejection of the null hypothesis when it is actually correct

Type II error: failure to reject the null hypothesis when it is actually incorrect

Underlying cause of death: (1) the disease or injury that initiated the train of morbid events leading directly to death or (2) the circumstances of the accident or violence that resulted in fatal injury

Unwarranted variation (in patient care): differences in medical practice that cannot be explained by patient preference, disease status, or the practice of evidence-based medicine

Utility: in decision analysis, a patient's preference for one outcome over another, usually graded on a scale of 0, representing death, to 1, representing perfect health

Validity: the extent to which a measurement or a study result correctly represents the characteristics or relationship of interest

Variability: the property of having a spread of values, which may arise from random sources (viz, the operation of chance) or from systematic influences (viz, bias)

Vital statistics: information concerning patterns of registered life events, such as births, marriages, divorces, and deaths

Warranted variation (in patient care): differences in medical practice based on differences in patient preference, disease prevalence, or other patient- or population-related factors

Weighted average: a summary measure in which some of the component data values are assigned greater influence than others; for example, precision-based weighting is the calculation of a summary measure in which the relative influence of individual results is based on statistical confidence in the respective results

Withdrawals: subjects who are initially included in a study but later voluntarily or involuntarily terminate participation

Years of potential life lost (YPLLs): a measure of total life lost to a particular age (e.g., 75 years) within a population because of premature deaths

FURTHER READING

www.cdc.gov/ophss/csels/dsepd/ss1978/Glossary.html

Index

Note: Figures are indicated by an *f* and tables by a *t*.